Management of Head and Neck Surgery Complications

Kwang-Jae Cho • Jun-Ook Park
Editors

Management of Head and Neck Surgery Complications

Pearls and Pitfalls

Springer

Korean Society of Head and Neck Surgery
KSHNS 1990
대한두경부외과학회

Editors
Kwang-Jae Cho
Department of Otolaryngology—Head and Neck Surgery
Uijeongbu St. Mary's Hospital,
The Catholic University
Uijeongbu-si, Republic of Korea

Jun-Ook Park
Department of Otolaryngology—Head and Neck Surgery
Seoul St. Mary's Hospital,
The Catholic University
Seoul, Republic of Korea

ISBN 978-981-96-1859-0 ISBN 978-981-96-1860-6 (eBook)
https://doi.org/10.1007/978-981-96-1860-6

This Springer imprint is published by the registered company Springer Nature Singapore Pte Ltd.
The registered company address is: 152 Beach Road, #21-01/04 Gateway East, Singapore 189721, Singapore

Preface

Head and neck surgery is one of the most complex and challenging fields in medicine, where unexpected complications often arise, even for experienced surgeons. Recognizing the critical need for practical guidance in managing such complications, *The Surgeon's Handbook: Expert Solutions for Head and Neck Surgery Complications* was developed to serve as an indispensable resource.

This handbook is a collaborative effort, bringing together the expertise of leading surgeons from the Korean Society of Head and Neck Surgery and international experts. It is designed to provide clear solutions to key questions that arise when complications occur during head and neck surgery. Each chapter is meticulously designed to offer guidance that junior surgeons and seasoned professionals can immediately apply in real-time surgical settings.

Comprising 20 chapters, this book covers a broad range of potential surgical complications. This handbook provides practical solutions based on both referenced literature and personal surgical experience. What sets this handbook apart is the inclusion of expert opinions in each chapter. World-renowned head and neck surgeons share their insights and strategies, grounded in years of specialized practice. This book also features detailed illustrations, clinical photographs, and summaries, rendering the information comprehensive, accessible, and easy to follow.

The collaborative efforts of our editorial team, led by Dr. Kwang-Jae Cho, president of the Korean Society of Head and Neck Surgery, and Dr. Jun-Ook Park, editor-in-chief, made this project possible. We also extend our deepest gratitude to the many contributors, including the authors, committee members, and associate editor, Dr. Doh Young Lee, for their dedication. Special thanks are due to Dr. Seung Heon Kang for his pivotal role as secretary and to Dr. Junsun Ryu for his invaluable contributions in providing illustrations for this handbook.

We hope that this handbook will become an essential guide to head and neck surgery complications for practicing surgeons, leading to improved outcomes and enhanced patient care.

Uijeongbu-si, Republic of Korea — Kwang-Jae Cho
Seoul, Republic of Korea — Jun-Ook Park
December 2024

List of Experts

Chung-Hwan Baek, Department of Otorhinolaryngology-Head and Neck Surgery, Sungkyunkwan University College of Medicine, Seoul, Republic of Korea

Seung-Kuk Baek, Department of Otorhinolaryngology-Head and Neck Surgery, Korea University College of Medicine, Seoul, Republic of Korea

Kwang Jae Cho, Department of Otorhinolaryngology-Head and Neck Surgery, The Catholic University College of Medicine, Uijeongbu, Republic of Korea

Eun-Jae Chung, Department of Otolaryngology-Head and Neck Surgery, Seoul National University College of Medicine, Seoul, Republic of Korea

Man Ki Chung, Department of Otorhinolaryngology-Head and Neck Surgery, Sungkyunkwan University College of Medicine, Seoul, Republic of Korea

Phil-Sang Chung, Department of Otorhinolaryngology-Head and Neck Surgery, Dankook University College of Medicine, Cheonan, Republic of Korea

David Eisele, Department of Otolaryngology-Head and Neck Surgery, Johns Hopkins University College of Medicine, Baltimore, Maryland

Antoine Eskander, Department of Otorhinolaryngology-Head and Neck Surgery, University of Toronto College of Medicine, Toronto, Canada

Gia Gill, Department of Otorhinolaryngology-Head and Neck Surgery, University of Manitoba College of Medicine, Winnipeg, Canada

Wei-Chung Hsu, Department of Otolaryngology-Head and Neck Surgery, National Taiwan University College of Medicine, Taipei, Taiwan

Han-Sin Jeong, Department of Otorhinolaryngology-Head and Neck Surgery, Sungkyunkwan University College of Medicine, Seoul, Republic of Korea

Young Hoon Joo, Department of Otorhinolaryngology-Head and Neck Surgery, The Catholic University College of Medicine, Bucheon, Republic of Korea

Yuh-Seog Jung, Department of Otolaryngology-Head and Neck Surgery, National Cancer Center, Goyang, Republic of Korea

Chul-Ho Kim, Department of Otorhinolaryngology-Head and Neck Surgery, Ajou University School of Medicine, Suwon, Republic of Korea

Dong Young Kim, Department of Otorhinolaryngology-Head and Neck Surgery, Gachon University College of Medicine, Incheon, Republic of Korea

Min Sik Kim, Department of Otorhinolaryngology-Head and Neck Surgery, The Catholic University College of Medicine, Seoul, Republic of Korea

Seong Keun Kwon, Department of Otorhinolaryngology-Head and Neck Surgery, Seoul National University College of Medicine, Seoul, Republic of Korea
Soon-Young Kwon, Department of Otorhinolaryngology-Head and Neck Surgery, Korea University College of Medicine, Ansan, Republic of Korea
Tack-Kyun Kwon, Department of Otolaryngology-Head and Neck Surgery, Seoul National University College of Medicine, Seoul, Republic of Korea,
Byung-Joo Lee, Department of Otorhinolaryngology-Head and Neck Surgery, Pusan National University College of Medicine, Busan, Republic of Korea
Jin-Choon Lee, Department of Otolaryngology-Head and Neck Surgery, Pusan National University College of Medicine, Yangsan, Republic of Korea
Joon Kyoo Lee, Department of Otorhinolaryngology-Head and Neck Surgery, Chonnam National University, Hwasun, Republic of Korea
Kang Dae Lee, Department of Otorhinolaryngology-Head and Neck Surgery, Kosin University College of Medicine, Busan, Republic of Korea
Myung-Chul Lee, Department of Otorhinolaryngology-Head and Neck Surgery, Korea Cancer Center Hospital, Seoul, Republic of Korea
Sang Joon Lee, Department of Otorhinolaryngology-Head and Neck Surgery, Dankook University College of Medicine, Cheonan, Republic of Korea
Sei Young Lee, Department of Otorhinolaryngology-Head and Neck Surgery, Chung-Ang University College of Medicine, Seoul, Republic of Korea
Seung Won Lee, Department of Otorhinolaryngology-Head and Neck Surgery, Soonchunhyang University College of Medicine, Bucheon, Republic of Korea
Yoon Se Lee, Department of Otolaryngology-Head and Neck Surgery, University of Ulsan College of Medicine, Seoul, Republic of Korea
Hok Nam Li, Department of Otorhinolaryngology-Head and Neck Surgery, The Chinese University of Hong Kong College of Medicine, Sha Tin, Hong Kong
Yun-Sung Lim, Department of Otorhinolaryngology-Head and Neck Surgery, Dongguk University College of Medicine, Goyang, Republic of Korea
Brett A. Miles, Department of Otolaryngology-Head and Neck Surgery, Zucker School of Medicine at Hofstra/Northwell, New York, New York
Il-Seok Park, Department of Otolaryngology-Head and Neck Surgery, Hallym University College of Medicine, Hwaseong, Republic of Korea
Jun-Ook Park, Department of Otorhinolaryngology-Head and Neck Surgery, The Catholic University College of Medicine, Seoul, Republic of Korea
Jung Je Park, Department of Otorhinolaryngology-Head and Neck Surgery, Gyeongsang National University College of Medicine, Jinju, Republic of Korea
Junsun Ryu, Department of Otolaryngology-Head and Neck Surgery, National Cancer Center, Goyang, Republic of Korea
Jatin Shah, Department of Surgery, Memorial Sloan Kettering Cancer Center, New York, New York

Jin Ho Sohn, Department of Otolaryngology-Head and Neck Surgery, Kyungpook National University College of Medicine, Daegu, Republic of Korea

Si-Youn Song, Department of Otolaryngology-Head and Neck Surgery, Yeungnam University College of Medicine, Daegu, Republic of Korea

Dong-Il Sun, Department of Otorhinolaryngology-Head and Neck Surgery, The Catholic University, Seoul, Republic of Korea

Chen-Chi Wang, Department of Otorhinolaryngology-Head and Neck Surgery, National Yang Ming Chiao Tung University College of Medicine, Taipei, Taiwan

Jeong-Soo Woo, Department of Otorhinolaryngology-Head and Neck Surgery, Korea University College of Medicine, Seoul, Republic of Korea

Che-Wei Wu, Department of Otorhinolaryngology-Head and Neck Surgery, Kaohsiung Medical University College of Medicine, Kaohsiung, Taiwan

Tsung-Lin Yang, Department of Otorhinolaryngology-Head and Neck Surgery, National Taiwan University College of Medicine, Taipei, Taiwan

Seiichi Yoshimoto, Department of Otorhinolaryngology-Head and Neck Surgery, National Cancer Center, Tokyo, Japan

Contents

Part I

Oral Cavity and Oropharynx

1 Oral Cancer Surgery

Young-Gyu Eun

1.1 KQ 1.1. How to Manage Orocutaneous Fistulas?

Young-Gyu Eun

1.1.1 Diagnosis

Orocutaneous fistulas occur most frequently after composite resection of the tongue, floor of the mouth, and mandible, with neck dissection. Orocutaneous fistulas are characterized by fever, pain, neck erythema, neck swelling, and an increased white blood cell count. Clinical vigilance and early recognition can lead to the rapid management and minimization of adverse sequelae. Occasionally, the use of perioperative antibiotics can blunt the usual signs and symptoms; therefore, systemic antibiotic treatment should be considered when making a clinical diagnosis.

When the diagnosis of fluid collection is suspected, a computed tomography scan may demonstrate its presence; however, more often, only tissue edema is observed on the computed tomography scan. The neck wound can be aspirated with a needle if there is fluctuation; however, often there is no evident collection in the fistula. Examination of an oral wound is likely to reveal dehiscence and an opening of the neck.

Expert Opinion

Early diagnosis and treatment are crucial in determining the treatment duration and prognosis, as most orocutaneous fistulas occur within 7 days post surgery. During this period, it is important to recognize the signs of a fistula.

Useful Methods for Identification:

1. CBC: Check if WBC count is continuously decreasing by monitoring CBC after operation. If WBC count initially improves but then worsens, or if it continues to rise, a fistula should be suspected.
2. Daily Neck AP & Lateral Soft Tissue View: Take daily images to check for changes in air shadow in the neck. An increase in air shadow indicates a potential fistula. This method is useful as CT scans are not feasible frequently, making it a simple and effective screening tool.

(continued)

Supplementary Information The online version contains supplementary material available at https://doi.org/10.1007/978-981-96-1860-6_1.

Y.-G. Eun (✉)
Department of Otolaryngology–Head and Neck Surgery, Kyung Hee University Medical Center, Seoul, Korea
e-mail: ygeun@khu.ac.kr

K.-J. Cho, J.-O. Park (eds.), *Management of Head and Neck Surgery Complications*,
https://doi.org/10.1007/978-981-96-1860-6_1

3. Check Changes of Drainage: Monitor the characteristics of the secretions. Normally, there should be no tissue debris. However, the presence of significant tissue debris or a foul smell in the drained secretions necessitates checking for a fistula.
4. Patient's Pain Response on Touching the Wound: Excessive pain when touching the surgical field may indicate a fistula. (Seung-Kuk Baek)

1.1.2 Management

The neck wound needs to be opened to allow the drainage of pus and saliva. The wound should be opened as anteriorly as possible, with adequate drainage of the area of inflammation to help prevent involvement of the carotid artery in the fistula tract and subsequent carotid rupture, which is often fatal. By diverting the fistula flow anteriorly, the carotid artery is spared from exposure to saliva. The opening of the wound needs to be sufficiently large to allow excellent drainage; it should be at least 2–4 cm, and frequently, a much larger opening is necessary. The goal is to ensure that the skin opening is larger than the oral opening, resulting in the fistula cavity assuming a conical shape with the tip facing upward.

Expert Opinion

When creating a fistula, it should be placed at the site with the shortest distance to the skin. To prevent the controlled fistula from dehiscence under tension due to neck movements, a tension-free suture technique should be employed. Additionally, careful effort must be made to construct the fistula properly and securely to avoid the need for reoperation. (Chul-Ho Kim)

It is important to position the wound opening at a distance from the carotid artery while also minimizing the distance between the wound opening (skin opening) and the oral opening. (Sei Young Lee)

However, it is not necessary to excessively resect the surrounding healthy tissue to enlarge the opening. (Sei Young Lee)

1.1.2.1 Conventional Wound Care (CWC)

Expert Opinion

In large irradiated wounds, complete closure through secondary healing may be challenging. Therefore, once the wound has stabilized and infection and inflammation have subsided, flap surgery should be considered to close persistent fistulas. (Chul-Ho Kim)

Even in non-irradiated patients, fistula may not usually heal within 7 days. (Soon-Young Kwon)

Conventional wound care consists of compressive dressings and the avoidance of oral feeding. In addition to wound opening, the patient must not receive anything orally; the wound should be cultured and irrigated (if necessary), and wound packing should be performed two to three times daily. Packing should reduce oral contamination of the fistula and facilitate inferior drainage. Strip packing is available in various sizes, and is ideal for this purpose. In case of the presence of necrotic tissue, it should be debrided. If there is a foul odor, a dakin solution of sodium hypochlorite on the packing can temporarily help sterilize the wound; however, it may inhibit healing if used for a markedly long time. Systemic antibiotics should be administered for 7–10 days or until there is no evidence of cellulitis or wound purulence.

Surgical closure of the skin is not helpful due to continued contamination from the mouth. Closing oral openings with sutures is rarely helpful. Flap reconstruction is not indicated unless there is major tissue loss or the recipient bed is clean. Careful wound care allows the fistula to heal for several weeks. The wound slowly granulates from a deeper aspect, and the skin closes. The packing was gradually reduced over time to allow closure. In non-irradiated patients, a small, well-cared-for fistula may heal within 7 days. However, large irradiated wounds may take weeks or months to granulate slowly.

Clinicians should be aware of the several reasons for non-healing fistulas. The most important factor is the presence of a tumor. Tumors at the edges of a wound never heal, and biopsies of non-healing fistulas are indicated to rule out cancer. Patients with a negative nitrogen balance heal very slowly. Therefore, adequate enteral nutrition through a tube is necessary. Distal obstruction of the pharynx diverts additional material into the fistula and prevents its closure. The presence of a foreign body (e.g., nonabsorbable suture material and exposed hardware) inhibits wound closure. An often-overlooked wound healing problem is low thyroid hormone levels, which are common among patients with a history of radiation treatment.

1.1.2.2 Negative Pressure Wound Therapy (NPWT)

In recent years, NPWT has shown promising results in addition to non-surgical treatments. NPWT can also be used as an adjunct to aid fistula closure or as prophylaxis in high-risk patients. The efficacy of NPWT is likely multifactorial. First, because of the constant negative pressure, NPWT is highly effective in eliminating dead space and salivary leakage around the fistula. This is particularly important in the neck region because prolonged soaking of neck tissues in saliva increases the risk of carotid artery blowout. Second, NPWT demonstrated wound adhesions capable of withstanding the high swallowing pressure necessary to ensure complete wound healing. This partly explains why the simple suture repair of fistulas often fails. In addition, NPWT promotes wound healing by increasing blood flow, improving bacterial clearance, and stimulating granulation tissue growth [1].

The NPWT system was set up to apply continuous negative pressure at the wound site. It consisted of a vacuum-assisted closure therapy machine, foam and occlusive dressings, and specialized suction tubing with a canister. The dressing used was black open-cell polyurethane foam, which promotes granulation tissue formation and is flexible, thereby allowing contouring for application to irregularly shaped wounds often encountered in complex, 3-dimensional head and neck wounds. Hydrogum dental paste was used as a sealant in conjunction with the NPWT system. Once a fistula with significant openings at either end was identified, gum was used to temporarily seal the end. The dry gauze was first soaked in gum. Subsequently, Hydrogum-laden gauze was inserted and molded into the shape of the end of the fistula. The Hydrogum was set up before applying the NPWT system. The use of gum allowed the wound-care team to create a form-fitting sealant. Moreover, the hydrogel exhibited excellent dimensional stability, allowing it to retain its shape and seal until the next dressing change unless the NPWT system failed or was overwhelmed by the amount of fluid. The dental paste was changed every time the NPWT dressings were reapplied (i.e., every 2–3 days). [2] Suction settings ranged from 50 to 125 mmHg for continuous suction. Complete fistula closure may take 10–36 days to completely close the fistula [2].

The use of NPWT in the head and neck region makes it difficult to seal the undulating wound surfaces without leakage. The movements of the mouth, eyelids, nose, and mandible make it difficult to maintain an airtight seal. If the sealing is insufficient and air leakage cannot be controlled, frequent reinforcement of the dressing is required, or NPWT must be stopped prematurely. In addition, incomplete sealing prevents the maintenance of an airtight environment, results in remnant saliva, and worsens the infection [3].

If the NPWT foam is placed shallowly in the fistula tract from the cutaneous opening, the lumen of the fistula collapses, and effective negative pressure can usually be applied. Bending the neck to the affected side and/or downward at the onset of negative pressure is also useful in preventing air leakage. If the fistula is large and the amount of saliva leakage is excessive, fistula closure can be strengthened, and the fistula tract can be narrowed by increasing the negative pressure (Fig. 1.1) [3].

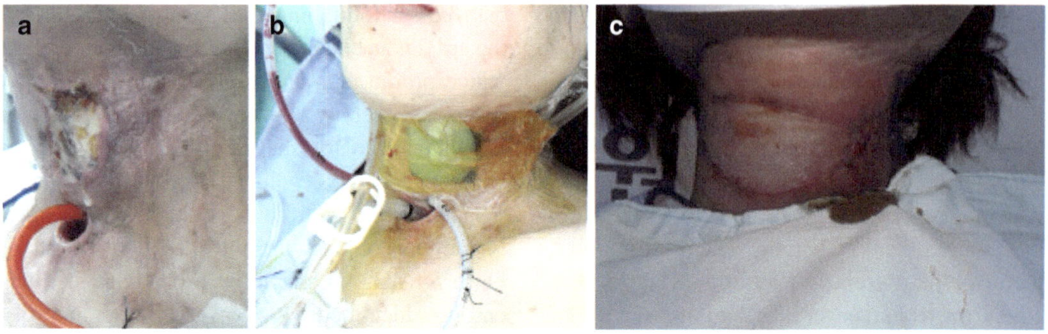

Fig. 1.1 (**a**) Pharyngeal fistula. (**b**) Application of negative pressure wound therapy (NPWT). (**c**) Evaluation on the 21st day after NPWT

The use of NPWT in patients whose fistula site requires a vacuum to be placed directly over the exposed blood vessels should be avoided because of concerns that it may lead to the erosion of the vessel walls [2]. If there is any suspicion of a remnant tumor, our review indicates a consensus that NPWT is contraindicated in these cases because of the risk of tumor seeding [1]. Complications associated with NPWT include pain, skin irritation, skin maceration, tissue necrosis, bleeding, infection, and hemodynamic instability when large volumes of fluid are removed [2].

1.2 KQ 1.2. How to Manage Unintended Oronasal Fistulas?

Young-Gyu Eun

1.2.1 Diagnosis

The diagnosis of an oronasal fistula was based on the patient's symptoms and oral examinations. Symptoms include dysarthria and regurgitation of food or water through the nose.

1.2.2 Management

Closure of the oronasal fistula is of great importance because untreated fistulas significantly reduce the patient's post-operative quality of life by causing oronasal regurgitation, dysarthria, and dysphagia. Oronasal fistulas can be managed through observation, obturation, and surgical repair. Therefore, it is reasonable to observe asymptomatic individuals. However, undetected fistulas can be exposed to orthodontic palatal expansion and become symptomatic. Symptomatic patients who are deemed non-ideal surgical candidates because of medical comorbidities, severe scarring, or multiple failed repairs can be managed using temporary or long-term prosthetic obturation [4]. The advantage of obturation, particularly for smaller defects, is its expediency. The procedure is much faster and requires far shorter hospitalization (important for patients with comorbidities); new dentition is immediate with restoration of appearance (allowing patients to resume their normal life), and the cavity can be clinically surveyed for recurrence. However, its use poses potential issues with radiation; as the defective area heals and contracts, the obturator requires numerous refinements. A dedicated prosthodontic team is required to prefabricate the device and optimize the postoperative prosthesis over time. The treatment of defects using an obturator has several disadvantages, including: (1) discomfort in wearing the prosthesis, (2) inconvenience in removing and cleaning the prosthesis, (3) inability to successfully retain the prosthesis when the defect is large or when dentition is lacking, and (4) frequent need for readjustments by a prosthodontist [5].

> **Expert Opinion**
> In cases of postoperative palatal perforation, symptoms and their severity vary depending on the size of the defect. For smaller perforations, many patients adapt well without significant issues. Therefore, surgeons often prefer to thoroughly discuss the necessity of reconstruction with the patient before deciding whether to proceed reconstruction surgery. (Chul-Ho Kim)
>
> Despite its various disadvantages, an obturator remains the most effective treatment method due to its simplicity and ease of application. (Sei Young Lee)

Several surgical maneuvers have been described for the closure of oronasal fistulas, but no single technique has been proven superior [6]. The ideal repair technique is usually determined by the fistula size and location, patient age, surgical history, and surgeon's experience.

1.2.3 Soft Palate

Two-layered closure using local advancement flaps is effective for small-to-medium-sized hard and soft palate fistulas. Velopharyngeal competence should be determined before soft palate fistula repair. In the absence of velopharyngeal insufficiency (VPI), a sharp incision/excision of the fistula edge, wide undermining of the adjacent tissue, and layered closure are sufficient. Care should be taken in the flap design to avoid anteroposterior shortening of the soft palate. This procedure was combined with revision palatoplasty (double-opposing Z-plasty or straight-line repair with intravelar veloplasty [IVVP]) for concomitant VPI.

1.2.4 Hard–Soft Palate Junction

This location has the highest rate of occurrence of oronasal fistulas. Small fistulas can be closed with local tissue advancement flaps, such as buccal fat flaps (BFF), as adjunctive tissues for both the oral and nasal layers. In most cases, complete epithelialization was observed after four weeks (Fig. 1.2).

1.2.5 Hard Palate

Surgical repair of the hard palate requires distinct tissue sources for the closure of the nasal and oral layers. (Video 1.1) The nasal mucosal lining sources include a turnover flap, vomer flap, nasal sidewall flap, inferior turbinate flap, buccal myomucosal flap, and buccal fat flap, and facial artery musculomucosal (FAMM) flap. The sources of the oral lining include the oral mucoperiosteal flap, buccal myomucosal flap, buccal fat, FAMM, and tongue flaps. For larger fistulas, regional tissue is recommended for the nasal layer, and FAMM or buccal myomucosal flaps are recommended for the oral layer. Although anterior-based tongue flaps have been reported to have a higher success rate than FAMM flaps, their association with greater pain, difficulty eating, and significantly longer operative time may limit their use. Despite a paucity of studies comparing the effectiveness of various flaps, these results suggest that buccal myomucosal flaps are superior to local and regional flaps.

> **Expert Opinion**
> Hard palate fistula is caused by unnecessary damage of the nasal side mucoperiosteum when resecting the palatal bone with tumor. Therefore, care should be taken to leave the intact nasal side mucoperiosteum in such cases.
>
> If the defect size of the nasal side is not large, repair can be done using only one oral flap with a certain thickness that can obliterate the fistula tract. Dissecting the nasal side mucoperiosteum from fistula bone margin and suturing the nasal mucoperiosteum and the upper portion of the obliterated oral flap with barbered suture device can promote the healing process.

(continued)

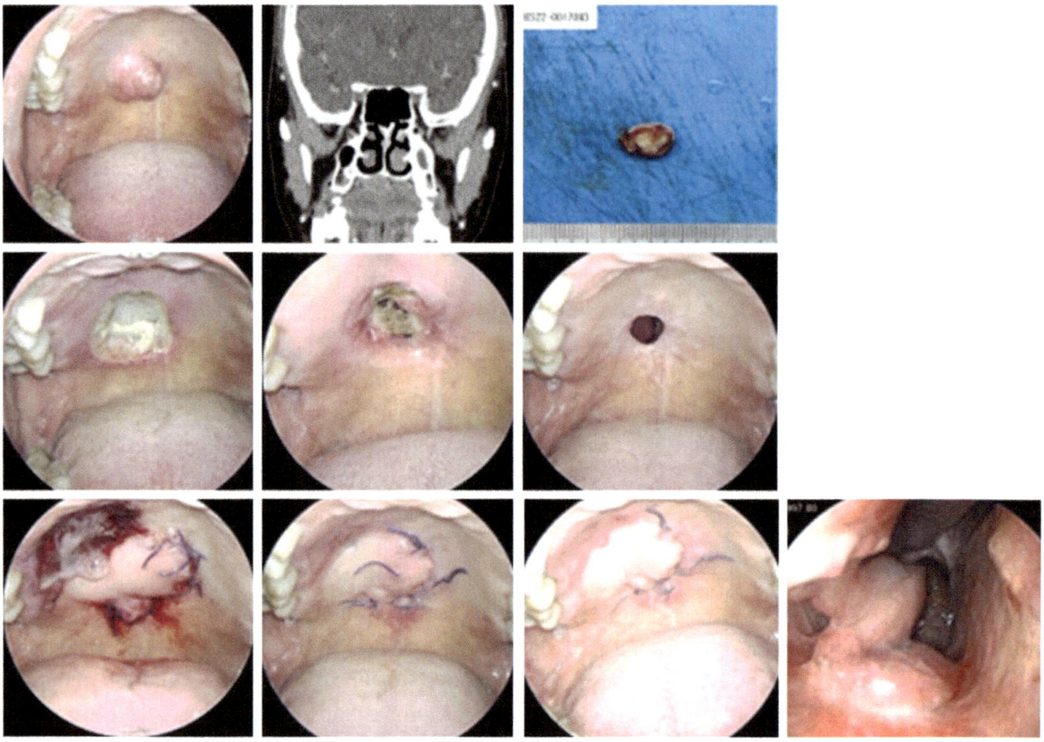

Fig. 1.2 Hard–soft palate junction reconstruction with palatal rotation flap (Copyright: Prof. Doh Young Lee)

> Even if the nasal side mucosa of the soft palate remained intact after tumor resection, fistulas may develop at the palatine-palatine junction several weeks later due to continuous movement of the soft palate. In most cases, it can be resolved with an oral flap. (Chung-Hwan Baek, Soon-Young Kwon)

In most cases, the size of palatal defects decreases during the healing period after maxillectomy using an obturator, and the defect margin is covered with the mucosa. Delaying the closure of the defect allows for epithelialization of the defect margin, and more mucosa is available for closure. In cases where the defect is too large to be reconstructed with a local flap at the time of maxillectomy, prosthetic obturation helps the patient until the defect margin is epithelialized [7].

1.3 KQ 1.3. How to Manage Salivary Leakage After Buccal Cancer Surgery?

Young-Gyu Eun

1.3.1 Diagnosis

Iatrogenic parotid duct injury is often unavoidable when buccal squamous cell carcinoma (SCC) is surgically treated because of the intimate anatomical relationship between the buccal mucosa, Stensen duct, and parotid gland. It is often difficult to achieve negative margins while preserving parotid duct integrity. Sialocele formation is a frequent and untoward complication caused by the extravasation of saliva into a surgical defect, which delays healing, creates fistulas, and causes painful facial swelling. Currently, there is no consensus regarding the management of parotid sialoceles.

Sialocele was diagnosed by aspiration of the swelling and was confirmed to have amylase levels of >10,000 U/L. A CT scan may depict a single or multiloculated collection of low-density tissue relative to the surrounding soft tissue of the face and neck. If left untreated, sialoceles can cause irreparable damage to the free, vascularized flap. Damage to the reconstruction can occur if the sialocele remains enclosed and generates pressure that causes ischemia to the skin paddle of the reconstruction, perforating vessels supplying the reconstruction, or can act as a nidus for infection. Such complications can delay the recovery time of patients who are indicated for adjunctive therapies such as radiation.

1.3.2 Management

Surgical and non-surgical approaches are available for treating parotid salivary gland duct injuries. The treatment type should be determined based on the extent of damage to the area. Non-surgical approaches are typically used when the parotid gland parenchyma is contused.

Expert Opinion

In cases where a surgeon performs a wide excision for buccal cancer, the primary focus is not on preventing injury to the parotid duct during surgery. The procedure is conducted with oncological safety as the priority, and if issues related to the parotid gland or duct injury arise postoperatively, they can be managed at that time. Moreover, since most patients undergo postoperative radiation therapy, which often results in reduced salivary gland function, complications specifically related to the salivary glands are rare. (Chul-Ho Kim)

1.3.3 Conservative Measures

The simplest method of controlling saliva is to divert the flow away from important structures. Lateralization of fistulas involves incising the skin flap in the lateral position and placing a Penrose drain in the wound to divert saliva away from the great vessels. A pressure dressing is applied to prevent fluid accumulation beneath the skin flap.

Local wound care measures consisting of repeated needle aspirations and pressure dressings have been employed for successful nonoperative management of parotid sialoceles and fistulas.

1.3.4 Pharmacological Interventions

There is no scientific evidence of the benefits of pharmacological intervention in perioperative or postoperative settings to reduce the incidence of saliva-related complications.

1.3.5 Anticholinergics

Anticholinergics are a class of drugs currently used to reduce salivary production by blocking the parasympathetic effects of the neurotransmitter acetylcholine on the salivary glands. *Banthine (methanthaline), pro-banthine (propantheline),* and *penztropine* are systemically administered anticholinergic agents. *Nebulized scopolamine* is another agent useful for controlling oral cavity secretions. Glycopyrrolate appears to be a better choice than scopolamine or atropine for the treatment of saliva-related complications because it does not have side effects on the central nervous system owing to its quaternary ammonium structure, which prevents it from crossing the blood–brain barrier. Side effects such as constipation, urinary retention, blurred vision, flushing, and delirium are unpleasant and may lead to discontinuation of therapy before any significant benefit is obtained.

1.3.6 Botulinum Toxin A

Injectable botulinum toxin A is a mechanistically different strategy for reducing the parasympathetic activity in the salivary glands. Botulinum toxin A is locally injected and inhibits the release of acetylcholine from the presynaptic membrane by interacting with intracellular SNARE proteins. The duration of the effects on saliva production and composition was approximately 3 months. Numerous methods for administering Botox have been described; however, currently, there is no consensus regarding the amount or approach used to prevent paralysis of the facial nerve or the masticatory methods. Two methods are described in the literature. The first involved a subcutaneous injection of 30–50 U, directly after aspiration of the sialocele [8]. The second approach involved the injection of 10–20 U at 2–3 sites under electromyographic control, without complications at 14–21 months of follow-up [9].

1.3.7 Surgical Treatment

Surgical options to reduce the salivary flow are recommended if conservative therapy and pharmacological interventions fail. Surgical treatment is permanent and thus utilized on a limited basis. Surgical approaches including gland denervation, duct repair, diversion, ligation, and parotidectomy have been described. Parotidectomy can help reduce salivary flow. However, excision of the major salivary glands is an invasive procedure that requires general anesthesia and is associated with a significant risk to the facial nerve in cases of surgery of the parotid gland and the marginal mandibular nerve in submandibular gland surgery.

Expert Opinion

When buccal cancer approaches the duct orifice, transposition of the orifice of the entire intact parotid duct with a meticulous frozen biopsy can be performed. In case of sacrifice of the orifice, proximal margin of the divided duct can be diverted to margin free buccal mucosa. When diversion is difficult, ductal ligation is necessary for prevention of saliva leakage and pooling to prevent delayed wound healing. Since most patients require postoperative radiotherapy, if saliva pooling is suspected, wound exploration at previous duct area can be performed to ligate the duct using hemoclip. This can be performed under local anesthesia if the patient cooperates well, and if not, under general anesthesia without using anticholinergics. (Chung-Hwan Baek)

References

1. Khoo MJW, Ooi ASH. Management of postreconstructive head and neck salivary fistulae: A review of current practices. J Plast Reconstr Aesthet Surg. 2021;74(9):2120–32. https://doi.org/10.1016/j.bjps.2020.12.096.
2. Tian B, Khoo D, Tay AC, Soo KC, Tan NC, Tan HK, et al. Management of orocutaneous fistulas using a vacuum-assisted closure system. Head Neck. 2014;36(6):873–81. https://doi.org/10.1002/hed.23393.
3. Inatomi Y, Kadota H, Yoshida S, Kamizono K, Shimamoto R, Fukushima S, et al. Utility of negative-pressure wound therapy for orocutaneous and pharyngocutaneous fistula following head and neck surgery. Head Neck. 2020;42(1):103–10. https://doi.org/10.1002/hed.25989.
4. Goiato MC, dos Santos DM, Moreno A, Santiago JF Jr, Haddad MF, Pesqueira AA, et al. Prosthetic treatments for patients with oronasal communication. J Craniofac Surg. 2011;22(4):1445–7. https://doi.org/10.1097/SCS.0b013e31821d17bd.
5. Triana RJ Jr, Uglesic V, Virag M, Varga SG, Knezevic P, Milenovic A, et al. Microvascular free flap reconstructive options in patients with partial and total maxillectomy defects. Arch Facial Plast Surg. 2000;2(2):91–101. https://doi.org/10.1001/archfaci.2.2.91.
6. Rothermel AT, Lundberg JN, Samson TD, Tse RW, Allori AC, Bezuhly M, et al. A toolbox of surgical techniques for palatal fistula repair. Cleft Palate Craniofac J. 2021;58(2):170–80. https://doi.org/10.1177/1055665620949321.
7. Jung S, Kook MS, Park HJ, Oh HK. Delayed closure of the palatal defect using buccal inversion and palatal rotation flaps after maxillectomy. J Craniofac Surg. 2013;24(2):660–4. https://doi.org/10.1097/SCS.0b013e31827c8611.

8. Vargas H, Galati LT, Parnes SM. A pilot study evaluating the treatment of postparotidectomy sialoceles with botulinum toxin type A. Arch Otolaryngol Head Neck Surg. 2000;126(3):421–4. https://doi.org/10.1001/archotol.126.3.421.
9. Marchese-Ragona R, Marioni G, Restivo DA, Staffieri A. The role of botulinum toxin in postparotidectomy fistula treatment. A technical note. Am J Otolaryngol. 2006;27(3):221–4. https://doi.org/10.1016/j.amjoto.2005.09.009.

2 Oropharyngeal Cancer Surgery

Doh Young Lee

2.1 KQ 2.1. How to Manage Massive Oral Bleeding After Oropharyngectomy?

Doh Young Lee

Bleeding from an artery in the surgical bed can be fatal. Although the bleeding starts from 'sentinel blood,' which is in the form of blood-tinged mucus, brown mucus, or red streaks, there can be no previous detection of small bleeding. A recent meta-analysis and systematic review of post-oropharyngectomy bleeding reported rates ranging from 3.1% to 19.7%, with pooled mean and median rates of 5.8% and 6.5%, respectively. The risk of bleeding is directly related to the highly vascular anatomy of the oropharynx, where an intricate network of vessels exists within the muscular and mucosal layers. Therefore, bleeding after oropharyngectomy can be unpredictable, and its severity may vary from mild to life-threatening.

Expert Opinion
The oropharynx, including the tonsils and the base of the tongue, receives blood supply from several vessels, such as the lingual artery, facial artery, ascending pharyngeal artery, and internal maxillary artery. Due to this extensive blood supply, any surgical procedure (whether open or transoral, minimal or extensive resection) in the oropharynx, including a simple tonsillectomy, carries a risk of intraoperative and postoperative hemorrhage. This risk should be clearly communicated during patient consultations prior to surgery. (Chen-Chi WANG)

Erosion of the exposed vessels within the surgical bed is a common cause of post-TORS bleeding and is associated with larger primary tumors, a greater extent of surgery, prior radiation, hypertension, salivary exposure/infection, and perioperative anticoagulation. In addition, the timing of secondary infection was consistent with that of postoperative hemorrhage, ranging from days 1 to 21, with a median time of 5–8 days. Most mortalities result from asphyxia due to aspirated blood rather than from blood loss. Therefore, immediate protection of the airway against postoperative bleeding is crucial.

D. Y. Lee (✉)
Department of Otorhinolaryngology Head and Neck Surgery, Seoul National University College of Medicine, Seoul, South Korea
e-mail: dohyoungishere@snu.ac.kr

K.-J. Cho, J.-O. Park (eds.), *Management of Head and Neck Surgery Complications*,
https://doi.org/10.1007/978-981-96-1860-6_2

◆ Bleeding after oropharyngectomy can also be unpredictable, and its severity may vary from mild to life-threatening. Because most mortalities result from asphyxia of aspirated blood rather than from blood loss, immediate protection of the airway in post-operative bleeding is important.

Ligation of branches of the external carotid artery may decrease the severity of bleeding but does not influence the rate of bleeding. From a personal perspective, if meticulous dissection and careful placement of surgical clips are performed during surgery (e.g., clips and suture ligature on vessels >2–4 mm in diameter) and the surgeon confirms complete bleeding control, transcervical artery ligation is not required. The ligation of larger arteries in the neck, such as the lingual and facial arteries, may result in delayed wound healing and infection, which can be the main etiology of postoperative bleeding. Ligation of the proximal stump of the external carotid artery is not recommended for this reason.

Expert Opinion

In my opinion, ligation of the cervical vessels could help prevent post-operative bleeding, and I do not agree with the notion that ligation of the branches of external carotid arteries impedes wound healing. (Min Sik Kim)

Expert Opinion

According to recent literature, the rate of bleeding in patients who underwent prophylactic transcervical arterial ligation was similar to that in those who did not, but the severity of postoperative bleeding was reduced. However, other complications, such as oro-cervical fistula formation, incidental injury to the hypoglossal nerve, or neurological events associated with retrograde clot propagation or vascular anomalies, should be taken into consideration. Instead, some commercially available hemostatic agents can be used on the oropharyngeal wound as an adjunct to achieve hemostasis after carefully checking for bleeding during the surgery. (Chen-Chi WANG)

2.1.1 Management of Bleeding

The following strategies for managing post-oropharyngectomy bleeding have been considered (Fig. 2.1).

1. Compression: This should be performed transorally and externally. Packing the surgical bed with a gauze pack or tonsillar gauze ball should be performed using fingers or forceps that can be firmly fixed to the surgical bed. Detecting the exact bleeding focus is difficult; therefore, transoral compression of the surgical bed with a broad base is necessary to minimize bleeding and protect the airway. The first step involved compressing the inferior portion of the surgical bed and suctioning blood from the superior portion of the surgical bed. This step enables the detection of bleeding from the superior or inferior portion of the surgical bed. External compression of the upper neck may effectively compress the surgical bed and cause bleeding. In addition, compression of the external carotid area can decrease the blood flow to the surgical bed and cause bleeding. Caution is needed to minimize the compression of the internal carotid artery.
2. Hemodynamic stability is important when selecting a sequential procedure for the definite treatment of bleeding. If the patient is hemodynamically stable and the bleeding focus is well-visualized or known, the patient

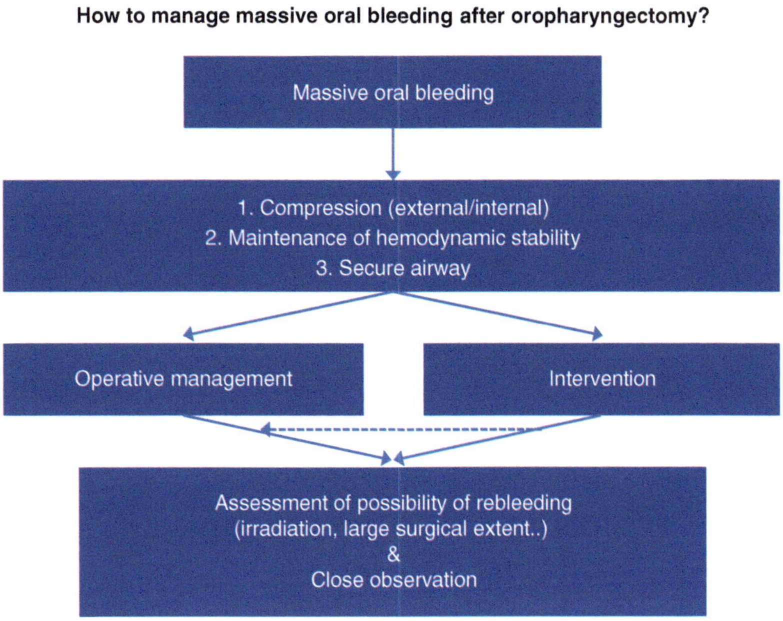

Fig. 2.1 Algorithm for management of unintended communication defect between oropharyngectomy surgical bed and neck

can be transferred to the operating room, and the artery can be ligated. However, if the patient is hemodynamically unstable or if the bleeding focus is unknown, transfer to an intervention room for an intravascular procedure is preferable.

3. Secure the airway: Airway protection is the most important procedure in patients with bleeding. Prophylactic tracheostomy may be indicated if a significant risk of postoperative bleeding is anticipated. If the patient has a tracheostomy tube or opening, insertion of a cuffed cannula or ballooning of the cuff is a simple method to protect the airway. If the patient does not have a tracheostomy tube or opening, minimizing bleeding from the surgical site by transoral external compression is important for securing the airway. Continuous bleeding of the blood clot in the laryngopharynx severely inhibits intubation; therefore, orotracheal intubation cannot be easily performed during bleeding. When bleeding decreases, intubation should be performed by experienced doctors with the support of many assistants.

Expert Opinion

Depending on the facility, Interventional Radiology (IVR) may not be immediately available. If hemodynamics are unstable, the lingual and facial arteries should be ligated first via a cervical approach. This can often reduce the force of bleeding and facilitate transoral hemostasis. (Seiichi Yoshimoto)

Expert Opinion

To allow intubation, blood clots must be scraped away with fingers after using a bite block or gauze placed between the upper and lower teeth until suction is ready. Once suction is ready, a large suction catheter should be used. Utilizing two suction systems is also effective. (Seiichi Yoshimoto)

If securing the airway through orotracheal intubation is difficult due to bleeding

(continued)

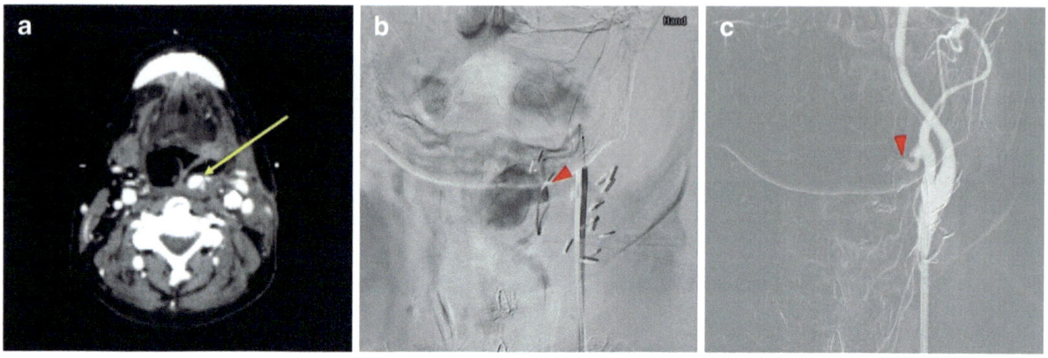

Fig. 2.2. A patient with post-oropharyngectomy bleeding. Aneurysmal change of bleeding focus in CT scan (**a**, yellow arrow), bleeding focus in angiography (**b**, red arrowhead), and plugging of bleeding focus (**c**, red arrowhead)

and oral pressure, an emergent tracheostomy or cricothyroidotomy should be performed promptly to secure the airway. (Kwang Jae Cho, Chen-Chi WANG)

During an interventional procedure, angiography is performed to detect the bleeding focus. If bleeding is minimized, transoral and external compressions are stopped to locate the bleeding focus easily. When a bleeding focus was found, arterial plugging was performed, followed by confirmatory angiography (Fig. 2.2). Patients were required to stay in the intensive care unit for a few days. Nasogastric and non-per-oral (NPO) tubes are required for proper nutritional support and to minimize irritation of the surgical bed.

Expert Opinion

After an interventional procedure or surgical treatment (such as ligation), I prefer TPN over an NG tube to avoid potential irritation from the surgical bed and to maintain NPO status. (Kwang Jae Cho)

2.2 KQ 2.2. How to Reconstruct the Unintended Communication Defect Between the Oropharynx and Neck During Transoral Lateral Oropharyngectomy?

Doh Young Lee

Unintended communication through surgical defects is significantly correlated with regenerative potential and the formation of dead space. The regenerative potential is associated with sufficient blood supply to the surgical bed and is significantly influenced by preoperative radiation therapy. In addition, patient comorbidities and nutritional status can affect the regenerative power of the surgical bed and surgical outcomes of unintended fistula formation. Dead space is correlated with the surgical extent, which indicates the size of the resected tissue and violation of the parapharyngeal fat pad. Moreover, if the extent of the neck dissection is far from the oropharyngeal level near the surgical bed, abundant tissue is lacking below the surgical bed, resulting in unintended communication. Therefore, to avoid ‘unintended’ communication, preoperative prediction is important, and surgical repair at the

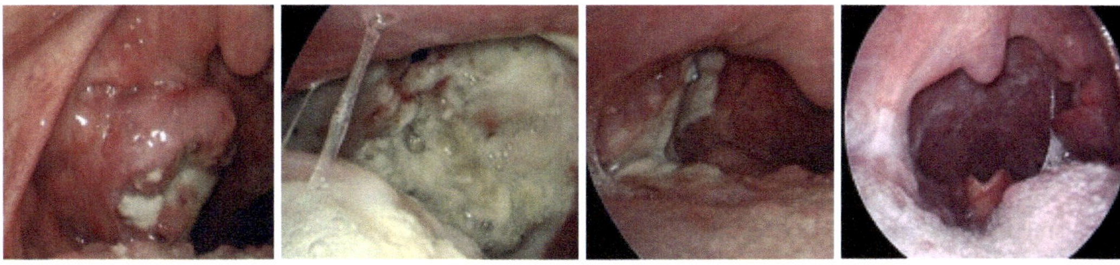

Fig. 2.3 Unintended communication defect healed by conservative management

time of resection should be considered in patients with a high risk of communication defects between the oropharynx and neck.

◆ Unintended communication defect is significantly correlated with regenerative potentials such as preoperative radiation and patients' comorbidities or nutritional status, as well as dead space of surgical defect, which is associated with size and surgical extent.

Expert Opinion

When performing oropharyngeal cancer surgery, it is very common to perform a neck dissection up to the area near the pharyngeal surgical bed, considering the location of the primary tumor. (Min Sik Kim)

When performing oropharyngectomy and neck dissection simultaneously, a communication defect usually occurs at neck level Ib. In cases of oropharyngeal cancer, even if there is cN+ disease, the rate of occult metastasis to level Ib is not high when there is no clearly identifiable metastatic lymph node at level Ib. Therefore, when performing oropharyngectomy along with a comprehensive neck dissection that includes level Ib, I usually choose to remove only the level Ib lymph nodes and leave the submandibular gland in place. Preserving the submandibular gland can help prevent communication defects. (Kwang Jae Cho)

Small defects often close spontaneously with conservative management (Fig. 2.3). If a communication defect is detected during surgery, a transcervical fibrin sealant, collagen membrane, or dermal substitute can be placed. A local rotational muscle flap, including the digastric, mylohyoid, and sternocleidomastoid muscles can reinforce the neck space.

Expert Opinion

Other muscles, such as the omohyoid muscle and sternohyoid muscle, can also be used to close the unintended communication between the oropharyngeal wound bed and the neck space. (Chen-Chi WANG)

Another effective method is to rotate the submandibular gland after ligating and transecting the facial artery, then place it in the parapharyngeal space. There is no concern about blood flow to the submandibular gland even after the main blood supply from the facial artery is cut off. Additionally, negative pressure drainage should be avoided as it may promote fistula formation. Instead, multiple Penrose drains should be used for open drainage in the neck, and the submandibular area should be compressed with a bandage. (Seiichi Yoshimoto)

"There have been cases where, despite good wound healing after surgery and completion of radiotherapy, carotid artery rupture occurred several months later due to impaired blood supply and tissue necrosis, nearly resulting in death. Although carotid

(continued)

artery rupture is rare, it is often fatal when it occurs, underscoring the importance of vigilance in such cases. (Min Sik Kim)

During the postoperative period, the following are suspicious signs of communication defect formation: (1) color change and foul odor of the negative suction drain; (2) air leakage of the negative suction drain; (3) pain/tenderness and reddish discoloration of the neck; (4) fever; and (5) elevation of WBC and CRP levels. Communication defects tend to develop approximately 7–12 days after post-oropharyngectomy.

Expert Opinion
In the early stages of suspected fistula formation, a suction tube can be inserted into the contralateral nostril and secured with tape, similar to a nasogastric tube. The tip of the suction tube is placed in the oropharynx to continuously suction the accumulated saliva and minimize the flow of saliva into the neck space. (Chen-Chi WANG)

The first step involves medical treatment and adequate nutritional support to minimize infections in the surgical bed and neck. If the symptoms and signs of communication defects are not severe and the surgical bed is not severely inflamed, conservative management is sufficient. As the approach to the surgical bed for oropharyngectomy is relatively easy, active debridement of dead tissue should be performed, and retention sutures can be helpful in decreasing surgical defects. Repetitive checks and application of negative pressure on the suction drain should be performed if the air leakage is intermittent, whereas continuous negative suction using wall suction should be considered in patients with continuous air leakage. Nasogastric tube feeding and maintenance of a non-peroral (NPO) status are necessary to prevent infection and provide proper nutrition.

◆ Minimizing surgical defects using retention sutures and maintenance of negative pressure can be applied to patients with relatively less severe conditions.

From a personal perspective, irradiated wounds have a minimal chance of spontaneously healing communication defects when continuous air leakage occurs through a negative suction drain. Therefore, in irradiated wounds, fresh tissue transfer, including local, pedicled, and free flaps, should be considered according to the defect size and patient status.

Expert Opinion
Once a fistula has formed, negative pressure drainage may actually hinder its healing. It seems that inserting Penrose drains into the neck and compressing the submandibular area with a bandage would facilitate the closure of the fistula. (Seiichi Yoshimoto)

◆ In an irradiated wound, surgical repair should be in consideration if the air leakage is continuous on the negative suction drain.

Surgical treatment includes wide debridement of necrotic tissue and covering of the surgical bed with healthy tissue, such as free-flap reconstruction. The flap type can be selected based on its extent and depth. The most frequently used flaps are anterolateral thigh (ALT) and RFFF, which are used to delay wound healing. A myomucosal flap can be applied to a small defect, but infection of the surgical bed may cause the failure of free tissue transfer.

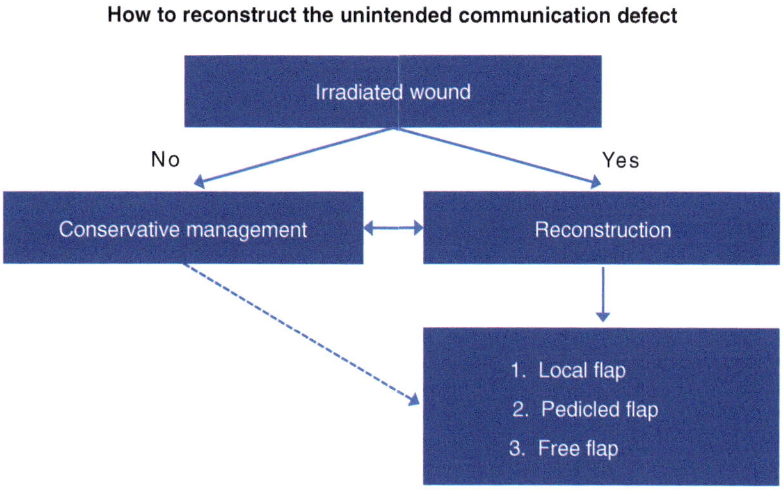

Fig. 2.4. Algorithm for management of unintended communication defect between oropharyngectomy surgical bed and neck

> **Expert Opinion**
> The simplest and easiest option to use is the trapezius latissimus dorsi island flap. It offers a similar size and reliability to a free flap and can be completed within about an hour during surgery, making it an effective option. (Min Sik Kim)

The overall management is summarized in Fig. 2.4.

2.3 KQ 2.3. How to Manage Infection or Delayed Healing After Transoral Oropharyngectomy?

Doh Young Lee

Mucosal regeneration was completed 3–4 weeks after the transoral oropharyngectomy (Fig. 2.5). The duration may vary according to the patient's age, medical condition, extent of surgery, and history of RT. The most intractable delayed wound healing occurs in patients with a history of radiation, while the remaining patients can be managed and treated conservatively. Synechia between the tonsil fossa and tongue base may occur frequently, especially when the surgical extent of the tongue base area is wide. However, delayed wound healing for >2 months may delay the start of adjuvant treatment after surgery and cause severe pain, leading to a vicious cycle in which wound healing is continuously delayed, with poor oral intake. This has the potential to cause necrosis of the surgical bed.

> ◆ Wound healing after transoral oropharyngectomy is generally completed 1 month post-surgery. A delay of more than 2 months required active intervention.

> **Expert Opinion**
> Delayed wound healing may indicate tumor recurrence. And in my experience, delayed wound healing increases the risk of vessel damage and wound infection and may require more tissue for reconstruction. Therefore, conservative treatment is monitored for up to one month. (Min Sik Kim)
>
> When radiation therapy is anticipated after oropharyngectomy, performing local flap reconstruction during surgery is useful in preventing postoperative infections, delayed healing, and soft tissue necrosis. (Kwang Jae Cho)

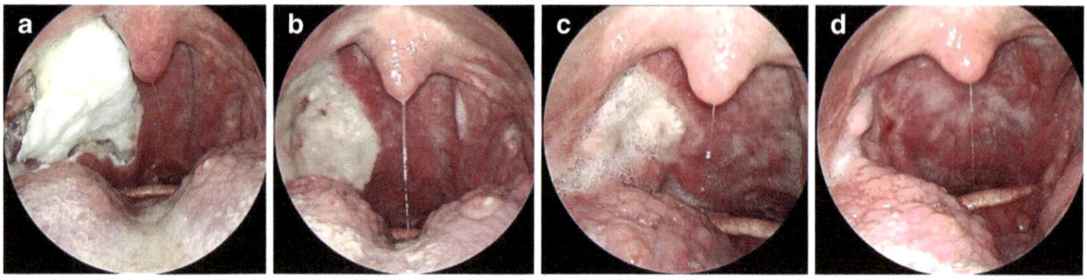

Fig. 2.5. Normal wound healing process after transoral oropharyngectomy. (**a**) Postoperative 1 week. (**b**) Postoperative 2 weeks. (**c**) Postoperative 3 weeks. (**d**) Postoperative 4 weeks

Medical treatment is essential to reduce symptoms such as pain, secondary infection, and inflammation. Medical treatments included antibiotics, NSAIDs, steroids, and oral gargles (hexamidine, betadine, or lidocaine). In patients with a history of radiation, antioxidants, including pentoxifylline, tocopherol, and humidifiers, can be considered for radiation necrosis. If the symptoms are severe and the patient cannot swallow food or maintain adequate oral nutritional intake, temporary hospitalization and parenteral nutritional support may be helpful. A necrotic tissue biopsy should be performed before treatment to rule out recurrence. Contrast-enhanced computed tomography should be performed to confirm the extent of delayed wound healing and the depth of safety of the internal carotid artery.

◆ The initial step for delayed wound healing is medical treatment and adequate nutritional support.

Expert Opinion

For patients with a history of significant acid reflux, potent anti-reflux medications, such as proton pump inhibitors, should be considered. (Chen-Chi WANG)

Because the surgical bed for oropharyngectomy is relatively easy, active debridement of dead tissue should be performed in patients undergoing wound healing. Generally, this procedure can be performed in an outpatient clinic under local anesthesia. General anesthesia may be applied only if the patient cannot tolerate the pain that occurs during the debridement procedure or if mouth opening is not sufficient for the procedure due to trismus. During debridement, all dead tissues are removed until healthy blood is visible on the surgical bed. Care should be taken in the deep surgical bed to prevent the internal carotid artery from passing through the neck. Debridement can be performed 1 or 2 times a week until the necrotic tissue ceases to develop.

◆ Debridement of dead tissue can be conveniently performed once or twice a week in the outpatient clinic using local anesthesia.

In patients with long-term intractable cases, hyperbaric oxygen therapy can be considered according to the institutional circumstances. Hyperbaric oxygen therapy is administered 1–2 times per week for 90 minutes. Treatment outcomes vary by 20–90%, and the combination of debridement and early application of hyperbaric oxygen therapy may increase the success rate. The effects of hyperbaric oxygen therapy include angiogenesis, epithelialization, and antibacterial effects on the surgical bed, which can delay wound healing.

◆ A combination of hyperbaric oxygen therapy can be considered in patients not responding to debridement for 2–3 weeks.

Expert Opinion
In the case of local recurrence, hyperbaric oxygen therapy may exacerbate the tumor. Therefore, it is necessary to perform a biopsy or other tests to confirm the absence of recurrence before initiating hyperbaric oxygen therapy. (Seiichi Yoshimoto)

Surgical treatment includes wide debridement of necrotic tissue and covering of the surgical bed with healthy tissue, such as free-flap reconstruction. The flap type can be selected based on its extent and depth. The most frequently used flaps were ALT and RFFF (Fig. 2.6). A myomucosal flap can be applied to a small defect; however, infection of the surgical bed may cause the failure of free tissue transfer.

Surgical repair of delayed wound healing should be considered in the following cases:

The overall management is summarized in Fig. 2.7.

A 66-year-old male with base of tongue (BOT) cancer underwent concurrent chemoradication therapy (CCRT) and reached CR. After 1 year, the tumor recurred in the right tonsillar pillar and was treated with a partial oropharyngectomy. Delayed wound healing occurred for 4 months, which did not respond to repeated debridement and consequently caused severe pain. Eventually, flap reconstruction was necessary, and the surgical bed was reconstructed using an ALT-free flap.

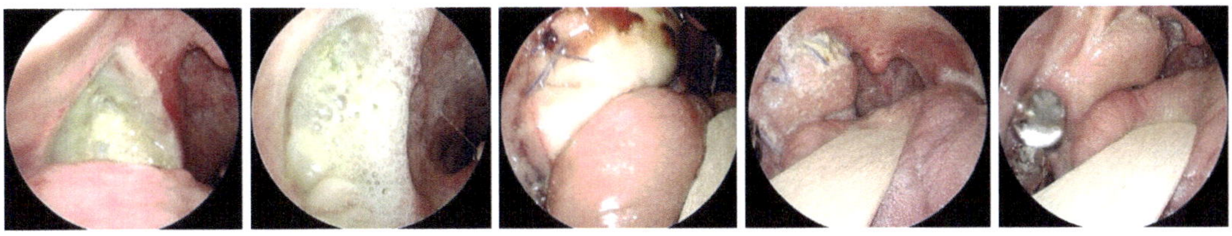

Fig. 2.6. Surgical approach for delayed wound healing after transoral oropharyngectomy

Fig. 2.7. Algorithm for management of delayed wound healing after transoral oropharyngectomy. *(1) Delayed wound healing over 3–4 months despite the active medical treatment and debridement of the wound. (2) Severe pain or trismus causing inadequate nutritional support. (3) Possibility of a carotid blowout

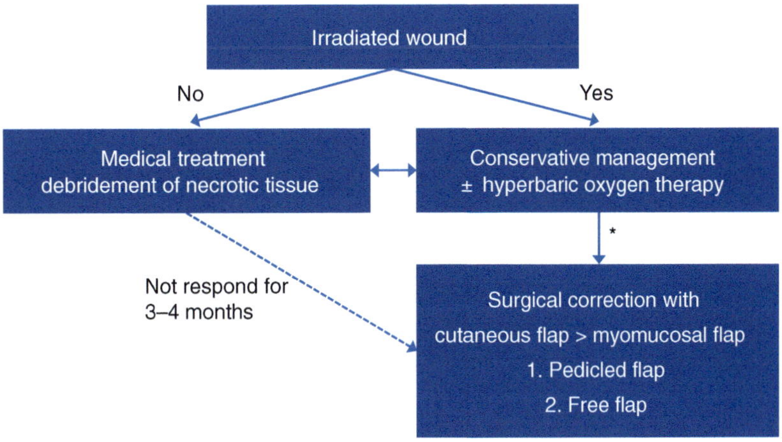

Part II

Salivary Glands and Parapharyngeal Space

Surgery of Parotid Gland Tumors

3

Eun-Jae Chung and Jae-Yol Lim

3.1 KQ 3.1. How to Manage Inadvertent Facial Nerve Transection During Parotidectomy?

Eun-Jae Chung

Facial nerve paralysis after parotidectomy can vary in severity depending on its extent; however, it can also lead to permanent physical and psychological disabilities. Furthermore, when patients and their caregivers are not clearly informed prior to the surgery, there is a high potential for medical disputes [1]. However, in various situations, unintentional or potential sacrifice of a patient's facial nerve may be unavoidable for head and neck surgeons. Therefore, understanding how such cases are treated is essential.

Supplementary Information The online version contains supplementary material available at https://doi.org/10.1007/978-981-96-1860-6_3.

E.-J. Chung (✉)
Department of Otorhinolaryngology–Head and Neck Surgery, Seoul National University Hospital, Seoul National University College of Medicine, Seoul, Republic of Korea
e-mail: voicechung@snu.ac.kr

J.-Y. Lim (✉)
Department of Otolaryngology, Gangnam Severance Hospital, College of Medicine, Yonsei University, Seoul, Republic of Korea
e-mail: jylimmd@yuhs.ac

The first important aspect that must be understood and familiarized with is the anatomical and functional details of the peripheral facial nerve, as well as the retrograde approach to the facial nerve during parotidectomy.

Expert Opinion
In situations where the main trunk of the nerve is displaced or difficult to locate, surgeons should focus more on osseous landmarks such as the bony external auditory canal, styloid process, mastoid tip and careful elimination of thin layers of gland and soft tissue which lie between these structures to facilitate finding the nerve in difficult situations. (Brett Miles)

Expert Opinion
Among the facial nerve branches, two branches are most important: (1.) zygomatic ("to protect the eye") and (2) mandibular ("to protect symmetry and cosmesis"). The least important branch is the cervical branch. (Yuh S Jung)

The facial nerve divides into upper and lower divisions within the parotid gland and travels through five peripheral branches (Fig. 3.1a) [2]. The five peripheral branches of the facial nerve

K.-J. Cho, J.-O. Park (eds.), *Management of Head and Neck Surgery Complications*,
https://doi.org/10.1007/978-981-96-1860-6_3

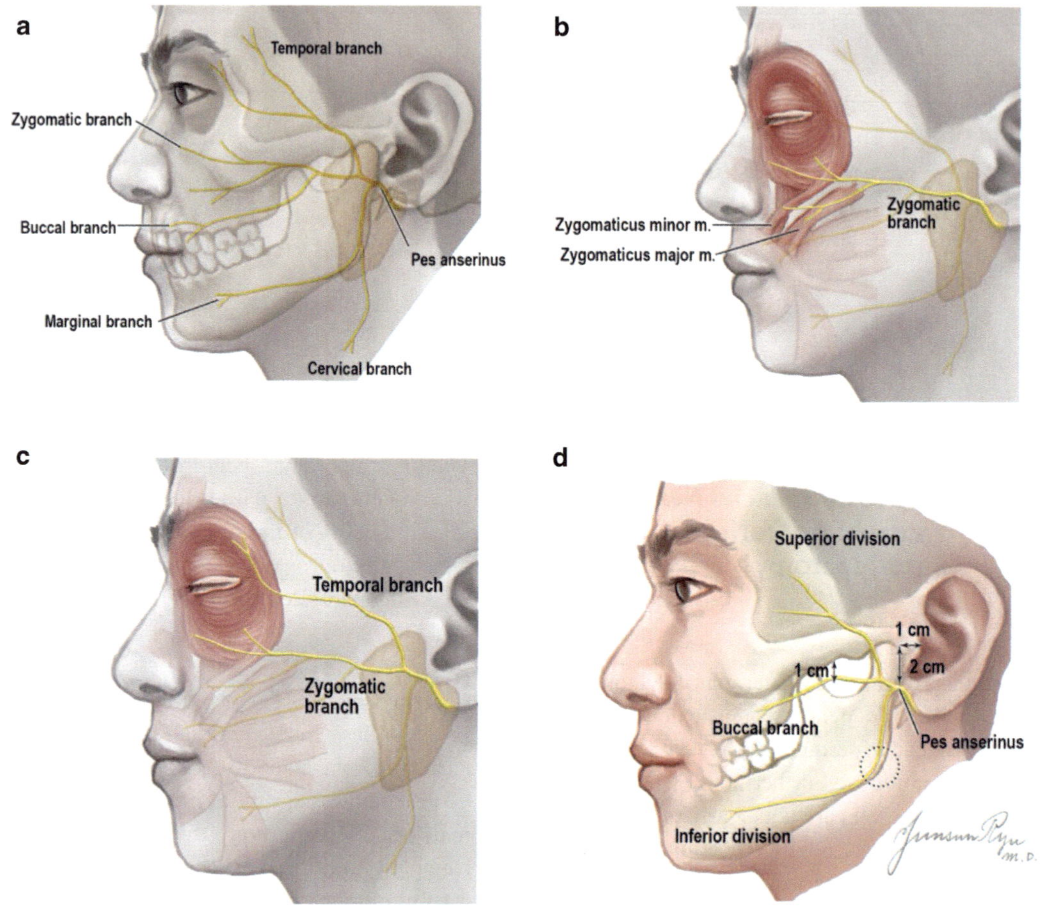

Fig. 3.1 (**a**) The five peripheral branches of the facial nerve; (**b**) The zygomatic branch of the facial nerve (nerve to orbicularis oculi and zygomaticus major muscle); (**c**) Orbicularis oculi muscle is innervated by both the zygomatic and temporal branches; and (**d**) Locating the peripheral branches of the facial nerve for retrograde facial nerve dissection

are not equally important for physiological functions. In many cases, selective restoration of the function of the most essential branch is crucial. The zygomatic branch is the most important peripheral branch (Fig. 3.1b), as it provides innervation to the orbicularis oculi and zygomaticus major muscles and plays a key role in eye closure and smiling movements. Because the orbicularis oculi muscle is innervated by both the zygomatic and temporal branches (Fig. 3.1c), reinnervation of the temporal branch is necessary not only to maintain muscle tone but also for eye closure. The lower division of the facial nerve controls movement to the lower corner of the mouth; therefore, reinnervating the lower division also helps maintain tension in the lower corner of the mouth for natural facial movement recovery.

In cases where the facial nerve is unintentionally or intentionally transected, reinnervating the damaged nerve yields the best results because no other reconstruction method could replicate the natural movement of the patient's own facial muscles. A key procedure for reinnervation is securing a healthy distal portion of the damaged facial nerve, which is often challenging in the same surgical field [3]. Surgeons should be familiar with the retrograde approach for locating the facial nerve in front of the parotid gland.

Expert Opinion
If possible, direct end-to-end anastomosis of the nerve without tension should be considered as the first reconstructive method. The sacrifice of the facial nerve in patients with parotid gland cancer, especially those with intact facial nerve function, must be carefully determined. All recent guidelines and meta-analyses recommend facial nerve preservation whenever possible, because there is no correlation between facial nerve sacrifice and oncological outcome. If facial nerve preservation is impossible, selective transection and rerouting of the peripheral branches is proper. If the patient's life expectancy is short, static reconstruction of the facial nerve is preferred to its dynamic reconstruction. (Han-Sin Jeong)

When surgeons cut the nerve while considering re-anastomosis, they should use the scalpel, not scissors. (Si-Youn Song)

The author's method of locating the peripheral branches of the facial nerve while conducting nerve exploration with nerve stimulation (Fig. 3.1d) is as follows [4].

- Zygomaticotemporal branch: the point where an imaginary line connecting the incisura of the external auditory canal and the lateral canthus meets the zygomatic arch.
- Buccal branch: the point where an imaginary line connecting the incisura of the external auditory canal and philtrum meets the anterior border of the parotid gland.
- Marginal mandibular nerve branch within 1 cm of the mandibular angle.

◆ The five peripheral branches of the facial nerve are not equally important for physiological function. In many cases, selectively restoring the function of the most essential branch is crucial.

◆ Familiarity with the retrograde approach for locating the facial nerve from the front of the parotid gland is essential for achieving optimal reinnervation.

3.1.1 Reconstruction Strategy Based on the Transection Site

3.1.1.1 Inadvertent Facial Nerve Transection at the Peripheral Branch Level

The further the peripheral branches of the facial nerve progress forward, the thinner they become, and the more they divide into numerous branches. Therefore, transection is more likely when the parotid tumor is located in the anterior region. It is generally advisable to perform reanastomosis when the facial nerve is transected. However, reanastomosis may not always lead to functional recovery based on the diameter of the nerve and the role of the transected branch. Moreover, in many cases, there may be no functional issues even when reanastomosis is not performed. Therefore, in such cases, the decision should be made considering factors such as the branch that has been transected, the ability to secure a healthy distal portion of the damaged facial nerve, and the presence of microscopic residual disease on frozen biopsy sections.

Expert Opinion
Intraoperative use of a nerve-stimulation probe may also give the surgeon an overview of the functional branches to target for repair. (Brett Miles)

In case of transection of the facial nerve medial to the connecting line between the lateral canthus and oral angle, re-anastomosis usually cannot recover the function of nerve. (Si-Youn Song)

The author considers two branches to be the most important among those originating from the upper division in terms of eye location as a reference point. These are (1) the zygomatic branch, which travels downward based on the location of the eye, supplying the nerve to the zygomaticus major muscle, and (2) the branch that travels upward based on the location of the eye, supplying the nerve to the orbicularis oculi muscle. Following these two important peripheral nerve branches, the marginal mandibular nerve is considered to have lower priority. Reanastomosis is often not essential during transection of the peripheral branches of the frontalis muscle. This represents a potential second stage of reanimation surgery. Reanastomosis of the buccal or cervical branches is typically not essential after transection.

When performing anastomosis on a transected nerve, it is crucial that the nerve ends are brought together without tension. Interpositional nerve grafts should be considered if tension exists between the nerves. In such cases, the great auricular nerve, which is located within the surgical field, may be used. The sural or antebrachial cutaneous nerves can also be used in cases requiring longer nerve grafts. The most important factor the author considers during nerve anastomosis is the contact between axons. To achieve this, the diameter and location of the target nerve are taken into account, and the epineurium and fascicle are included in the stitch either individually or together to increase the contact between axons. Although it varies depending on the thickness of the nerve, the author performed four sutures for the main branches of the facial nerve and two to four sutures for the nerves, such as the marginal mandibular or masseteric nerves.

Expert Opinion

The sural nerve is used because not only it is long it also has a similar branching pattern to the facial nerve, which makes it easier to reconstruct multiple branches simultaneously. (Han-Sin Jeong)

In case of extensive parotid gland malignancy, surgeon should have concerns about oncological safety using the great auricular nerve. In some reports, motor nerve grafting shows better results than sensory nerve graft. (Si-Youn Song)

Although transection of the buccal branch often results in food leakage during swallowing, this is largely transient. Buccal branches communicate with adjacent branches of the facial nerve in 70%–90% of patients. Reanimation is mostly unnecessary.

After 2–4 stitches, the neurorrhaphy site should be covered with tissue glue to enhance stabilized healing and regeneration.

Reanimation targeting the zygomatic and mandibular trunks separately might decrease the risk of synkinesis. Comparative trials endpointing this might be needed. (Yuh S Jung)

3.1.1.2 Inadvertent Facial Nerve Transection at the Upper or Lower Division Level

Transection at or above the level of the upper or lower main division of the facial nerve can result in various forms of permanent disability, making appropriate reconstruction essential. As previously mentioned, the peripheral branches originating from the upper division play the most critical role in facial movement. Therefore, establishing a reconstruction strategy based on this function is valuable.

Similar to the peripheral regions, a linear transection is managed with an end-to-end anastomosis whenever possible. If tension exists between the nerves, an interpositional graft should be considered. However, synkinesis is inevitable when a single main division is connected to multiple peripheral branches of the upper division. Moreover, in such cases, there is often a lack of post-surgical movement or dissatisfaction with the degree of movement. A nerve transfer technique using the masseteric or hypoglossal nerve as the power source for reinnervation rather than the proximal facial nerve has been successfully applied. It is essential to confirm the absence of residual tumors using a frozen biopsy prior to nerve anastomosis.

3.1.1.3 Inadvertent Facial Nerve Transection at the Main Trunk Level

When transection occurs at the main trunk level, simple end-to-end anastomosis is the most efficient approach for unintentional simple linear transection. However, in many advanced cases, the extent of transection is extensive, where the proximal end is part of the main trunk and the distal end includes individual peripheral branches. In cases where multiple peripheral branches are anastomosed to a single main trunk, there is a much higher likelihood of unsatisfactory movement. Moreover, synkinesis cannot be avoided. The author prefers the dual or triple reinnervation techniques, which use different power sources for each facial movement (Fig. 3.2).

(1) Eye closure movement

Proximal facial nerve stump (exploration of the facial nerve stump in the temporal bone if necessary): Anastomosis between the facial nerve peripheral branch and the orbicularis oculi muscle using an interpositional nerve graft (7-7)

(2) Smiling movement

Masseteric nerve in the masseter muscle: direct end-to-end anastomosis of the facial nerve peripheral branch to the zygomaticus major muscle (5-7)

(3) Reconstruction of marginal mandibular nerve reconstruction (optional).

Hypoglossal nerve (ansa cervicalis or interpositional graft for end-to-end anastomosis): marginal mandibular nerve (12-7)

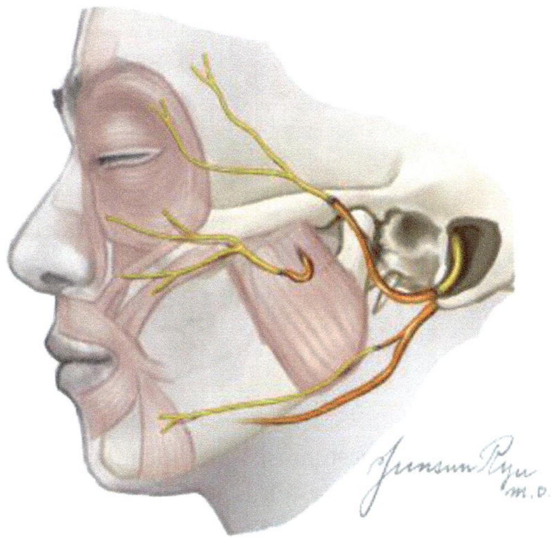

Fig. 3.2 Dual or triple reinnervation technique, which uses different power sources for each facial movement

> ◆ When transection of the facial nerve occurs, performing a simple end-to-end anastomosis is the most efficient approach for simple linear transection. However, there is often a lack of postoperative movement or dissatisfaction with the degree of movement in case the transection occurs at or above the level of the upper or lower main divisions. Moreover, synkinesis is inevitable.
>
> ◆ The dual or triple reinnervation technique using the masseteric or hypoglossal nerve as power sources for reinnervation rather than the proximal facial nerve has been successfully applied.

3.1.2 Masseteric Nerve Transfer

The masseteric nerve is currently one of the most highly regarded nerves during reinnervation surgery to restore facial movements [5]. It allows for strong and natural movements, and, when used in conjunction with the facial or other cranial nerves, dual or triple reinnervation can be performed while minimizing synkinesis. The masseteric nerve is particularly useful in restoring the movement of raising the corner of the mouth, as chewing is similar to raising the corner of the mouth, resulting in a natural smile movement. Furthermore, complications arising from sacrificing the masseteric nerve are minimal.

As mentioned previously, it is advisable to focus on reconstructing smile movements. However, if the proximal facial nerve root cannot be secured for eye closure, the entire upper division can be anastomosed to the masseter nerve.

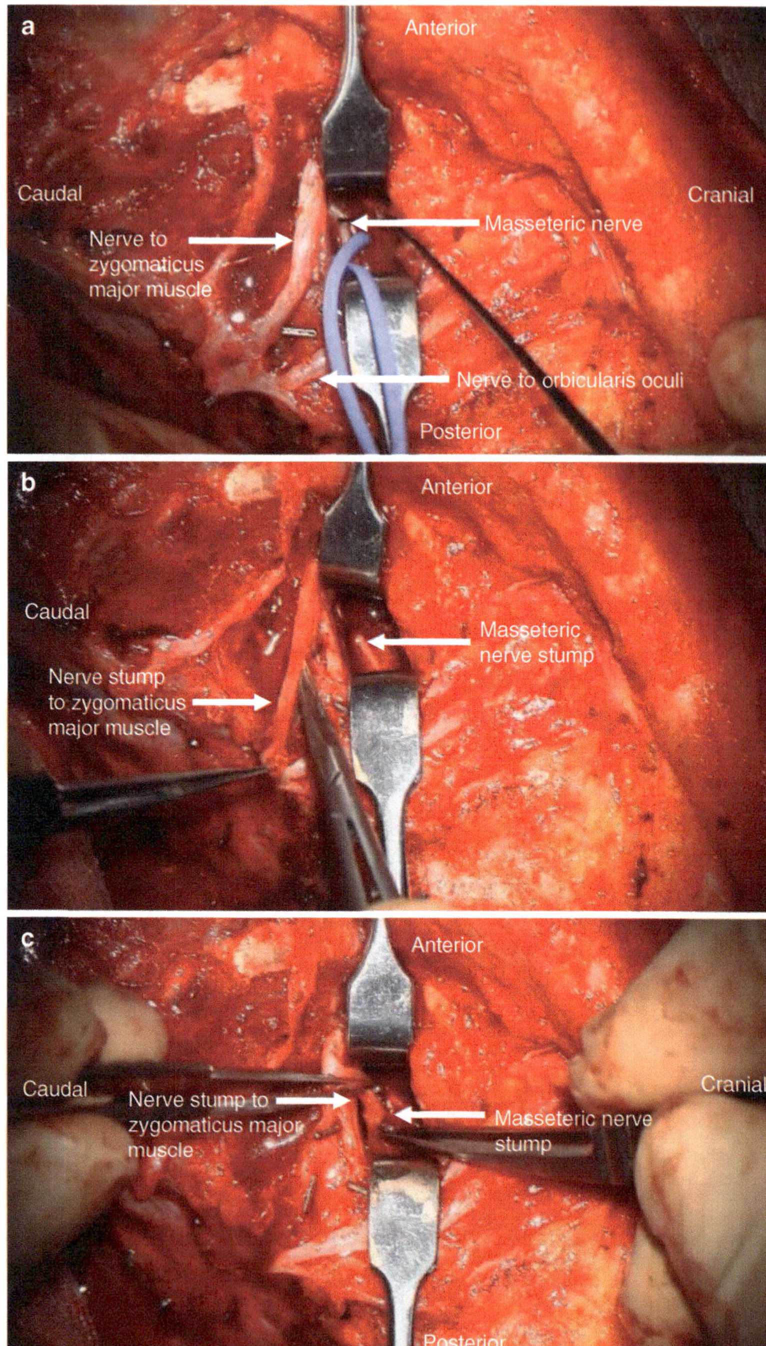

Fig. 3.3 (**a**) The masseteric nerve can be identified at 3 cm anterior to the tragus and 1 cm inferior to the zygomatic arch. (**b**, **c**) The masseteric nerve and facial nerve peripheral branch intended for anastomosis were adequately released and subsequently anastomosed together without tension

The masseteric nerve can be identified 3 cm anterior to the tragus and 1 cm inferior to the zygomatic arch within the masseter muscle using a nerve stimulator (Fig. 3.3a). Once the masseteric nerve and facial nerve peripheral branch intended for anastomosis are identified, they should be adequately released and subsequently anastomosed together without tension (Figs. 3.3b, c).

◆ The masseteric nerve is currently one of the most highly regarded nerves during reinnervation surgery for restoring smiling movements.
◆ The masseteric nerve can be identified at 3 cm anterior to the tragus and 1 cm inferior to the zygomatic arch within the masseter muscle using a nerve stimulator.

3.2 KQ 3.2. How Should the Tumor Be Managed If It Encases the Facial Nerve During Surgery for Parotid Cancer?

Eun-Jae Chung

Facial nerve paralysis after parotidectomy can vary in severity depending on its extent; however, it can also lead to permanent physical and psychological disabilities. Although medical disputes have high potential when patients and their caregivers are not clearly informed before surgery, in complicated situations, unintentional or potential sacrifice of a patient's facial nerve may be unavoidable for head and neck surgeons.

Although fine-needle aspiration (FNA) biopsies of salivary neoplasms have proven extremely useful for preoperative planning, interpreting these biopsies can be challenging and may result in diagnostic ambiguity and inaccuracy. Malignant salivary gland tumors can only be diagnosed using surgical specimens. Malignant tumors are commonly misdiagnosed as benign.

Therefore, there are situations in which the surgeon has no choice but to sacrifice the facial nerve, even if the tumor is not diagnosed as malignant, despite the absence of facial paralysis before surgery. Typical cases occur when the tumor has clearly invaded or completely encased the facial nerve, even in the absence of direct invasion. It is crucial to be able to predict these possibilities before surgery and explain them to the patients and their caregivers. In these cases, efforts also need to be made to minimize postoperative disabilities.

3.2.1 Preoperative Considerations

Tumors encasing the facial nerve can sometimes be easily predicted; however, in some cases, this may not be straightforward. When tumors are located around the stylomastoid foramen or are anteriorly positioned in contact with the masseter muscle, although malignancy is not confirmed through preoperative imaging or biopsy, the possibility of malignancy and the potential need to sacrifice the facial nerve must be considered (Fig. 3.4).

Expert Opinion
In cases of deep-seated parotid tumor or parotid tumor adjacent to stylomastoid foramen, Double Echo Steady State (DESS) MRI sequence is helpful to visualize facial nerve directly. It provides critical information about the contact, invasion, or displacement between the tumor and facial nerve, which can help determine if further surgical approach, such as a mastoidectomy, is necessary. (Han-Sin Jeong)

Precise cytopathologic diagnosis is essential both medically and legally. (Yuh S Jung)

In cases where a schwannoma is suspected based on a preoperative biopsy and even when the diagnosis is not definitive, the presence of spindle cells in the specimen, particularly if the tumor is positioned around the stylomastoid foramen along the course of the facial nerve, highlights the likelihood of a facial nerve schwannoma. Careful attention is essential to prevent irreversible, permanent postoperative paralysis in asymptomatic patients.

In these cases, it is paramount to inform patients without preoperative facial paralysis about the possibility of sacrificing the facial nerve if the tumor cannot be separated from the facial nerve or if complete encasement necessitates nerve splitting. In such cases, regardless of the reconstruction method, the structure cannot be restored to its original state.

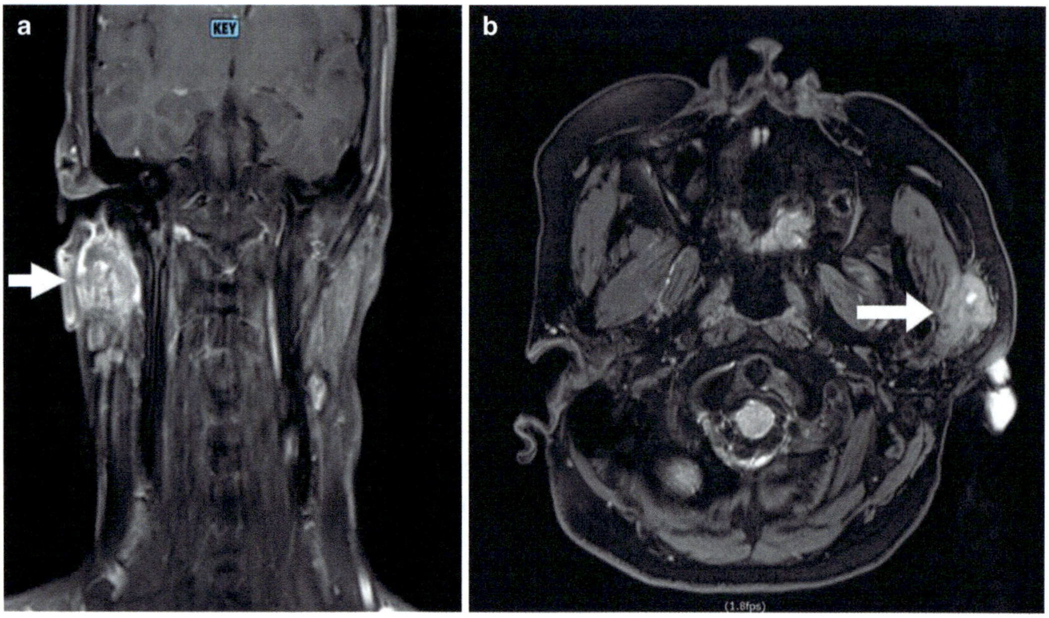

Fig. 3.4 (**a**) Cases where tumors (arrow) are located around the stylomastoid foramen. (**b**) Cases where tumors (arrow) are located anteriorly with contact toward the masseter muscle

It is also vital to accurately inform patients and their families about the expected results of optimal reconstruction. When it is highly unlikely that facial nerve preservation is possible or there is a high risk of facial paralysis after surgery, capturing photographs of the surgical field and providing an adequate explanation to the guardian before proceeding to the next steps is recommended. Allowing them to enter the operating room for an explanation may also be a good option.

Expert Opinion
Facial palsy is seen only or mostly in malignant diseases, but there could be some exceptions. (Yuh S Jung)

Malignant tumors should be considered if accompanied by facial paralysis before surgery. Although adenoid cystic carcinoma is the most well-known type, many high-grade salivary gland cancers exhibit perineural spread through the facial or trigeminal nerves. This can be easily overlooked on preoperative imaging or clinical findings. Any lesions that are overlooked during surgery or postoperative radiation therapy may lead to treatment failure as residual lesions. Therefore, multidisciplinary treatment planning is essential.

3.2.2 Intraoperative Considerations

If the tumor encases the facial nerve and the facial nerve plane cannot be secured, there is a high likelihood of malignancy. In the present case, the benign tumor may have been an extensive recurrent pleomorphic adenoma or facial nerve schwannoma. If there is no facial paralysis before surgery, it is generally recommended to excise the tumor while preserving the facial nerve to the maximum possible extent without leaving any visible lesions and to perform adjuvant treatment after tumor removal. If the tumor cannot be separated from the facial nerve or must be split because of complete encasement, the decision regarding the sacrifice of the facial nerve, even in the absence of preoperative facial paralysis, depends on various considerations. Is it a high-grade malignancy? What were the patients' ages and social activities? What is the feasibility of the adjuvant treatment? What are the opinions of the patients and their families? In such situations, it is highly recommended that such decisions be made through preoperative consultations. Radical radiation therapy may also be an option if patients and their families refuse surgical treatment due to the possibility of postoperative facial paralysis or other serious surgical complications.

If facial paralysis occurs preoperatively (including incomplete paralysis) or if there is clear evidence of facial nerve invasion or complete encasement, sacrifice of the facial nerve is inevitable in most cases [2, 3]. The extent of facial nerve invasion must be accurately assessed, and immediate reconstruction should be performed.

Expert Opinion
Even in cases of incomplete paralysis, there are reports showing that there is no direct (pathological) facial nerve invasion in about 1/3 of cases. Therefore, the facial nerve should be preserved as much as possible if it is separated from the tumor. (Han-Sin Jeong)

In these cases, retrograde facial nerve dissection can be combined with the classical approach described in the previous section (Fig. 3.5). Retrograde facial nerve dissection was performed while accurately assessing whether facial nerve sacrifice was necessary and to what extent. A surgical drape was prepared to extend the incision into the temporal area and improve the exposure. When facial reanimation surgery, other than reinnervation, is performed simultaneously, the entire face is draped for various reanimation procedures.

- ◆ Tumors encasing the facial nerve can sometimes be easily predicted. However, there are cases where it may not be so straightforward, especially in cases where tumors are located around the stylomastoid foramen or anteriorly positioned with contact toward the masseter muscle.
- ◆ If the tumor cannot be separated from the facial nerve or if it has to be split due to complete encasement, the decision regarding facial nerve sacrifice, even if there is no preoperative facial paralysis, depends on various considerations.
- ◆ Retrograde facial nerve dissection is performed while accurately assessing whether facial nerve sacrifice is necessary and to what extent it is required.

3.2.3 Cases Where Facial Nerve Sacrifice Is Inevitable Without Preoperative Facial Paralysis

Expert Opinion
Careful dissection of the facial nerve attached to tumors should be attempted with a cold knife. Place vessel loops on the proximal facial nerve and the distal facial nerve, and pull them carefully. Sacrifice of the facial nerve is performed when definite invasion to the facial nerve is identified. (Han-Sin Jeong)

These reanimation or reconstructive procedures are thought to be durable to postoperative radiation, in limited literatures.

Frequent use of nerve stimulation critically helps through the dissection or reconstruction process. (Yuh S Jung)

In these cases, reinnervation is recommended, as described in the previous section, simultaneously with facial nerve sacrifice. If reinnervation cannot be performed simultaneously owing to various conditions during surgery, reinnervation should be performed in the operating room as soon as possible, even the following day.

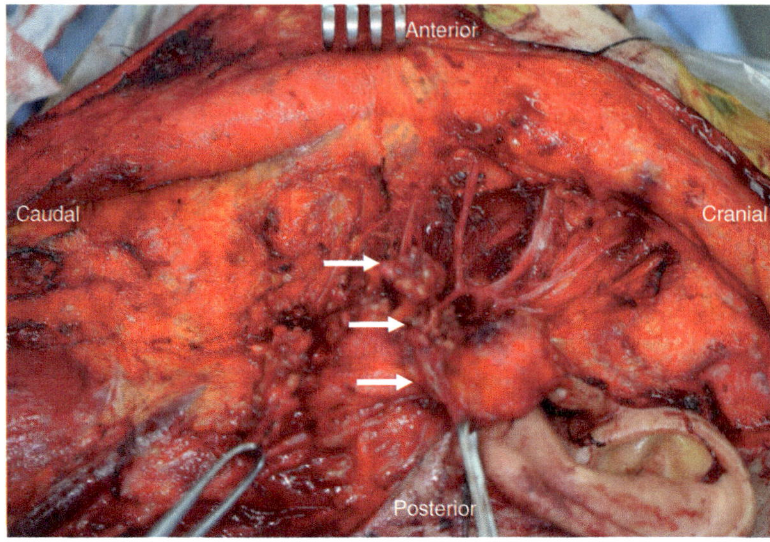

Fig. 3.5 Combined retrograde facial nerve (arrows) dissection with the classical approach

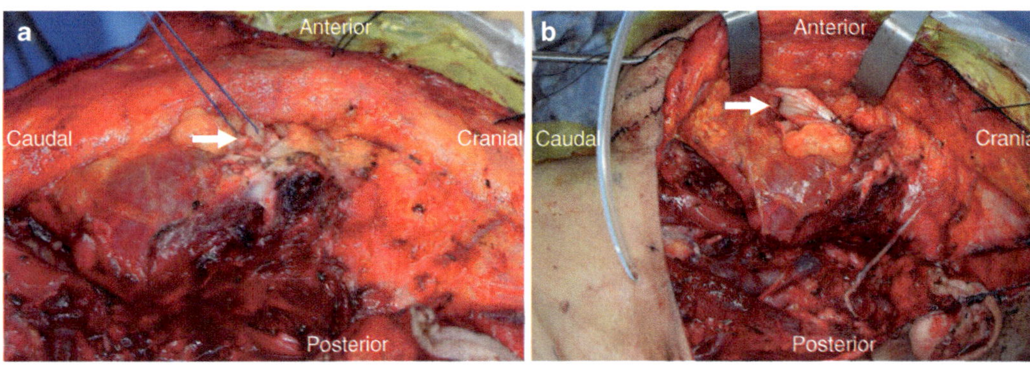

Fig. 3.6 Orthodromic temporalis tendon transfer. (**a**) Securing the coronoid process (arrow) in the surgical field tenotomized. (**b**) The palmaris longus, plantaris tendon, or fascia lata harvested are firmly fixed above the secured coronoid process (arrow) and surrounding soft tissue. Below, they are divided into two or three strips, and through mucosal tunneling, they are pulled to ensure that the entire strip is removed

Securing a healthy segment of the proximal facial nerve may be impossible in cases of facial nerve schwannoma and parotid cancer with extensive perineural spread. In such cases, nerve transfer using alternative power sources such as the masseteric or hypoglossal nerves at the proximal end should be considered [4]. For the distal end of the facial nerve, a single-stage temporalis muscle transfer is preferred for simultaneous smile reanimation. In contrast, reanimation surgery for eye closure or the marginal mandibular nerve is preferred in the second stage [6]. The temporalis muscle transfer surgical technique for parotid tumors begins with opening a portion of the masseter muscle attached to the zygomatic arch to access and secure the coronoid process in the surgical field [7]. Blunt dissection can help achieve further lengthening after the coronoid process is secured and osteotomized. The harvested palmaris longus, plantaris tendon, and fascia lata were firmly fixed above the secured coronoid process and surrounding soft tissue (Fig. 3.6). The strips were then divided into two or three sections. These undergo mucosal tunneling to ensure complete removal of the strip rather than just a point, thus preventing an unnatural mouth corner due to excessive tension (resembling a joker's face). Fixation points were created by making vertical incisions of approximately 3 mm in the midline of both the upper and lower lips and securing them to the mucosal tissue.

Expert Opinion

The management of facial nerve schwannoma is quite complex and while MRI can be classical in findings, the diagnosis often is made during surgery. Tumors that stimulate the nerve monitor regardless of where the probe is placed are highly suspicious for schwannoma. Management requires extensive patient/family counseling, and is dependent on age, affected branches, growth rate. Keep in mind alternative approaches, such as observation or stereotactic radiation, where possible. (Brett Miles)

In the case of facial nerve schwannoma, close follow-up and the wait-and-see strategy is needed in the patient with no symptoms. Non-surgical options, such as radiation, can be considered for older patients.

To maintain a healthy stump of the proximal facial nerve, mastoid surgery is also necessary when definite invasion to the facial nerve is identified. (Han-Sin Jeong)

It is better to dissect the proximal facial nerve with a clear margin to enhance reconstruction. Mastoidectomy is occasionally essential. (Yuh S Jung)

3.2.4 Case with the Pre-existing Facial Paralysis Before Surgery

Facial nerve-encasing tumors with pre-existing facial paralysis before surgery, particularly high-grade tumors, are more likely to be malignant. In most cases, facial paralysis is unlikely to improve or worsen over time. Therefore, even in cases of partial paralysis, suspected areas of facial nerve invasion should be excised. First, all peripheral facial nerve branches were exposed, and retrograde facial nerve dissection was performed. Normal and paralyzed nerves can be differentiated by nerve stimulation.

The duration of paralysis is crucial when treating nerves that have lost their function. Reinnervation is recommended if paralysis occurs within 1 or 1.5 years. If paralysis persists, facial reanimation procedures, such as brow lift, gold plate insertion, lower eyelid sling, temporalis muscle transfer, and free flap transfer (gracilis or latissimus dorsi muscle), can be considered.

Typically, a combination of various surgical techniques is considered whenever possible (Fig. 3.7).

◆ Simultaneous reinnervation should be the first reconstructive option for inevitable facial nerve sacrifice.

◆ If securing a healthy segment of the proximal facial nerve is not possible, nerve transfer using alternative power sources, such as the masseteric nerve, should be considered.

◆ Single-stage temporalis tendon transfer is one of the preferred options for smile reanimation.

◆ Reinnervation is recommended if paralysis occurs within 1 or 1.5 years. If the paralysis persists over time, facial reanimation procedures should be considered instead.

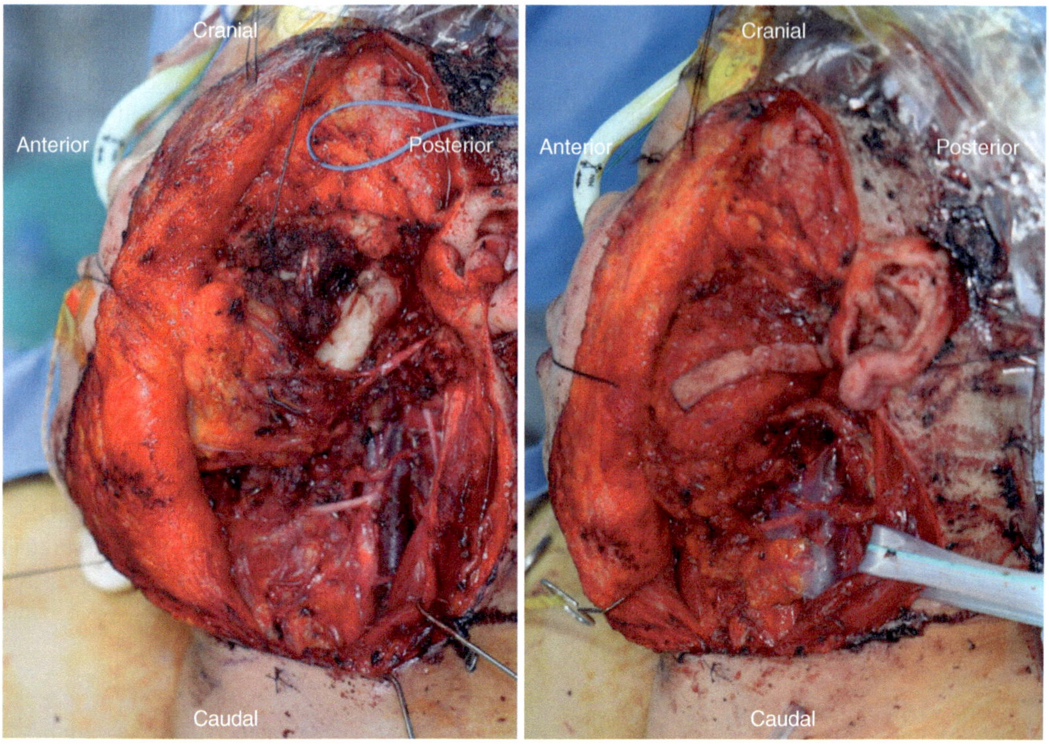

Fig. 3.7 Combination of various surgical techniques. (1) Eye closure: proximal facial nerve stump—facial nerve peripheral branch to orbicularis oculi muscle anastomosis using interpositional nerve graft. (2) Smile: orthodromic temporalis tendon transfer. (3) Facial nerve lower division preserved. (4) Adipofascial radial forearm free-flap covered the facial contour and grafted nerve

3.3 KQ 3.3. How Can Other Neurological Complications, Such as Auricular Sensory Change or Frey Syndrome, Be Prevented and Managed?

Jae-Yol Lim

3.3.1 Auricular Paresthesia or Anesthesia

The great auricular nerve transmits sensory fibers from the cervical plexus to the lower lateral face, ear pinna, and postauricular skin. It is divided into anterior and posterior branches as it travels along the lateral aspect of the sternocleidomastoid muscle (Fig. 3.8). Previously, the great auricular nerve was often sacrificed during parotidectomy because of its proximity to the glands. However, this has been linked to complications such as numbness, decreased sensation, and the risk of damage from heat or cold insults. Preserving the posterior branch of the nerve is important to minimize the risk of cutaneous anesthesia. However, some degree of numbness or tingling may persist, particularly in the earlobes.

◆ If possible, preserving the posterior branch of the great auricular nerve is recommended to reduce the risk of cutaneous anesthesia after parotidectomy.

◆ Surgeons must be aware that the anterior branch cannot be spared, and sparing the posterior branch results in limited cutaneous anesthesia.

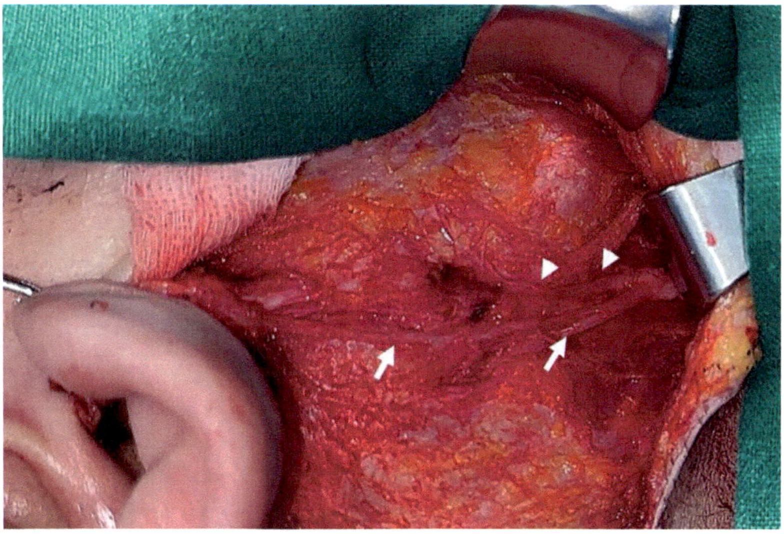

Fig. 3.8 Greater auricular nerve's trajectory. It splits into anterior (arrowheads) and posterior (arrows) branches, the latter of which should be preserved if possible

> **Expert Opinion**
> Monopolar dissection for flap elevation can damage the great auricular nerve. (Han-Sin Jeong)
>
> Patients need to be informed, especially about precautions for freezing weather. The risk of frostbite in the auricles may be increased. (Yuh S Jung)

Although opinions in the literature may differ, systematic reviews generally agree on the importance of preservation efforts [8]. However, the results of these studies vary. Even when the great auricular nerve is sectioned, it can show signs of recovery; however, patients with completely preserved nerves may continue to experience some level of anesthesia [9]. This variability may be due to the branching pattern of the great auricular nerve and its connections with other cutaneous nerves, such as the posterior auricular, auriculotemporal, and facial nerves [10]. Surgeons need a nuanced understanding of these factors to find a balance between therapeutic intervention and the potential sensory repercussions of parotid gland surgery.

3.3.2 Frey Syndrome

Frey syndrome is a medical condition characterized by sweating and flushing of the skin on the lateral side of the face and upper neck during meals. It is mainly observed around the parotid region and does not disappear independently but persists for many years. This condition is related to damaged sweat glands and skin vessels, resulting from skin flap elevation and subsequent abnormal reinnervation by parasympathetic fibers originating from the auriculotemporal nerve (Fig. 3.9). It can occur during various procedures involving the parotid region, although it is typically associated with the extent of parotidectomy. The incidence of Frey syndrome after parotidectomy varies widely, ranging from 50% to 100%, depending on the evaluation method, unless preventive measures are diligently employed [11].

> **Expert Opinion**
> Fortunately, severe, symptomatic Frey's syndrome is relatively rare in clinical practice and can be managed with topical antiperspirants, or botulinum toxin. (Brett Miles)
>
> If possible, sparing parotid fascial structures not separating from subcutaneous layer might help. Separating parotidectomy bed from subcutaneous tissue using implants or even muscle flaps could be preventive in theory. However, there is few well designed comparative data yet. (Yuh S Jung)

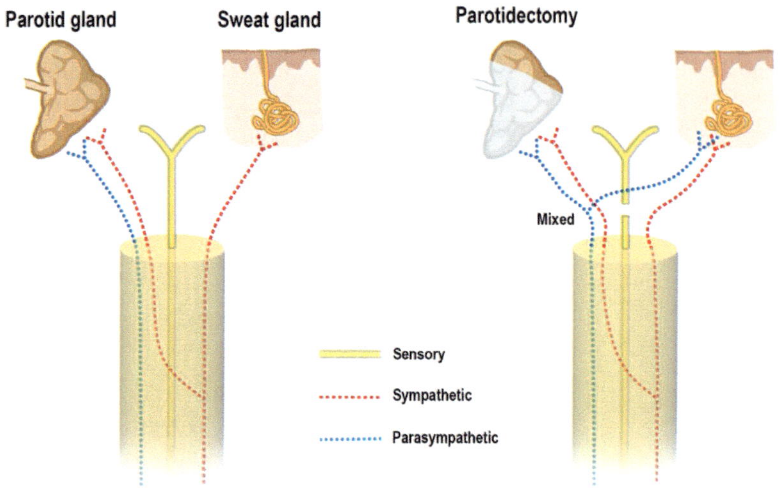

Fig. 3.9 Schematic representation of the pathophysiology of Frey syndrome. The reinnervation of parasympathetic fibers after parotidectomy leads to facial sweating and flushing during meals, known as Frey syndrome

◆ Preventive strategies are crucial in reducing the incidence of Frey syndrome, although the most effective technique remains debatable.

◆ Elevating thick skin flaps has shown promise in reducing the incidence; however, the results have been inconsistent.

◆ Dissecting and closing the superficial muscular aponeurotic system (SMAS) significantly decreases the occurrence of Frey syndrome (Fig. 3.10).

◆ The role of muscle interposition, such as the sternocleidomastoid muscle, remains uncertain owing to conflicting data.

◆ Using implant materials, while seemingly effective, poses a risk of associated infections, sialoceles, or both.

Patients who experience gustatory sweating and flushing typically have mild-to-moderate symptoms. However, approximately 20% of patients experience frustrating symptoms requiring treatment [12]. The preferred treatment involves injecting botulinum neurotoxin (Botox) into the dermal area. Before administering Botox, a starch-iodine test is performed to locate the affected skin. Botox is then injected intradermally at a dosage of 5 U/0.1 mL at every 1 cm corner, up to 50 U for the entire gland lesion. Complications associated with intradermal Botox injections are rare. The effectiveness of the treatment lasts for an average of 15–18 months before repeated injections are required. This approach aims to prevent and treat Frey syndrome and enhance the quality of life of the affected individuals.

Expert Opinion

Considering the degradation time, the effects of botulinum neurotoxin (Botox) treatment for Frey syndrome can last up to 6 months. (Han-Sin Jeong)

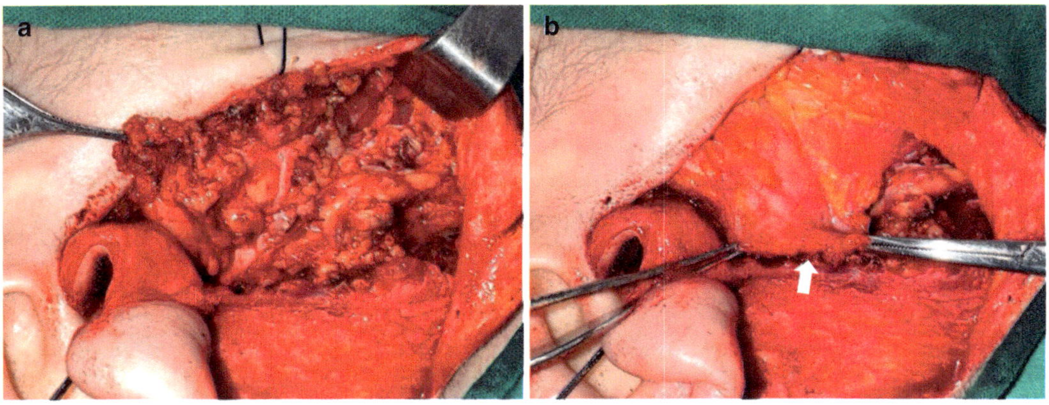

Fig. 3.10 Superficial muscular aponeurotic system (SMAS). SMAS is used to cover the surgical field after a partial parotidectomy. (**a**) Surgical field after partial parotidectomy. (**b**) Coverage of surgical field using SMAS (arrow)

3.4 KQ 3.4. How to Manage Inadvertent Injury of the Stensen's Duct During Parotid Gland Surgery?

Jae-Yol Lim

During parotid gland surgery, it is crucial to take preventive measures such as meticulous dissection, identification, and protection of the Stensen's duct to avoid inadvertent injuries. Injuries to the Stensen's duct during surgery can lead to complications such as salivary leakage, sialocele formation, and an increased risk of infection if not addressed promptly [13]. Therefore, successfully managing Stensen's duct injuries is paramount for preserving salivary function and minimizing postoperative complications. To effectively manage such injuries, surgeons must possess surgical expertise, pay attention to details, and provide meticulous postoperative care. A concise guide outlining the practical ways to navigate and manage such injuries is as follows:

(1). Immediate identification: Swift recognition of injury is crucial. The intraoperative identification of this issue enables prompt intervention and reduces the risk of subsequent complications.

(2). Isolation and protection: Isolate the injured segment of the Stensen's duct to prevent contamination from oral flora and minimize the risk of infection. Gentle retraction and protection are essential to avoid exacerbating damage.

(3). Microsurgical repair: Microsurgical repair is the gold standard for managing Stensen's duct injuries. Delicate suturing with fine absorbable materials aids in accurately approximating the duct's edges. Suturing of Stensen's duct injuries should be performed with meticulous precision to ensure tight and secure closure. The use of a microscope or magnifying loupes enhances precision.

(4). Stent placement: For salivary duct injuries, stent placement involves careful positioning of a temporary or permanent stent to support structural integrity and maintain duct patency. The choice of stent type depends on the extent of the injury, availability, and the surgeon's preference.

(5). Saliva diversion: In scenarios where direct repair poses challenges, diverting saliva away from the injured duct may be a viable option. This can be achieved by creating a new route for saliva drainage by connecting it to another healthy salivary duct or oral mucosa or using a drainage tube to guide the saliva away from the injured area. The goal is to provide an alternative and functional pathway for saliva to prevent complications and promote healing.

(6). Postoperative monitoring: Close postoperative monitoring is essential for assessing the success of the repair and detecting any signs of complications. Regular follow-ups, including imaging studies, may be necessary to evaluate the integrity of the repaired duct.

(7). Patient education: Educate patients about potential postoperative complications and emphasize the importance of adhering to postoperative care instructions. Highlight the need to report unusual symptoms promptly.

◆ Swift identification during surgery is crucial for effectively managing Stensen's duct injuries.
◆ Microsurgical repair with delicate suturing is the gold standard for addressing these injuries.
◆ Consider stent placement for structural support and patency maintenance.
◆ Saliva diversion is an option when direct repair is challenging.
◆ Close postoperative monitoring is essential for assessing success and detecting complications.
◆ Patient education should emphasize adherence to care instructions and prompt reporting of symptoms.

Expert Opinion

In high-risk cases, the Stensen's duct can be cannulated with a lacrimal probe, which can be placed prior to the sterile preparation. This allows for a palpable landmark during parotid gland surgery and can facilitate duct repair. (Brett Miles)

After superficial parotidectomy, most of the parotid gland is removed (70%), so Stensen's duct ligation is often performed. In cases where much of the salivary gland remains, such as in partial parotidectomy, efforts are made to preserve the Stensen's duct.

If a leak occurs in the main or first branches of the Stensen's duct, the surgical method described in the text is used. Ligation of the main branch of the Stensen's duct is also a suitable method. However, a leak in the second branch or smaller can be resolved with conservative management.

A stent is not useful because it is not well anchored to the duct. (Han-Sin Jeong)

The Stensen's duct is located anteriorly to the parotid gland and runs horizontally on the masseter muscle before turning medially on its medial border, piercing the buccinator muscle. Anteriorly located tumors around buccal branches are high risk. (Yuh S Jung)

3.5 KQ 3.5. How Can Miscellaneous Wound Problems Such as Seromas, Sialoceles, and Sunken-Down Skin Deformities Be Managed After Parotidectomy?

Jae-Yol Lim

Postoperative wound complications such as hematoma and sialocele can lead to further complications such as infection, salivary fistula, flap necrosis, and adverse scarring. To proactively mitigate risks, it is essential to understand the contributing factors. Surgeons should exercise caution when patients are taking anticoagulant medications, maintain meticulous control during hypertensive episodes, and adopt strategies to minimize wound stimulation. Additionally, careful wound handling and avoiding extensive or careless dissection can significantly reduce the likelihood of hematoma and sialocele formation.

3.5.1 Hematoma

Hematoma is a critical concern in parotid gland surgery because of the proximity of small vessels to the facial nerve branches. The risk of hematoma formation increases with the use of anticoagulants, hypertension, coughing, extensive or careless dissection, and vigorous wound scrubbing. Ensuring hemostasis in parotid gland surgery is a delicate task, given the proximity of small vessels to the facial nerve branches, which raises the possibility of postoperative hematoma. Several factors increase this risk, including anticoagulant medications, hypertension, coughing episodes, vigorous wound scrubbing, and extensive or careless dissection.

Immediate attention and intervention are crucial when a hematoma is identified, particularly within the critical postoperative window. Timely recognition and emergency surgical treatment can prevent complications associated with uncontrolled swelling and hematoma progression. This intervention should occur in the operating room, which provides a controlled environment for meticulous management. The choice of anesthetic depends on the nature of the hematoma and the patient's condition. Local anesthesia may be adequate when the primary finding is skin ecchymosis, which is indicative of superficial bleeding. In contrast, situations involving massive arterial bleeding or uncooperative patients may require general anesthesia for effective bleeding control.

Expert Opinion

Care should be taken for vessels penetrating the parotid gland, such as the facial vein and superficial temporal artery. (Yuh S Jung)

3.5.2 Seroma, Sialocele, and Salivary Fistula

After surgery, fluids commonly accumulate in the body; this process is known as seroma formation. In parotidectomy, which involves the removal of the parotid gland from the face, fluid can accumulate and form a pseudocyst called a sialocele (Fig. 3.11). The pseudocysts lack a lining and are composed of pools of mucus that are not well defined. The incidence of sialoceles after parotidectomy ranges from 10% to 40%, and the use of energy devices and implants to prevent adhesions or bleeding increases their occurrence [14]. A study of 771 parotidectomies reported that limited parotid resection was associated with higher sialocele rates [15]. Therefore, a tailored approach is necessary to manage seromas, sialoceles, and salivary fistulas after parotid surgery. Understanding the contributing factors, implementing preventive measures, and considering targeted interventions can help optimize patient outcomes [14].

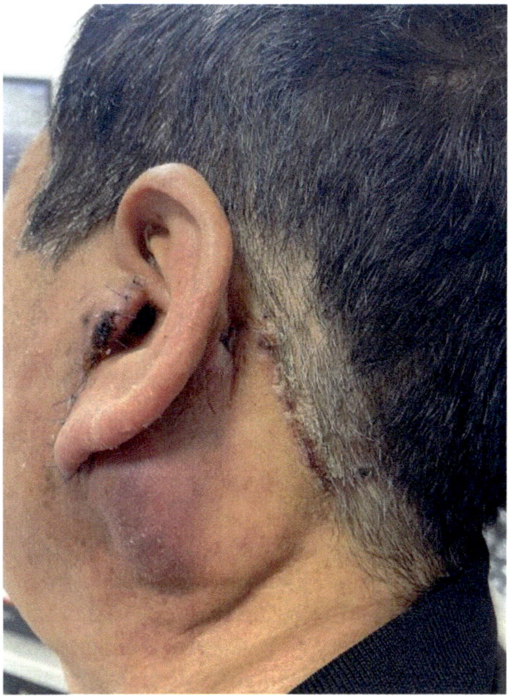

Fig. 3.11 Post-parotidectomy seroma. An elevated lesion in the postauricular area is observed after discharge following parotidectomy

Compression, sustained drainage, and aspiration effectively decrease salivary output and manage sialoceles when a Stensen's duct laceration is not suspected. Pressure dressings are simple and effective treatment options for this condition. If parotid swelling continues for an extended period and is accompanied by persistent wound complications, such as infection and unyielding drain output, despite repeated aspiration and compression, a more targeted intervention may be necessary. Botox injections, which aim to reduce saliva production and secretion from resected or injured salivary ducts, can be a viable option [16]. The dosage typically ranges from 5 units per 0.1 mL at every 1 cm corner to 50 units for the entire gland lesion. Percutaneous aspiration of leaked fluid and Botox injection can help avoid the need for invasive sialoadenectomy. Although a deep injection into the gland is required, it is associated with a low complication rate. It is crucial to address the persistence of sialoceles as they can lead to the development of salivary fistulas. Even after administering a Botox injection deep into the gland, a sustained compressive dressing is required during follow-up. Additionally, ancillary treatments such as somatostatin analogs or anticholinergic drugs can complement management strategies.

Expert Opinion

To prevent sialoceles, patients should avoid meals that are too hot, spicy, salty, sour, or hard. (Song Si Youn)

Adhesion barriers should be tailored. Making barriers with smaller sizes and pores for drainage may help to prevent seromas.

Adjuncts, such as a scopolamine patch, somatostatin injection, or both, can be readily applied to prevent seromas, sialoceles, and salivary fistulas. (Yuh S Jung)

- ◆ After a parotidectomy, fluid buildup can form a pseudocyst called a sialocele. These can occur in 10%–40% of cases and are more common with energy devices and implants.
- ◆ Limited parotid resections are also associated with higher sialocele rates.
- ◆ Compression, sustained drainage, and aspiration can help manage sialoceles.
- ◆ If complications persist, Botox injections or ancillary treatments may be necessary. It is crucial to address sialoceles to prevent salivary fistula development.

3.5.3 Skin Flap Necrosis

Skin flap necrosis is a rare complication after parotidectomy that is influenced by various factors such as smoking, prior radiation exposure, diabetes, thin skin flaps, prolonged surgical procedures, and inappropriate skin incisions. It typically manifests in the retroauricular portion (Fig. 3.12) and requires a comprehensive approach for effective management. The rarity of skin flap necrosis post-parotidectomy highlights the importance of a thorough preoperative assessment and strategic intraoperative measures to minimize risks. Rapid identification and intervention are important for successful management. Debridement, skin repositioning, and grafting may be required in severe cases.

Expert Opinion

Patients with an active and significant smoking history are at particularly high risk for skin necrosis. (Brett Miles)

Considering the vertical length of the ear, ensure that the retroauricular incision does not rise higher than half the height of the ear (especially if there is a preauricular incision). (Han-Sin Jeong)

Gentle manipulation of the skin flap, gentle retraction, and preservation of sound cutaneous tissue are essential to prevent skin flap necrosis. (Yuh S Jung)

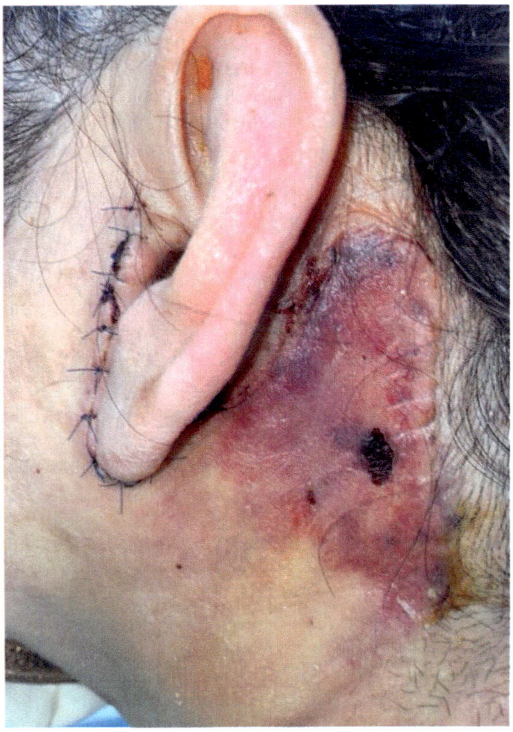

Fig. 3.12 Skin flap necrosis. Inadequate skin flap thickness poses challenges to sustained blood flow, exacerbating the risk of necrosis

Treating skin flap necrosis after parotidectomy involves several key steps. First, meticulous wound care is essential for routine management of the affected area and infection prevention. Regular attention to wounds is crucial for optimal healing. Second, the necrotic tissue is debrided to remove damaged or dead tissue, thereby facilitating healthy tissue regeneration. This step is fundamental for promoting the overall recovery of the surgical site. Third, in cases of extensive necrosis, the procedure involves using a rotational muscle flap. This technique strategically moves the surrounding muscle to replace the necrotic area, ensuring a continued blood supply and promoting successful tissue integration. Finally, in severe cases, the procedure involves skin grafting or transposition to restore the form and volume of the skin, particularly when larger areas are affected.

Expert Opinion

Negative pressure wound therapy after superficial soft tissue debridement is a good option in cases of skin flap necrosis. (Han-Sin Jeong)

3.5.4 Sunken-Down Skin Deformity

Although sunken-down skin deformity is rare, it requires a thorough understanding and strategic intervention. It is characterized by a depressed or hollow skin flap behind the ear. The development of this deformity can be attributed to several factors, including patient characteristics and surgical variables. Factors contributing to sunken-down skin deformities include heavy smoking, prior radiation treatment, diabetes, use of a thin skin flap during surgery, and total parotidectomy. Prolonged operative times and poorly designed incisions can also increase the risk of complications.

Preventive measures are crucial to avoid the development of sunken-down skin deformities. These include meticulous surgical techniques, consideration of patient risk factors, and close monitoring of the postoperative progress. Managing sunken-down skin deformities involves muscle rotation flaps, fat grafting, or fat injections in severe instances. The muscle rotational flap method was designed to strategically address volumetric deficits in muscle tissue. Fat grafting involves harvesting fat from another location and precisely injecting it into the affected region, yielding natural-looking outcomes while minimizing complications. Fat injection entails administering small amounts of fat into the sunken-down area to restore volume. The extracted fat is intricately injected to maintain consistent shape and volume. These treatment options are selected based on the patient's condition and the severity of the sunken-down area. Choosing an optimal treatment method tailored to each patient is crucial to achieving desirable outcomes and minimizing postoperative complications.

Expert Opinion

Extracapsular parotidectomy, while preserving uninvolved parotid tissue, helps to prevent sunken-down skin deformity. (Yuh S Jung)

References

1. Shindo M. Management of facial nerve paralysis. Otolaryngol Clin North Am. 1999;32(5):945–64. https://doi.org/10.1016/s0030-6665(05)70183-31.
2. AO Surgery Reference. Anatomy of the facial nerve https://surgeryreference.aofoundation.org.
3. Lu GN, Villwock MR, Humphrey CD, Kriet JD, Bur AM. Analysis of facial reanimation procedures performed concurrently with total parotidectomy and facial nerve sacrifice. JAMA Facial Plast Surg. 2019;21(1):50–5. https://doi.org/10.1001/jamafacial.2018.1057.
4. Sahovaler A, Yeh D, Yoo J. Primary facial reanimation in head and neck cancer. Oral Oncol. 2017;74:171–80. https://doi.org/10.1016/j.oraloncology.2017.08.013.
5. Terzis JK, Noah ME. Analysis of 100 cases of free-muscle transplantation for facial paralysis. Plast Reconstr Surg. 1997;99(7):1905–21. https://doi.org/10.1097/00006534-199706000-00016.
6. Terzis JK, Kalantarian B. Microsurgical strategies in 74 patients for restoration of dynamic depressor muscle mechanism: a neglected target in facial reanimation. Plast Reconstr Surg. 2000;105(6):1917–31.
7. Martin T, Sury F, Goga D, Parmentier J, Rozen A, Laure B. Reconstruction of large defects of the lips and commissure using a composite radial forearm palmaris longus free flap associated with a lengthening temporalis myoplasty. Ann Plast Surg. 2012;69(2):169–72.
8. George M, Karkos PD, Dwivedi RC, Leong SC, Kim D, Repanos C. Preservation of greater auricular nerve during parotidectomy: sensation, quality of life, and morbidity issues. A systematic review. Head Neck. 2014;36(4):603–8. https://doi.org/10.1002/hed.23292. Epub 2013 Jun 14.. PMID: 23766239.
9. Grosheva M, Shabli S, Volk GF, Sommer B, Ludwig L, Finkensieper M, Wittekindt C, Klussmann JP, Guntinas-Lichius O, Beutner D. Sensation loss after superficial parotidectomy: a prospective controlled multicenter trial. Head Neck. 2017;39(3):520–6. https://doi.org/10.1002/hed.24647. Epub 2017 Jan 9.. PMID: 28067982.
10. Yang HM, Kim HJ, Hu KS. Anatomic and histological study of great auricular nerve and its clinical implication. J Plast Reconstr Aesthet Surg. 2015;68(2):230–6. https://doi.org/10.1016/j.bjps.2014.10.030. Epub 2014 Oct 31.. PMID: 25465135.
11. Dulguerov N, Makni A, Dulguerov P. The superficial musculoaponeurotic system flap in the prevention of Frey syndrome: a meta-analysis. Laryngoscope. 2016;126(7):1581–4. https://doi.org/10.1002/lary.25895. Epub 2016 Feb 24.. PMID: 26915301.
12. Dulguerov P, Quinodoz D, Cosendai G, Piletta P, Lehmann W. Frey syndrome treatment with botulinum toxin. Otolaryngol Head Neck Surg. 2000;122(6):821–7. https://doi.org/10.1016/S0194-59980070008-8. PMID: 10828793.
13. Van Sickels JE. Management of parotid gland and duct injuries. Oral Maxillofac Surg Clin North Am. 2009;21(2):243–6. https://doi.org/10.1016/j.coms.2008.12.010. PMID: 19348990.
14. Britt CJ, Stein AP, Gessert T, Pflum Z, Saha S, Hartig GK. Factors influencing sialocele or salivary fistula formation postparotidectomy. Head Neck. 2017;39(2):387–91. https://doi.org/10.1002/hed.24564. Epub 2016 Aug 22. PMID: 27550745.
15. Witt RL. The incidence and management of siaolocele after parotidectomy. Otolaryngol Head Neck Surg. 2009;140(6):871–4. https://doi.org/10.1016/j.otohns.2009.01.021. Epub 2009 Apr 1. PMID: 19467406.
16. Pantel M, Volk GF, Guntinas-Lichius O, Wittekindt C. Botulinum toxin type b for the treatment of a sialocele after parotidectomy. Head Neck. 2013;35(1):E11–2. https://doi.org/10.1002/hed.21778. Epub 2011 Jun 17. PMID: 21688341.

4 Surgery of the Parapharyngeal Space

Dahee Kim

4.1 KQ 4.1. How to Prevent and Manage Neurological or Vascular Complications When Using the Transoral and Transcervical Approach for a Parapharyngeal Tumor or Retropharyngeal Lymph Node Resection?

Dahee Kim

The parapharyngeal space (PPS) is an inverted pyramid-shaped space extending from the cranial base of the skull to the apex of the greater cornu of the hyoid bone. It is located lateral to the buccopharyngeal fascia over the superior pharyngeal constrictor muscle and medial to the mandibular ramus, medial pterygoid, and parotid deep lobes. This space is divided into pre- and post-styloid compartments by the fascia, which extends from the styloid process to the tensor veli palatini muscle. The pre-styloid compartment includes the deep lobe of the parotid gland, minor salivary glands, and the mandibular branch of the trigeminal cranial nerve (V3), whereas the post-styloid compartment includes the internal carotid artery, internal jugular vein, cranial nerves (IX, X, XI, and XII), and sympathetic chain. Therefore, post-styloid compartment lesions may compress cranial nerves IX to XII, leading to cranial neuropathy such as impaired vocal cord mobility or Horner's syndrome [1–4].

The retropharyngeal space (RPS) extends from the skull base to the tracheal bifurcation level and is bounded anteriorly by the buccopharyngeal fascia (the middle layer of the deep cervical fascia) and posteriorly by the alar fascia (the deep layer of the deep cervical fascia). The carotid sheath exists laterally in this space with complex neurovascular structures in close anatomical proximity (Fig. 4.1).

The PPS and RPS nodes can be surgically resected using various approaches. For example, both can be removed using the transcervical, transcervicoparotid, transmandibular, transpalatal, or transoral approaches. Larger tumors, tumors close to the cranial base or neurovascular bundle, highly vascularized lesions, or those at a high risk of malignancy typically require a more extensive and/or invasive approach. The ideal surgical approach is decided based on the tumor size, location, histopathology, and the surgeon's preference.

Indications for the transoral approach to PPS or RPS lymph nodes are limited to small neoplasms in the pre-styloid compartment. The transoral approach avoids the risk of tumor spillage and nerve/vessel injury. Recently, the indications of robot-assisted surgery have

D. Kim (✉)
Department of Otolaryngology—Head and Neck Surgery, Severance Hospital, College of Medicine, Yonsei University, Seoul, Republic of Korea
e-mail: dhk@yuhs.ac

K.-J. Cho, J.-O. Park (eds.), *Management of Head and Neck Surgery Complications*,
https://doi.org/10.1007/978-981-96-1860-6_4

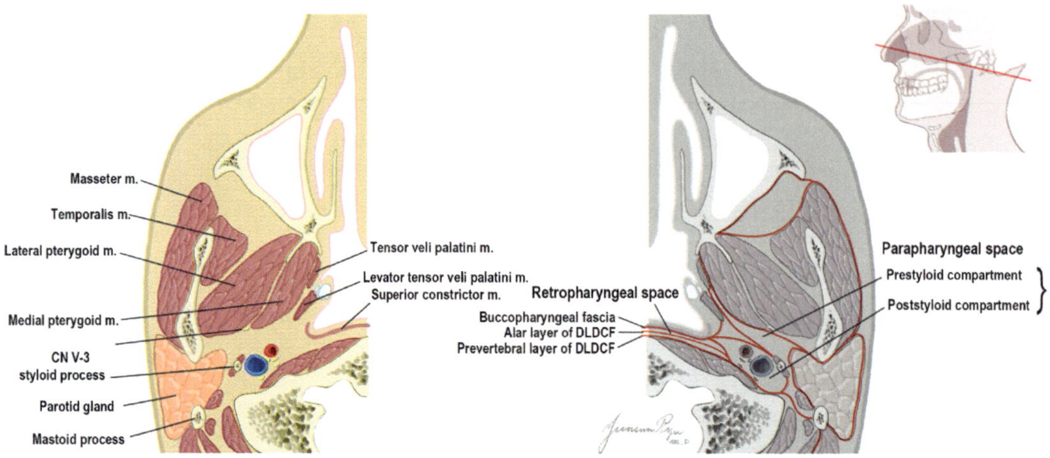

Fig. 4.1 Axial view of the parapharyngeal and retropharyngeal spaces. The parapharyngeal space is divided into the pre-styloid and post-styloid compartments. The retropharyngeal space is behind the buccopharyngeal fascia and in front of the alar fascia. m, muscle; DLDCF, deep layer of the deep cervical fascia

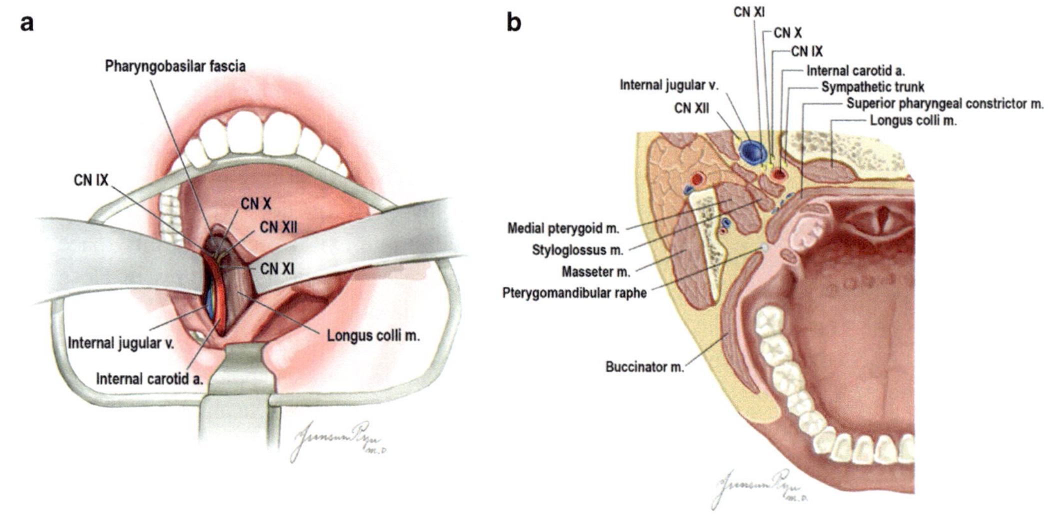

Fig. 4.2 Surrounding neurologic structures of the parapharyngeal and retropharyngeal space. Cranial nerves (IX, X, XI, and XII) and sympathetic trunk nerves are within close proximity to the parapharyngeal and retropharyngeal spaces and thus can be injured during surgeries in these spaces. (**a**) The transoral approach to the parapharyngeal space. (**b**) Three-dimensional view of the neurological structures. v, vein; a, artery; m, muscle

expanded to include angled visualization capabilities. The superior dexterity of robotic instruments has increased the resection of PPS and RPS lymph nodes using the transoral approach [5–7].

Regardless of the approach selected, various neurological and vascular complications can occur in the parapharyngeal and retropharyngeal lymph nodes after surgery. To prevent these complications, selecting the most appropriate approach is imperative. An ideal approach is to provide sufficient visualization to avoid injury to nearby structures (Figs. 4.2 and 4.3).

◆ Selection of the optimal approach to ensure adequate visual access to the tumor or lymph node is most important for avoiding injury to the surrounding structures.

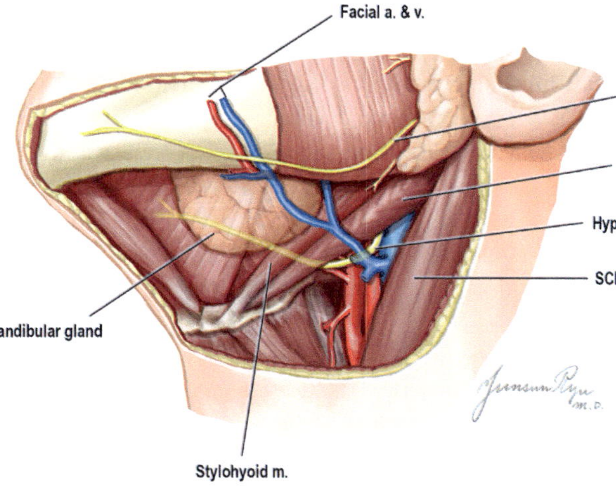

Fig. 4.3 Anatomy of the parapharyngeal space involved in the transcervical or transparotid approach. In deep parapharyngeal space tumors or retropharyngeal nodes requiring transcervical or transparotid approaches, the hypoglossal and marginal mandibular nerves can be exposed and injured. a, artery; v, vein; n, nerve; m, muscle

4.1.1 First Bite Syndrome

> **Expert Opinion**
> Botulinum toxin A injections into the parotid gland are performed under sonographic control in patients who have first bite syndrome. 33U of the toxin, fractionated into 3 doses of 11U, is administered without local anesthesia. (Jin-Choon Lee)

Following surgery in the parapharyngeal or retropharyngeal space, some patients may experience severe pain in the periauricular area during their first bite or meal. This is thought to originate from the abnormal responses of myoepithelial cells in the parotid gland due to the loss of signals or damaged cervical sympathetic innervation. With gustatory stimuli and salivation, the parasympathetic neurotransmitter co-stimulates sympathetic receptors, causing supramaximal contraction of myoepithelial cells, resulting in pain. The pain gradually subsided with the subsequent masticatory movements. The primary treatment for first bite syndrome is dietary modification to avoid stimulating foods (e.g., sweet, acidic, or sour) and medical therapy, including carbamazepine, amitriptyline, pregabalin, and neurotropic agents. In severe cases that are refractory to medication, a botulinum toxin A injection into the salivary gland or a stellate ganglion block may be performed [8].

4.1.2 Vagal Palsy

> **Expert Opinion**
> When performing the transoral approach, velopharyngeal insufficiency can occur even without nerve injury. Therefore, meticulous layer-by-layer repair of the constrictor and palatal muscles is necessary. (Junsun Ryu)

Owing to the anatomical proximity of the carotid sheath, surgery in the parapharyngeal or retropharyngeal spaces (e.g., tumor removal) can injure the vagus nerve. Vagal nerve injury can cause voice changes, aspiration, dysphagia, or gastrointestinal (GI) discomfort (e.g., nausea, vomiting, and reflux), and the severity of the symptoms depends on the level of injury. The pharyngeal branch of the vagus nerve, or the superior laryngeal nerve, contributes to most swallowing functions. Thus, preservation of these two branches is important for postoperative function. In cases where the injury occurs near the skull base or superior to the inferior (nodose) ganglion of the vagus nerve, severe dysphagia symptoms appear along with ipsilateral palatal palsy, causing velopharyngeal insufficiency. When injuries occur below this level, voice problems occur in the absence of severe dysphagia.

Nerve injuries are irreversible. Functional recovery depends on time, lung function, and patient age. Younger patients tended to adapt better than younger patients. Importantly, elderly patients with poor lung function require special care owing to the risk of aspiration or malnutrition. Patients with vocal cord palsy may require a thyroplasty or injection laryngoplasty for voice rehabilitation. Surgical treatment for severe velopharyngeal insufficiency, such as pharyngoplasty, may improve swallowing or decrease hypernasality.

Videoendoscopic swallowing assessment may assist in determining whether patients with dysphagia require swallowing rehabilitation, cricopharyngeal myotomy, or gastrostomy (in severe cases) [3, 9].

◆ Personalized functional rehabilitation following vagal nerve injury is indicated. The type of rehabilitation required depends on the severity of the neurological damage, the presence of voice and/or swallowing disorders, and any accompanying symptoms.

4.1.3 Sympathetic Plexus Injury: Horner's Syndrome

When the PPS or RPS lymph nodes are deep, the nerves of the sympathetic trunk can be injured during surgery, causing Horner's syndrome. Horner syndrome is characterized by ipsilateral ptosis, myosis, and anhidrosis. Some patients experienced enophthalmos, facial flushing, or headaches. No specific treatment is required for this condition. However, surgical management may be useful in treating severe ptosis.

4.1.4 Hypoglossal Nerve Palsy

During dissection of parapharyngeal space tumors, the hypoglossal nerve can be injured by traction or direct injury at a higher level. Injury to the hypoglossal nerve alone did not significantly impair the pharyngeal phase of swallowing. Moreover, the oral phases of swallowing and articulation can be obtained over time during rehabilitation. However, if hypoglossal palsy is present with vagal nerve palsy, it can result in severe swallowing and articulation disorders requiring gastrostomy, tracheostomy, and long-term rehabilitation.

Expert Opinion
Care should be taken to avoid hypoglossal nerve injury when cutting the stylohyoid muscle, digastric muscle, or stylomandibular ligament for visualization of the parapharyngeal space. (Jin-Choon Lee)

4.1.5 Marginal Mandibular Nerve Palsy

Marginal mandibular nerve palsy is mostly treated with transcervical and transparent approaches. Staying close to the platysma muscle during flap elevation can prevent injury to the marginal mandibular nerve. Special caution is required to avoid the cranial elevation of the flap.

Most injuries are temporary and recover within 3–4 months postoperatively. However, some injuries are permanent and can result in resting asymmetry. In cases in which the nerve is transected during surgery, primary anastomosis without tension or nerve grafts may be performed to facilitate recovery. In severe cases, reanimation procedures include repositioning of the contralateral nerve and muscle transfer.

Expert Opinion
When dissecting the submandibular gland, use of a cold knife, metzenbaum, or mosquito can reduce hypoglossal nerve injury and marginal mandibular nerve injury, compared to that of using monopolar cautery. (Jin-Choon Lee)

4.1.6 Vessel Injury: Common Carotid Artery (CCA), Internal Carotid Artery (ICA), External Carotid Artery (ECA), and Ascending Pharyngeal Arteries

During parapharyngeal or retropharyngeal space surgery, vessels may be injured. The ICA, ECA, internal jugular vein, and vertebral artery may also have been affected. Injury to the CCA or ICA at the base of the skull can be lethal and should be avoided. Preoperative imaging was performed to prevent vessel injury. Careful radiological inspection of the skull base/vertebral bony erosion and tortuous ICA course are important. In cases of hypervascular tumors such as paragangliomas, preoperative angiography or a balloon occlusion test should be performed. In some cases, selective embolization may be necessary.

When the ICA is tractioned during surgery, a minor intimal injury can occur, with delayed embolism, causing neurological complications. To prevent this complication, prolonged pressure on the ICA should be avoided, with intermittent release of traction during the operation.

> ◆ Preoperative caution of the possibility of vascular damage is important. Careful inspection of the parapharyngeal or retropharyngeal areas beforehand can prevent irreversible and potentially lethal damages.

Complications associated with transoral or transcervical approaches for parapharyngeal or retropharyngeal space surgery include permanent swallowing and voice problems, which affect the patient's quality of life. Generally, most complications improve over time. However, some complications may be fatal, and some may require secondary surgery. Meticulous intraoperative dissection is the most important preventive strategy. However, determining the optimal approach for excellent visual access to the tumor and surrounding structures is important.

Preoperative informed consent was obtained from all patients. The consequences of each type of neurological injury were explained to the patients. This is particularly important to improve postoperative understanding and rehabilitation compliance.

References

1. Tae K. Diagnostic and Surgical Approaches of Parapharyngeal space tumors. Korean J Otorhinolaryngol-Head Neck Surg. 2008;51:441–6.
2. Andersen PE. Parapharyngeal space tumor. James I. Cohen GLC, editor: Elsevier; 2011.
3. Baek CH. Parapharyngeal space tumors: Iljogak; 2009.
4. Ferrari M, Schreiber A, Mattavelli D, Lombardi D, Rampinelli V, Doglietto F, et al. Surgical anatomy of the parapharyngeal space: multiperspective, quantification-based study. Head Neck. 2019;41(3):642–56.
5. Lim JY, Park YM, Kang MS, Kim DH, Choi EC, Kim SH, et al. Comparison of surgical outcomes of robotic and conventional approaches in patients with pre- and poststyloid parapharyngeal space tumors. Ann Surg Oncol. 2020;27(11):4535–43.
6. Wu C, Xu C, Shi X, Liu H, Liu Q, Wu H, et al. Indications for resection of parapharyngeal space tumors by transoral robotic surgery and prevention and treatment of complications. Lin Chuang Er Bi Yan Hou Tou Jing Wai Ke Za Zhi. 2022;36(6):429–35.
7. Zhu X, Shi X, Zhou L, Zhang M, Cheng L, Shi Y, et al. Trends in the surgical management of parapharyngeal space tumors: a single-center retrospective analysis. Eur J Surg Oncol. 2023;49(1):47–54.
8. Chiu AG, Cohen JI, Burningham AR, Andersen PE, Davidson BJ. First bite syndrome: a complication of surgery involving the parapharyngeal space. Head Neck-J Sci Spec. 2002;24(11):996–9.
9. Moore EJ, Olsen KD. Complications of surgery of the parapharyngeal space. In: Eisele DW, Smith RV, editors. Complications in head and neck surgery. Mosby; 2009.

5 Surgery for Submandibular and Sublingual Gland Tumors

Woo-Jin Jeong and Han Su Kim

5.1 KQ 5.1. How to Prevent and Manage Nerve Injuries, Including the Lingual, Hypoglossal, and Facial Nerves, When Performing Submandibular Gland Resection?

Woo-Jin Jeong

Submandibular gland resection may lead to nerve damage, particularly injury to the lingual, hypoglossal, and facial nerves. The risk of nerve injury increases in the presence of severe adhesions caused by chronic inflammation. Because these nerves are responsible for controlling the movements and sensations of the tongue, mouth, and face, damage to these nerves can have significant consequences for patients. The most commonly injured nerve is the marginal mandibular branch of the facial nerve (7.7–9%), followed by the hypoglossal (2–2.9%) and lingual nerves (1.4%) [1, 2]. Given that there are limited options once paralysis occurs, injury prevention is paramount. To prevent nerve injury, it is crucial to thoroughly understand the pertinent anatomy and ensure that appropriate surgical techniques are employed.

Supplementary Information The online version contains supplementary material available at https://doi.org/10.1007/978-981-96-1860-6_5.

W.-J. Jeong (✉)
Department of Otorhinolaryngology—Head & Neck Surgery, Seoul National University Bundang Hospital, Seoul National University College of Medicine, Seongnam, South Korea
e-mail: safar@snubh.org

H. S. Kim (✉)
Department of Otolaryngology, Head and Neck Surgery, College of Medicine, Ewha Womans University, Seoul, South Korea
e-mail: sevent@ewha.ac.kr

> **Expert Opinion**
> When performing surgery for benign submandibular gland tumors, using a cold knife and bipolar cautery is preferred over monopolar cautery, in order to avoid injury to the marginal mandibular branch of the facial nerve. (Han-Sin Jeong)

The marginal mandibular branch of the facial nerve (MMFN), which is responsible for the movement of the lower lip, is the most commonly affected. This branch lies deep in the platysma muscle and superficial to the submandibular gland within the superficial layer of the deep cervical fascia. This nerve typically runs near the crossing point of the inferior border of the mandible and facial vessels. However, in some cases, particularly in elderly patients, the nerve may loop down the neck or form multiple branches.

K.-J. Cho, J.-O. Park (eds.), *Management of Head and Neck Surgery Complications*,
https://doi.org/10.1007/978-981-96-1860-6_5

Therefore, a skin incision of at least two fingerbreadths (2–3 cm) below the inferior border of the mandible should be made. Premature flap elevation should be avoided, and the fascia should be incised at the level of the inferior border of the submandibular gland to expose its capsule. As the marginal mandibular branch of the facial nerve lies superficial to the anterior facial vein, it can be protected from damage by ligating the inferior portion of the anterior facial vein and elevating the superior flap together with the ligated anterior facial vein directly on the gland capsule (Fig. 5.1).

Expert Opinion

When the skin incision is made along the inferior border of the submandibular gland and the dissection is deep along the lower border of the gland, it is easy to identify the posterior belly of the digastric muscle. Then, with a careful extracapsular dissection, you can remove the gland whilst preserving the facial vessels and nerve. (Dong Young Kim)

The lowest portion of the marginal mandibular nerve may run around the notch on the inferior border of the mandible, created by the facial vein. The notch can be identified easily by palpation and is a good landmark for identification of the marginal mandibular nerve. (Soon Young Kwon)

◆ Ligating the anterior facial vein and elevating the upper flap, along with ligating the posterior facial vein, can prevent injury to the marginal mandibular branch of the facial nerve.

During submandibular gland resection of malignant tumors, lymph node dissection is mandatory around the marginal mandibular branch of the facial nerve. Submandibular gland resection for malignant tumors carries a higher risk of nerve injury compared to that for benign tumors. Nerve identification may help prevent nerve injury in cases of malignancy. Notably, intraoperative nerve integrity monitoring (IONM) has been shown to significantly reduce marginal mandibular nerve injury during neck dissection [3]. Moreover, it may help prevent injury during submandibular gland resection.

◆ Intraoperative nerve monitoring (IONM) may help prevent injury to the marginal mandibular branch of the facial nerve.

The lingual nerve is typically identified when the mylohyoid muscle is carefully retracted anteriorly. This maneuver allows for clear visualization and helps prevent accidental damage to the

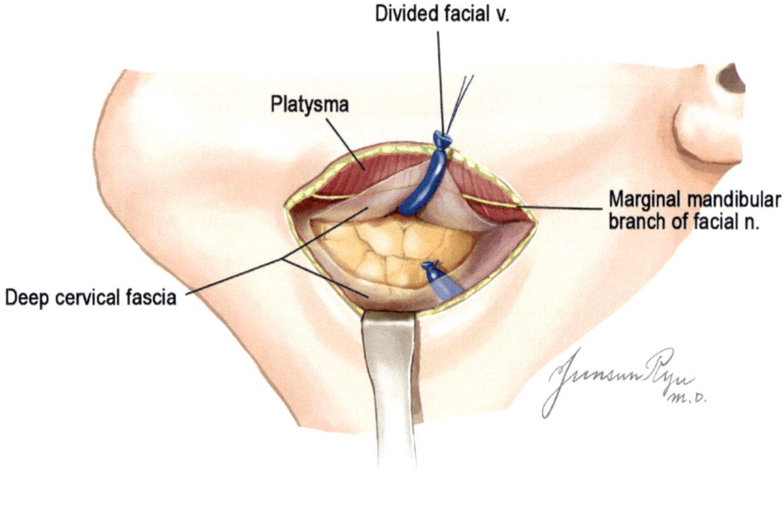

Fig. 5.1 During subplatysmal flap elevation, the facial vein is retracted superiorly to protect the marginal mandibular branch of the facial nerve. v, vein; n, nerve

nerve during surgical procedures. To further prevent inadvertent injury to the lingual nerve, the secretomotor pathways running from the submandibular ganglion to the gland should be meticulously ligated (Fig. 5.2). It is crucial to distinguish these pathways from the lingual nerve and ensure that they are securely tied off. Additionally, electrothermal devices such as Bovie can cause thermal injury to the lingual nerve and surrounding tissues.

Expert Opinion
The mylohyoid muscle is identified at the antero superior portion of the posterior belly of the digastric muscle. After ligating the branches of the nerve & vessels passing over the mylohyoid muscle, pulling the muscle anteriorly using a retractor ensures clear visualization of the lingual nerve. (Dong Young Kim)

Because it lies in the plane beneath the digastric muscle, identification of the hypoglossal nerve is typically unnecessary during standard submandibular gland resection. However, accurate identification may be required to ensure safe dissection. The nerve should be approached only after submandibular gland resection, and the digastric muscle should be identified. Subsequently, the hypoglossal nerve can be readily identified in the submandibular triangle through gentle dissection, as it is positioned deep and posterior to the junction of the anterior belly of the digastric muscle.

Expert Opinion
The hypoglossal nerve and sublingual vein travel together beneath the posterior belly of the digastric muscle. Therefore, care should be taken to avoid ligating the vein passing under the digastric muscle. (Dong Young Kim)

If nerve injury is identified during surgery, immediate repair should be performed. Primary repair should be attempted if a tension-free anastomosis can be achieved. Otherwise, an interposition graft may be performed, potentially utilizing segments of the greater auricular nerve that can be harvested within or near the operative field. Intraoperative steroid administration may be considered, although the evidence supporting this practice is limited. Postoperatively, if the nerve is preserved or repaired, nimodipine, a calcium channel blocker, may be administered to accelerate nerve recovery; however, evidence supporting its efficacy remains limited.

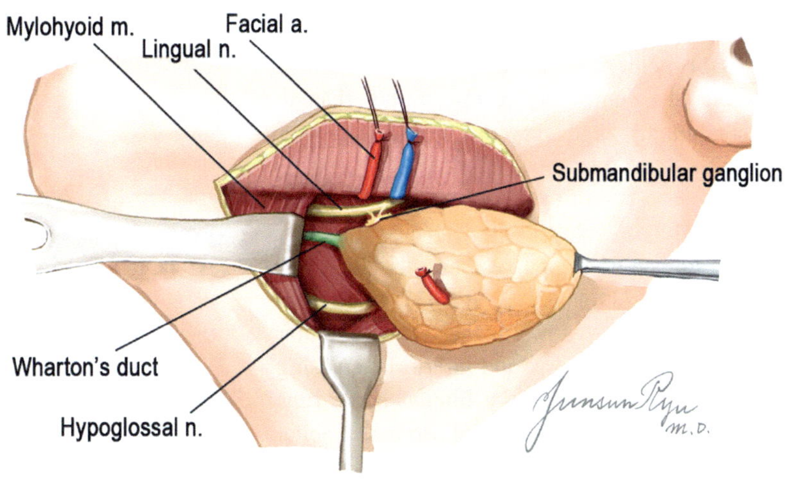

Fig. 5.2 In the ensuing dissection of the SMG, the facial artery or its branches entering the gland is ligated while preserving the trunk. The lingual and hypoglossal nerves are identified and preserved. The secretomotor fibers of the lingual nerve to the gland are divided. Wharton's duct is ligated after anterior retraction of the mylohyoid muscle. m, muscle; n, nerve; a, artery

◆ Preventing and managing nerve injury during submandibular gland resection surgery requires a standardized approach with meticulous dissection that considers the unique anatomy and function of the nerves in this area.

5.2 KQ 5.2. How to Prevent and Manage Inadvertent Injury of Wharton's Duct During Sublingual Gland Resection?

Woo-Jin Jeong

To ensure successful surgery of the sublingual glands, it is crucial to accurately identify Wharton's duct orifices and understand the anatomical relationships between the lingual nerve and Wharton's duct. During surgery, an incision is made on the floor of the mouth, extending from just posterior to the duct orifice to the retromolar trigone. Submucosal dissection reveals the sublingual gland, which is situated in the areolar tissue beneath the mucosa of the mouth floor and above the mylohyoid muscle, with Wharton's duct and lingual nerve positioned between the gland and the genioglossus muscle.

Expert Opinion
When performing sublingual gland resection, I prefer to make the mucosal incision along the course of the duct rather than horizontally as this can aid in wide exposure. (Soon-Young Kwon)

The lingual nerve courses beneath Wharton's duct from lateral to medial (Fig. 5.3). As the duct moves proximally toward the submandibular gland, it runs posteriorly and inferiorly, crossing the lingual nerve. Here, the lingual nerve runs superior to the Wharton's duct. Therefore, tracing Wharton's duct and lingual nerve to the deepest point is essential to prevent inadvertent injuries.

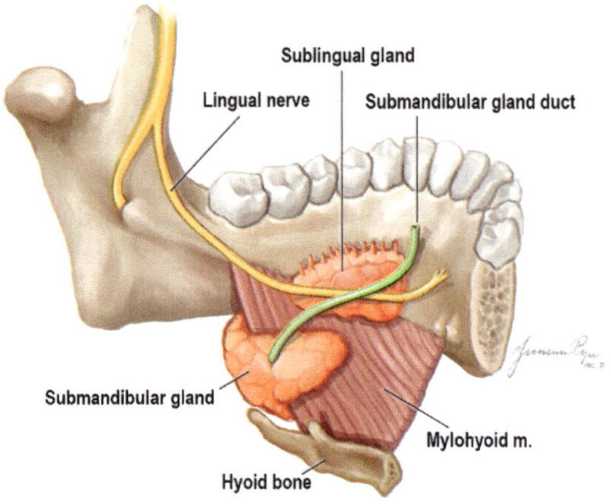

Fig. 5.3 Anatomy of the sublingual gland, submandibular duct, and lingual nerve. Note the crossing of the duct and nerve. m, muscle

If locating the duct is challenging, starting dissection from the posterior aspect of the sublingual gland is an option. The proximal portions of the duct and nerve are thicker in this area, reducing the risk of injury. Distinguishing the duct from the nerves or vessels can be difficult. However, if the duct orifice has already been located, a lacrimal probe can help identify the duct. Because lacrimal probes are relatively rigid, performing surgery with the probe in situ may result in duct damage. Thus, a cut-down tube is a better option (Fig. 5.4).

◆ A thorough understanding of the anatomy of Wharton's duct and its surrounding structures is essential for preventing complications.

Expert Opinion
A large incision along the sublingual crest will facilitate locating the duct behind the sublingual gland. Careful separation and ligation of the sublingual duct (Bartholin's duct), which connects to the submandibular duct, can also prevent injury to the submandibular duct. (Dong Young Kim)

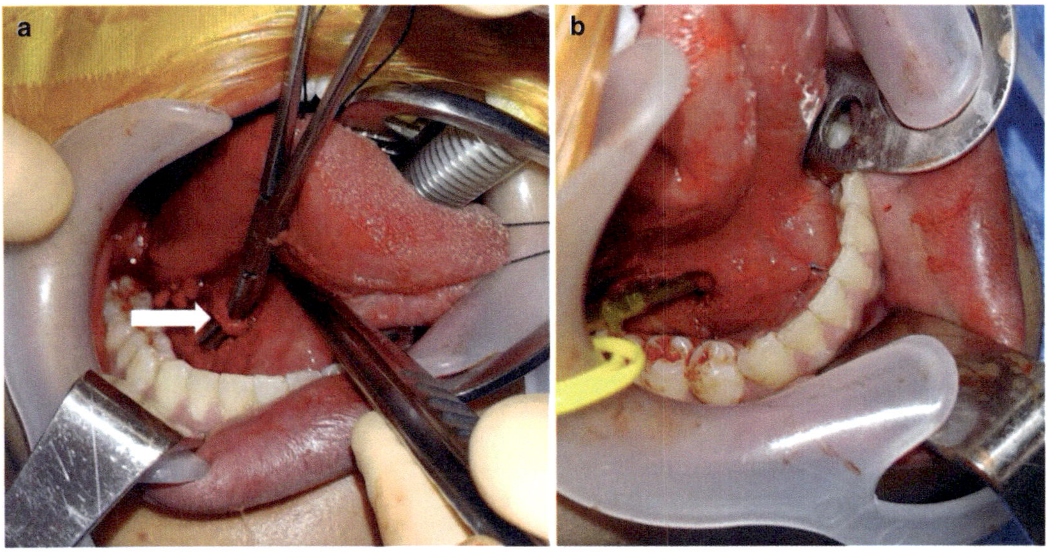

Fig. 5.4 (**a**) Wharton's duct (arrow). (**b**) Insertion of a cut-down tube for cannulation

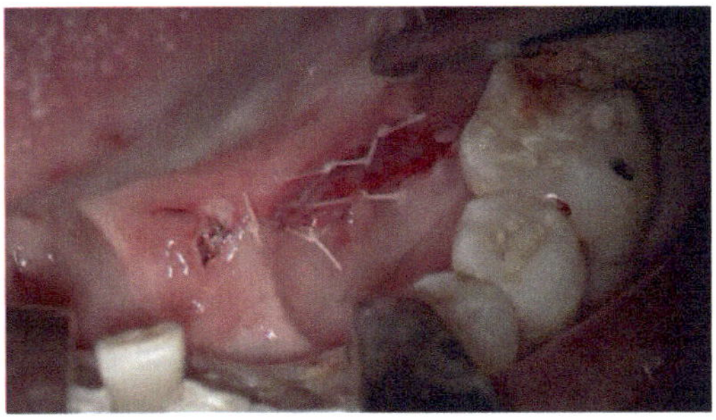

Fig. 5.5 Sialodochoplasty (copyright: Prof. Hyun Jun Hong)

If an inadvertent injury of the Wharton's duct occurs during sublingual gland resection, the management approach depends on the extent of the injury, whether the orifice is involved, and whether repair is possible. In cases where the orifice remains intact and primary repair is achievable, ductoplasty, a form of primary repair, may be attempted. This applies to partial injuries and transections. Ensure that the cut is clean and that tension-free anastomosis is possible. Typically, a thin-diameter (7-0, 8-0) monofilament suture (e.g., Nylon, Prolene) is used. Since restenosis is common, it is advisable to prepare materials for stenting, such as a cut-down tube, for insertion if needed (Fig. 5.5) [4]. Even when primary repair is possible, sialodochoplasty may be performed together with ductoplasty (described below) to facilitate saliva passage.

If primary repair is not achievable, the orifice cannot be identified, or the stump is too short or thin for primary repair, sialodochoplasty is required. This procedure entails sacrificing the distal portion of the duct and orifice and redirecting the proximal portion to the mid- to posterior floor of the mouth. The lumen of the duct is exposed and the duct wall is incised with sharp iris scissors and sutured to the adjacent oral mucosa to create a new orifice. The same suture material as that used in ductoplasty is preferable. Ensuring a tension-free anastomosis is crucial. Stenting is recommended due to the high risk of stenosis in the neoorifice.

Expert Opinion

When performing sialodochoplasty, the duct should be cut at an angle to widen the lumen. Only 2–4 stitches should be used and placed sparsely. Frequent salivary gland massage postoperatively helps maintain intact salivary flow, reducing stenosis. A stent is not useful in these circumstances because it would not anchor well to the duct. (Han-Sin Jeong)

◆ In cases of Wharton's duct injury, ductoplasty (primary repair), sialodochoplasty, or a combination of both, may be performed.
◆ Since restenosis is common, stenting with a cut-down tube and maintaining it for a certain period is worth considering.

5.3 KQ 5.3. How to Prevent and Manage Nerve Injuries in Intraoral Stone Removal?

Han Su Kim

Sialolithiasis is the primary cause of salivary gland obstruction and occurs predominantly in the submandibular gland (90% of cases are in the submandibular gland and 10% in the parotid gland) [5]. Based on the location, sialolithiasis is categorized as proximal (hilar/intraglandular and proximal ducts) or distal (middle and distal ducts) (Fig. 5.6).

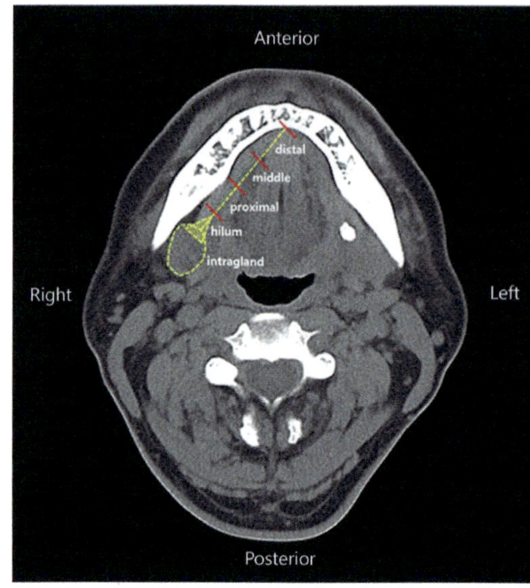

Fig. 5.6 The location of submandibular gland stones. Stones within the submandibular gland are classified based on their location. The distal part consists of both the distal and middle sections of the salivary gland duct, which runs over the mylohyoid muscle. The proximal part comprises the proximal salivary duct and the glandular region (intraglandular and hilum areas)

Approximately 40% of submandibular stones are situated in the distal part of Wharton's duct, which can be removed intraorally with a transmucosal incision near the duct orifice [5]. However, when dealing with proximal stones, the intraoral removal technique can present challenges owing to their relatively deep positioning and the potential risk of damaging critical anatomical structures. The prevention and effective management of nerve injuries during intraoral stone removal are essential for patient safety and well-being. The lingual and hypoglossal nerves are vital components of the oral cavity, and damage to these nerves can result in significant complications.

There is wide consensus that proximal stones cause lasting structural damage to the gland, which can predispose it to recurrent infections. Consequently, numerous sialadenectomies are performed annually, primarily to address duct problems without directly addressing the gland itself. However, increasing evidence suggests that the submandibular gland can regain its function after stone removal, raising questions regarding the role of sialadenectomy as an optimal treatment for proximal calculi [5].

Several steps can be taken to prevent and manage nerve injuries during intraoral stone removal.

5.3.1 Comprehensive Preoperative Assessment

I strongly recommend that all patients undergo an unenhanced computed tomography (CT) scan before the procedure. This imaging modality is highly efficient for the preoperative evaluation of stone quantity and location. Notably, while cone-beam CT (CBCT) provides valuable insights into stone detection, it may be inadequate for visualizing soft tissues [6]. A conventional CT scan also allows the evaluation of the contralateral side, which is essential because the presence of multiple sialolithiasis is frequently observed. The removal of all stones in a single session remains the gold standard in salivary gland surgery.

◆ A conventional CT scan is helpful for the preoperative evaluation of the location and number of stones.

Expert Opinion

Since contrast-enhanced CT can confirm the presence of pathology in the salivary glands, it is recommended to take non-contrast and contrast-enhanced images together if the patient has swelling of the salivary glands. (Dong Young Kim)

Contrast-enhanced CT is preferred for evaluating the pathology of the salivary gland. (Han-Sin Jeong)

5.3.2 Proper Anesthesia and Analgesia

With patient cooperation, distal stones can be removed under local anesthesia. It is important not to inject medication into the sublingual veins or directly into the lingual nerves.

In the case of a proximal stone, the patient may experience significant difficulties such as a gag reflex caused by pressure on the tongue, and surgery may take more time. Therefore, general anesthesia is highly recommended for proximal stone removal. To avoid obstruction of the surgical site by an intubation tube, transnasal intubation is preferred when general anesthesia is used.

Expert Opinion

When manipulating the proximal lesion with local anesthesia, bleeding can cause airway obstruction even with hematoma formation or compression, so attention should be paid to hemostasis. (Dong Young Kim)

Orotracheal intubation with contralateral fixation does not interfere with the visualization of the surgical field. (Han-Sin Jeong)

I prefer general anesthesia in all the cases, even in cases of distal stones, because the location of the stone can be changed and the swelling caused by the injection agent causes difficulty in identifying the stone. (Soon-Young Kwon)

5.3.3 Understanding the Anatomical Relationships and Landmarks

Most proximal stones are located in the hilum of the submandibular gland, which is not easily accessible during surgery. The deep locations of the hilum and submandibular gland ducts are often concealed by the crossing of the lingual nerve and the sublingual gland. However, the dynamics of the relationship between the duct and the other anatomical structures change. In the proximal space, the duct of the submandibular gland passes beneath the lingual nerve shortly after its emergence from the salivary glands. The duct traverses the lingual nerve as it progresses distally. Consequently, the gland duct is positioned between the lingual nerve medially and the sublingual gland laterally (Fig. 5.7) [7]. Therefore, it is essential to become familiar with the precise anatomical relationships among the nerves, glands, and sublingual vessels through a transoral approach.

5.3.4 Choice of the Surgical Approaches

Surgeons should consider adopting different approaches based on the location of the stone. I prefer to first identify the salivary gland duct rather than the stone itself because the stone is always located within the salivary gland duct. If the stone is located distally (superficially), the "medio-lingual" approach is recommended (Video 5.1). For stones located in the distal part of the duct, a mucosal incision was made between

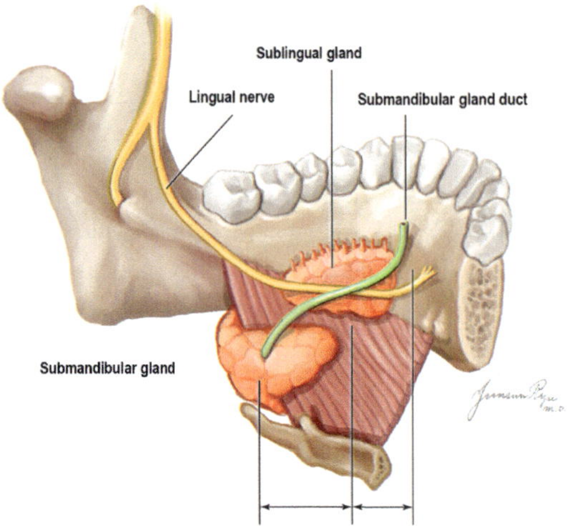

Fig. 5.7 The anatomical relationship between the duct and other anatomical structures. At the proximal space, the submandibular gland duct passes beneath the lingual nerve shortly after emerging from the salivary gland. As it progresses to the distal space, the duct traverses over the lingual nerve. Consequently, the gland duct is positioned between the lingual nerve medially and the sublingual gland laterally

the medial side of the sublingual gland and the tongue. Following the mucosal incision, the gland was exposed and gently pushed laterally to identify the duct situated just medial to the gland.

> **Expert Opinion**
> Salivary duct stones that occur in the hilum are often large. Therefore, it is necessary to locate them by palpation during procedure. In order to identify the duct, distinguishing it is difficult with the naked eye; therefore, approaching it from the distal part and check the duct is helpful. (Dong Young Kim)
>
> Lingual nerve retraction using finger rather than cotton swab is preferred because it does not slip and can properly adjust the pressure on the nerves. (Han-Sin Jeong)

When a stone is located in the proximal or deeper part of the duct, the "surgical triangle" is highly effective for exposing the hilum of the submandibular glands. The "surgical triangle" is defined by retracting the sublingual gland anteriorly, the posterior border of the mylohyoid muscle laterally, and the lingual nerve medially (Fig. 5.8). The surgical triangle has been modified from its original version [8]. The lingual nerve traverses the duct from the lateral to the medial side within the confines of the surgical triangle. Therefore, a mucosal incision was made near the gingiva. A linear incision was created from the premolar, running along the floor of the mouth toward the third molar tooth, leaving a 1.0 cm-wide cuff of normal lingual mucosa to facilitate wound closure.

> ◆ If stones are located distally (superficially), the "medio-lingual" approach is recommended. In contrast, the "latero-gingival" approach is more suitable for stones located proximally.

After a mucosal incision, the lingual nerve becomes readily identifiable beneath the sublingual gland and connective tissues. Upon exposure, the nerve can be gently pushed "medially" using a cotton swab to complete the surgical triangle (latero-gingival approach) (Video 5.2). Depending on the situation, it may be necessary to mobilize the lingual nerve from the duct and retract it medially to visualize stones within the duct or hilum of the gland. The duct is then incised, and the stone was retrieved. At this juncture, manual pressure is applied to elevate the submandibular gland if the hilum is located deep within it. This approach is valuable in preventing injury to the lingual and sublingual glands while accessing the hilum of the duct and gland [8].

5.3.5 Surgical Steps

After local or general anesthesia, a self-lip retractor is used to retract the lips. The mouth is held open using a Denhardt mouth gag, placed on the contralateral molars. The tongue is retracted using

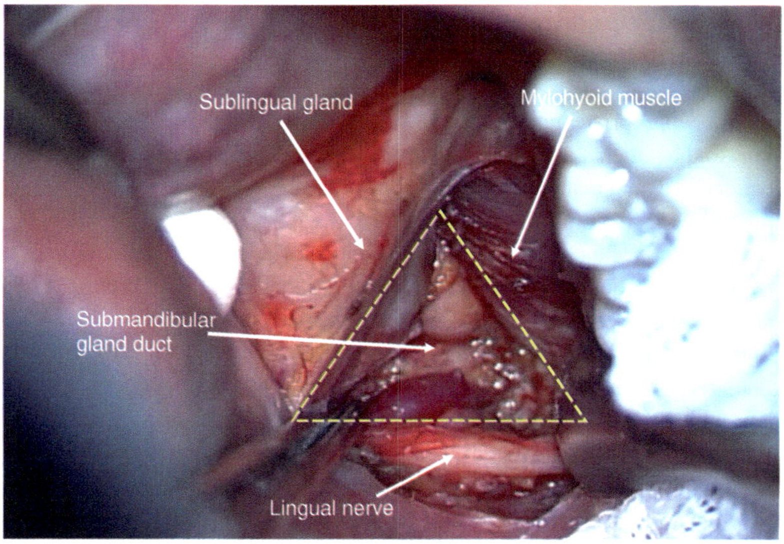

Fig. 5.8 The surgical triangle (right). The surgical triangle is defined by retracting the sublingual gland anteriorly, the posterior border of the mylohyoid muscle laterally, and the lingual nerve medially

a gauze swab or tongue retractor, thereby exposing and tensing the mouth floor. Personally, we opted to use monopolar cautery for mucosal incisions to minimize bleeding from the incised mucosa.

Expert Opinion
The sublingual crest is where saliva is secreted from the sublingual gland, so an incision parallel to the posterior approximately 5 mm or more helps to find the sublingual gland and prevent the occurrence of mucocele. (Dong Young Kim)

I prefer the mouth gag to be placed ipsilaterally for better exposure.

Incision at the duct is preferred just proximal to the location of the stone to avoid the stone moving into the proximal part of the duct. (Soon-Young Kwon)

Loose areolar connective tissue is meticulously dissected using bipolar cautery to minimize the risk of incidental injury to the nerves and glands. As the deeper tissues are released, the sublingual gland can be retracted laterally to expose the distal part of the salivary gland duct or medially to reveal the proximal part of the duct and hilum. An assistant can hold the sublingual gland in place using a gauze swab. The distal part of the duct becomes easily identifiable after retracting the sublingual gland, and an incision is made in the duct at the location of the stone. To remove the proximal stones, it is crucial to expose the course of the lingual nerve. Once the nerve is exposed, it is gently retracted medially to complete the surgical triangle. The proximal parts of the duct and hilum are positioned at the center of the surgical triangle, allowing easy identification of the stone within the duct.

The duct is then thoroughly irrigated with saline after stone removal. The floor of the mouth is loosely closed with 4-0 polyglactin (Vicryl™) without marsupialization or ductotomy. Meticulous hemostasis was necessary for all procedures to obtain a clear surgical field and visualize important structures such as the lingual and submandibular ducts [8].

Expert Opinion
I do not close the mucosa and prefer to marsupialize the duct and tether it to the adjacent mucosa because the closure of the mucosa reportedly causes more postoperative duct stenosis, even though this is debatable. (Soon-Young Kwon)

5.3.6 Postoperative Care and Monitoring

Provide appropriate postoperative care instructions to the patients, including guidelines for oral hygiene and pain management. Nerve injuries are a major concern for both surgeons and patients. The incidence of iatrogenic injury following conventional sialadenectomy is surprisingly high, and it may be considered a standard operative procedure. Temporary injury to the ramus mandibularis branch of the facial nerve occurs in approximately 10% of cases, whereas permanent injuries occur in 3% of cases. Injury to the lingual and hypoglossal nerves is less common (less than 4%); however, approximately half of these injuries are permanent [9]. In contrast, intraoral removal of stones from the hilum of the gland is associated with low morbidity. Injuries to the lingual nerve are typically temporary and resolve within 6 months [8].

Several non-neural complications, such as hemorrhage, infection, and ranula formation can occur. Most vessels in the floor of the mouth can be managed using bipolar cautery. However, injury to a larger lingual vein can cause severe and complicated bleeding. Therefore, if such injury is suspected during surgery, the vessels should be ligated using a tie or vessel clip.

Acute sialadenitis occurs in approximately 5% of the patients after the procedure [9]. Therefore, prophylactic oral antibiotics should be prescribed for 7 days, and the use of a chlorhexidine mouthwash is recommended. Patients were encouraged to consume plenty of oral fluids in the evening of the operation and resume a normal diet as soon as possible.

> **Expert Opinion**
> Soft diet is recommended postoperatively rather than normal diet. (Han-Sin Jeong)

5.4 KQ 5.4. How to Prevent and Manage Recurrent Ranula?

Han Su Kim

5.4.1 Identifying and Preventing Damage to the Sublingual Gland

Traditionally, exposing the entire course of the duct and separating it from the lingual nerve have been recommended [10]. Other authors have recommended removal of the sublingual gland during stone removal [11].

However, we believe that this traditional procedure increases the risk of injury to the sublingual gland, leading to postoperative ranula formation. Instead, I prefer applying different mucosal incisions based on the location of the stone. For distal stones, an incision is made on the floor of the mouth, on the lingual side of the salivary crest, medial to the sublingual gland, to avoid damage to the sublingual gland (medio-lingual approach). For proximal stones, a latero-gingival mucosal incision is preferred to facilitate easy identification and medial mobilization of the gland.

> ◆ Preserving the sublingual gland is one of the most crucial steps in preventing postoperative ranula.

> **Expert Opinion**
> In cases of multiple submandibular gland stones located across entire duct, a sublingual gland resection can be performed, which helps prevent ranula. (Han-Sin Jeong)

The oral mucosa is rich in blood vessels. I prefer using a monopolar device for mucosal incisions rather than a cold knife, as it helps decrease bleeding. Once the mucosa is parted, the loose areolar tissue on the floor of the mouth is carefully dissected using bipolar cautery. Upon dissection, the sublingual gland is visible upon dissection. In cases of distal stones, it should be mobilized along its medial margin and gently retracted laterally using a cotton swab to expose the duct. By contrast, for proximal stones, the sublingual gland is retracted medially, allowing easy identification of the lingual nerve beneath it. By preserving the sublingual gland during the procedure, unnecessary disruption of the anatomy and function of the gland can be avoided, which could help prevent complications such as ranulas without performing additional procedures (marsupialization) at the operation site.

5.4.2 Is Marsupialization of the Salivary Gland Duct Necessary?

Mounting clinical and experimental evidence suggests that salivary glands regain useful functions after stone removal [5]. Marsupialization of the salivary gland duct is generally not a standard procedure for salivary gland stone removal for two primary reasons. First, the transoral marsupialization of the proximal duct is challenging because of its deep position within the floor of the mouth. Secondly, when the stone is removed, the normal flow of saliva can be restored. Roh et al. reported that symptom recurrence and the recovery of salivary function after stone removal were unaffected by the presence or absence of a neo-ostium [12]. Additionally, they found that sialodochoplasty had no effect on the postoperative outcomes, suggesting that the presence of a neo-ostium might have a minimal effect on preventing symptom recurrence after complete stone removal. Moreover, several reports indicated that meticulous closure of the ductal incision may not be necessary to restore ductal patency or prevent recurrence [5].

5.4.3 Management of Recurrent Ranula

The proper treatment of recurrent ranulas remains controversial. Numerous surgical and non-surgical treatment modalities have been developed. If the lesion does not resolve after 6 months of observation or recurs persistently, surgical treatment is recommended [15].

Since the sublingual gland is responsible for ranula development, radical excision of the sublingual gland is considered the most effective treatment modality for both primary and recurrent ranulas [13]. Sublingual gland resection requires general anesthesia and may lead to complications such as lingual nerve or Wharton's duct injury. Therefore, less invasive surgical procedures that are feasible under local anesthesia in outpatient clinics have also been utilized. These include marsupialization and micro-marsupialization, using sutures to drain the pseudocyst while preserving the sublingual gland. The micro-marsupialization technique was described by Silva et al., who recommended the maintenance of sutures for up to 30 days after the procedure [14].

Micro-marsupialization should be considered as the primary treatment for recurrent ranulas. However, radical excision of the sublingual gland should be considered in patients with refractory recurrent ranulas.

- Micro-marsupialization is a simple, low-cost therapeutic modality for recurrent ranulas, which patients typically tolerate well.

Expert Opinion

When Bartholin's duct, the sublingual gland duct which opens into submandibular gland duct, is identified during sublingual gland resection, ligation of the duct is necessary. (Han-Sin Jeong)

References

1. Preuss SF, Klussmann JP, Wittekindt C, Drebber U, Beutner D, Guntinas-Lichius O. Submandibular gland excision: 15 years of experience. J Oral Maxillofac Surg. 2007;65(5):953–7.
2. Berini-Aytes L, Gay-Escoda C. Morbidity associated with removal of the submandibular gland. J Craniomaxillofac Surg. 1992;20(5):216–9.
3. Tirelli G, Bergamini PR, Scardoni A, Gatto A, Boscolo Nata F, Marcuzzo AV. Intraoperative monitoring of marginal mandibular nerve during neck dissection. Head Neck. 2018;40(5):1016–23.
4. Carlson ER, Ord RA. Salivary gland pathology: diagnosis and management. Newark, NJ: Wiley; 2015.
5. McGurk M, Makdissi J, Brown JE. Intra-oral removal of stones from the hilum of the submandibular gland: report of technique and morbidity. Int J Oral Maxillofac Surg. 2004;33(7):683–6.
6. Gardon MA, Foletti JM, Avignon S, Graillon N, Chossegros C. CT scan assessment in salivary gland lithiasis diagnosis. J Stomatol Oral Maxillofac Surg [Internet]. 2018;119(2):110–2. https://doi.org/10.1016/j.jormas.2017.11.012.
7. Iwai T, Sugiyama S, Oguri S, Mitsudo K. Anatomical relationship between the lingual nerve and submandibular duct. J Craniofac Surg. 2022;33(3):949–50.
8. Park HS, Pae SY, Kim KY, Chung SM, Kim HS. Intraoral removal of stones in the proximal submandibular duct: usefulness of a surgical landmark for the hilum. Laryngoscope. 2013;123(4):934–7.
9. Combes J, Karavidas K, McGurk M. Intraoral removal of proximal submandibular stones—an alternative to sialadenectomy? Int J Oral Maxillofac Surg. 2009;38(8):813–6.
10. Seward GR. Anatomic surgery for salivary calculi. Oral Surg Oral Med Oral Pathol [Internet]. 1968;25(4):525–31. Available from: https://linkinghub.elsevier.com/retrieve/pii/0030422068902946.
11. Eun YG, Chung DH, Kwon KH. Advantages of intraoral removal over submandibular gland resection for proximal submandibular stones. Laryngoscope. 2010;120(11):2189–92.
12. Roh JL, Park CI. Transoral removal of submandibular hilar stone and sialodochoplasty. Otolaryngol Head Neck Surg. 2008;139(2):235–9.
13. Gontarz M, Bargiel J, Gąsiorowski K, Marecik T, Szczurowski P, Zapała J, et al. Surgical treatment of sublingual gland ranulas. Int Arch Otorhinolaryngol. 2023;27(02):e296–301.
14. Silva DFB, Neves GDV, De MRQ, De Carvalho SHG, Pereira JV, Gomes DQDC. Modified micromarsupialization as treatment of ranula in a pediatric patient. J Craniofac Surg. 2020;31(3):E230–2.
15. Zhi K, Wen Y, Ren W, Zhang Y. Management of infant ranula. Int J Pediatr Otorhinolaryngol. 2008;72(6):823–6.

Part III

Larynx and Hypopharynx

Transoral Laser or Robotic Surgery

6

Seung Hoon Woo, Sang Joon Lee,
Hyun Jun Hong, and Young Ho Jung

6.1 KQ 6.1 How to Prevent and Respond to a Fire During Transoral Laser Surgery?

Seung Hoon Woo and Sang Joon Lee

Diagnostic and surgical lasers are generally safe and effective [1]. However, laser devices present significant hazards, particularly in surgical settings, posing risks to doctors, nurses, other medical staff, and patients. Laser-related dangers span a spectrum from minor injuries to severe, irreversible damage and even fatalities. Contrary to common belief, laser hazards extend beyond the laser beams and are typically categorized into beam and non-beam hazards. Beam hazards originate from the laser beam itself, which can cause ocular and cutaneous-related injuries: (1) Direct or reflected rays can harm the skin, hair, cornea, and retina, leading to permanent damage. (2) Improper handling of a laser beam can ignite the surgical drape, endotracheal tube, and patient's hair. (3) Non-beam hazards arise from laser devices or their interactions with materials in the surgical environment [2]. These include fire, plume, and electrical hazards. For example, laser–tissue interaction produces smoke with an irritating odor and particulate matter that irritates the eyes, nose, and lungs and induces vomiting. The use of lasers has also raised concerns about the potential transmission of viral and bacterial infections. This can occur when blood, interstitial fluids, and intracellular fluids are aerosolized, potentially carrying viral and bacterial pathogens that can be forcefully expelled into the operating room environment. Such risks are not limited to patients, laser users, and laser handlers, but also to passersby or those in the waiting room. Since the use of laser technology has spread beyond hospital settings, the risk of laser-related accidents is increasing. In South Korea, it is estimated that many non-hospital cases of laser-related accidents exist, even in the absence of officially reported cases. This could be attributed to the operation of laser devices by untrained nonmedical users in beauty salons and other nonhospital settings. Laser-related accidents can be prevented by ensuring safe laser environments, the use of

Supplementary Information The online version contains supplementary material available at https://doi.org/10.1007/978-981-96-1860-6_6.

S. H. Woo (✉) · S. J. Lee
Department of Otolaryngology—Head and Neck Surgery, Dankook University College of Medicine, Cheonan, South Korea

H. J. Hong (✉)
Department of Otorhinolaryngology, Yonsei University College of Medicine, Severance Hospital/Yonsei Cancer Center, Seoul, Republic of Korea
e-mail: hyunjun.hong@yuhs.ac

Y. H. Jung
Department of Otolaryngology, Head and Neck Surgery, Asan Medical Center, University of Ulsan College of Medicine, Seoul, South Korea

K.-J. Cho, J.-O. Park (eds.), *Management of Head and Neck Surgery Complications*,
https://doi.org/10.1007/978-981-96-1860-6_6

protective equipment, and safe laser operation. However, reports have indicated that laser users do not always follow precautionary measures: 67% of accidents that occur when using a medical laser reportedly result from improper handling of laser devices. This highlights the need for the development and implementation of safety measures, particularly in response to fires, during transoral laser surgery.

6.1.1 Fire and Electrical Hazards

An unpredictable fire resulting from an incorrect laser shot or an electric shock caused by high-voltage electricity can lead to horrific accidents during laser treatment (Fig. 6.1). According to experts, approximately 100 fires occur annually in operating rooms in the United States, with 10–20 of them causing severe injury to patients and resulting in 1–2 deaths [3]. The drape that covers the patient in the operating room is easily ignited by the laser because of the high oxygen levels in the operating environment. Drapes with weak ignition qualities must be used to prevent this phenomenon. In addition, the cover of the laser site should always be kept wet [4]. Endotracheal tube fires are described separately. Many lasers are high-voltage electric devices that can easily shock handlers, particularly when the protection plates are removed. Additionally, a risk of unnecessary disruption when the devices come in contact with water exists; this can result in short-circuits of the system wiring. Therefore, users must receive appropriate training from manufacturers.

6.1.1.1 Management of Anesthesia in Laser Surgery

The two most popular lasers, CO_2 and Neodymium-doped Yttrium Aluminum Garnet (Nd:YAG) use different wavelengths and are applied to different body parts. CO_2 lasers can be used for upper respiratory tract surgeries via direct firing or rigid bronchoscopy. Nd:YAG and Potassium Titanyl Phosphate (KTP) lasers are suitable for peripheral airway surgery using flexural endoscopy because their beams are effectively transmitted using fiber optics [5]. In addition to preoperative evaluation, the otolaryngologist and anesthesiologist should discuss each team's plan and come to a common understanding prior to surgery.

6.1.2 Upper Respiratory Tract Surgery

Several surgical techniques can be considered for laser ablation of pharyngeal and laryngeal lesions. Insufflation techniques can be used if intubation is not necessary and have the advantage of providing a wide surgical site. However, if the anesthesiologist is unable to regulate the patient's breathing, a high risk of aspiration pneumonia ensues. In

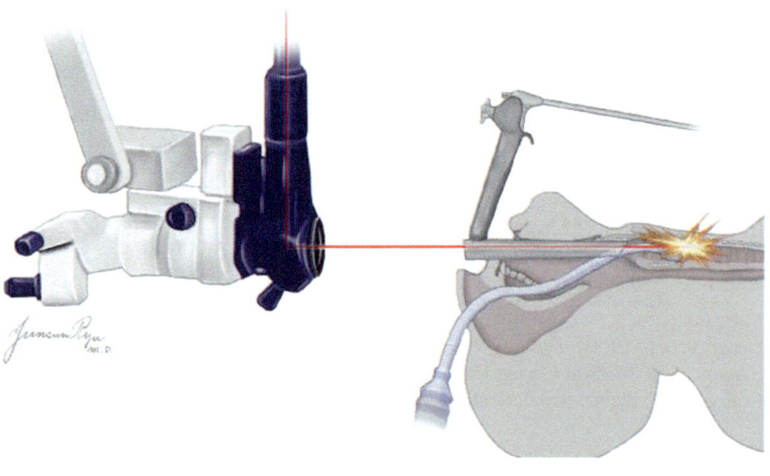

Fig. 6.1 An airway fire results when a laser strikes the polyvinyl chloride endotracheal tube

addition, anesthesia gas fills the operating room because the depth of anesthesia cannot be adjusted. Because of these drawbacks, this method has not been widely used [6, 7].

Jet ventilation can be installed using a laryngoscope; however, if the laryngoscope is not positioned accurately, oxygen will not enter the bronchi, and the esophagus and stomach can be dilated. This can lead to pneumothorax, pneumomediastinum, and barotrauma; thus, it is rarely used as a primary anesthetic [7].

Endotracheal intubation is a commonly used method. It narrows the practitioner's field of view and requires working with the anesthesiologist through a smaller endotracheal tube. A tube with an inner diameter of 5–6 mm is moderately adjusted and is suitable for surgeries around the tube. The use of endotracheal tubes increases the risk of an intratracheal laser fire. This risk can be reduced using an intra-metal tissue tube. However, solid tubes can cause trauma to the tracheal mucosa and can rupture the bronchi because the laser beam can be reflected by the tube, and the metal tube does not seal the bronchi [8]. The use of cuffs creates the risk of laser fire; therefore, metal tubing, which requires cuffs, is not commonly used [9].

Expert Opinion

When using a small-diameter tube, tube dislodgement may occur during laryngoscope manipulation for improved visibility, neck extension, or removal of the laryngoscope after the procedure, making continuous communication with the anesthesiologist important. (Jung Je Park).

Soft endotracheal tubes include red rubber, silicone rubber, and polyvinyl chloride (PVC), all of which are flammable. According to a comparative study of the flammability of these tubes, PVC melts and ignites at a relatively low temperature as compared with the other two substances [10]. The black letters on the tube and the radiopaque lines absorb the heat of the laser and can be the point of ignition. The cuff of the endotracheal tube has the thinnest wall and is vulnerable to ignition [11]. To reduce the risk of ignition, the cuff is filled with saline and methylene blue dye (Fig. 6.2), or the endotracheal tube is wrapped with a metal bandage. However, the disadvantage of applying excessive pressure to the bronchi remains.

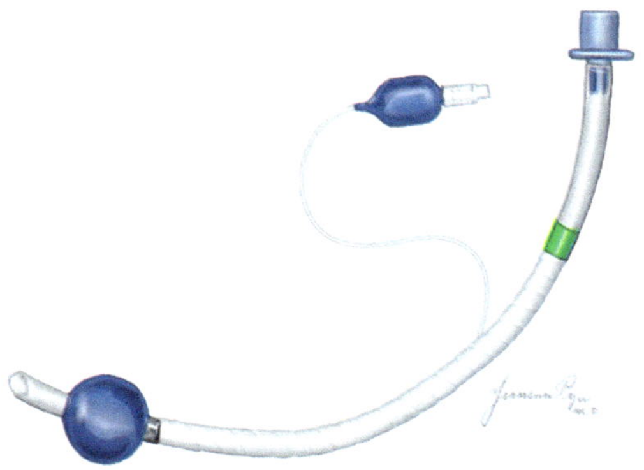

Fig. 6.2 The endotracheal tube cuff is filled with saline and methylene blue dye

To address these challenges, Xomed (silicone endotracheal tubes with non-reflective metal coatings), Bivona (silicone metal tubes), and Mallinckrodt (metal tubes in PVC tubes) were recently introduced. When the PVC tube burns, the gas pressure spreads to the flame; however, the metal tube prevents this phenomenon. When it completely passes through the wall of the laser tube, the gas leaks out and begins to ignite, and the pressure of the gas creates a blowtorch effect. Therefore, oxygen tension is important and must be kept at 40% or less. Based on the results of tube stability experiments for several types of tubes in South Korea, no type of tube is absolutely safe during laser surgery; however, the Xomed Laser Shield IITM and Rusch red rubber tube wrapped with aluminum foil have been reported to be relatively safe [12].

In a German survey, 59–86 hospitals used special laser endotracheal tubes. Fifteen endotracheal tube fires were reported in 20,000 laser surgeries performed at these hospitals. Six of the fifteen fires occurred despite the use of a special laser tube [13].

Expert Opinion
To reduce the risk of airway fire, it is important for the anesthetist to minimize FiO_2 (to around 30%) to prevent a blowtorch effect if the oxygen in the airways ignites (Jung Je Park).

6.1.3 Lower Respiratory Tract Surgery

CO_2 lasers via a rigid bronchoscope can be used to remove lesions in the lower respiratory tract, where anesthetic gas is supplied via the side port of the endoscope. In this case, the risk of endotracheal tube ignition is mitigated. Efficient ventilation in a sealed state can be achieved by covering the bronchoscope with wet gauze. In addition, the use of a bronchoscope makes it possible to operate deeper into the periphery. However, the Nd:YAG and KTP lasers are operated through a flexible bronchoscope that uses an endotracheal tube such that the tip of the bronchoscope is at the bottom of the tube, resulting in a high risk of ignition (Fig. 6.3).

6.1.4 Jet Ventilation and High-Frequency Ventilation

Jet ventilation can be performed using various tubes and ventilation catheters, wherein catheters can be inserted via the vocal cords, bronchi, and tracheostoma. Jet ventilation can achieve a normal respiratory rate of up to 60–120 beats per minute. High-frequency jet ventilation (HFJV) can be performed using a laryngoscope or a rigid or flexible bronchoscope. Although HFJV is helpful in several cases, it is limited by smoke and debris blown out during the procedure. Patient safety depends on the ability to measure airway pressure and immediately stop the HFJV. Hyperinflation of the lungs can be avoided through proper monitoring.

6.1.5 Tracheal Fire Management

Once a tracheal fire breaks out, the following measures should be taken to reduce morbidity and mortality: 1. Immediately remove the endotracheal tube. 2. Take precautions to avoid the fire spreading to the drape. 3. Mask ventilate until the endotracheal intubation can be reconstructed. Apart from high temperatures, lung damage also results from smoke, toxic fumes, and tissue fragments from the fire. Damage to the larynx and bronchi should be assessed using bronchoscopy. The carbonized tissue fragments must be removed. Lavage can push the tissue pieces deep into the bronchi and should be avoided. Mechanical ventilation, bronchodilators, and antibiotics should be administered for several days. When an endotracheal tube (particularly PVC) ignites, it emits toxic smoke, causing lung alveolar damage and adult respiratory distress syndrome.

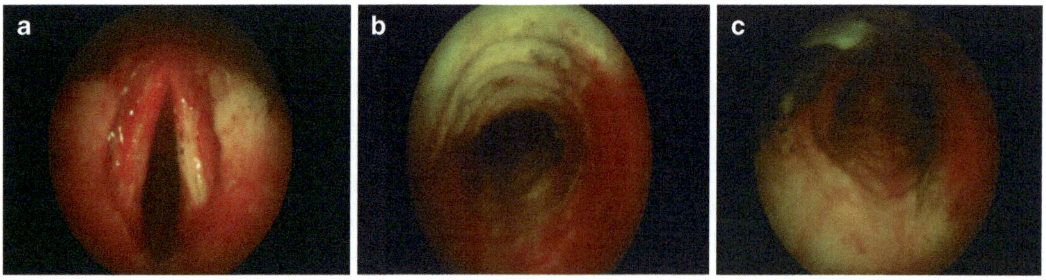

Fig. 6.3 Airway damage from laser ignition. (**a**) Vocal cord. (**b**) Upper trachea. (**c**) Lower trachea

6.1.5.1 Safe Laser Use by Medical Institutions and Medical Personnel

Since 1990, the popularity of laser technology has been growing in South Korean medical institutions. However, as mentioned previously, many risks limit their use. Medical institutions must implement administrative, medical, and mechanical protective measures. Unfortunately, these measures have not yet been implemented in Korean medical institutions. The American National Standards Institute (ANSI) has issued guidelines for the safe use of lasers in all medical institutions, and many institutions have adhered to these guidelines [14]. The Joint Commission on the Accreditation of Healthcare Organizations (JCAHO), a US hospital review agency, also uses ANSI guidelines for hospital review.

6.1.6 Laser Committee Installation and Role

The primary purpose of the Laser Committee is to provide medical and technical support for the use of lasers in hospitals. The committee is obliged to adopt and amend policies and procedures regarding the use of lasers, formulate guidelines and protocols for laser safety, determine the appropriate equipment and personnel, and vet doctors who qualify for laser technology. In addition, the committee is mandated to establish training guidelines for laser practitioners, anesthesiologists, and nurses, and to set standard qualifications to be used in screening during the personnel hiring process. The committee can also regularly review the quality of care for laser patients and provide the necessary advice. Laser safety officers (LSOs) rather than doctors should be appointed and should report to the Laser Committee. Laser physicists, medical engineers, nurses, and other medical professionals can act as LSO. The individual should have considerable knowledge of laser technology and should take responsibility for all laser safety issues in the hospital. The LSO must perform daily follow-ups to ensure that the safety guidelines are followed.

6.1.7 Laser Training and Personnel Composition

Hospitals are responsible for the quality of their laser procedures; therefore, they should have their own protocols to verify their doctors and other relevant medical personnel. Doctors are updated with information on laser education and practical training. Exemption should be applied to doctors who have sufficient knowledge of the diseases and lesions being treated and the basic properties of lasers and laser safety. The requirements for the surgical use of lasers are 16–20 h or more of formal education, 8–0 h or more of hands-on practice using laser equipment, hands-on practice with patients, and continuous medical education on laser technology. In addition, the use of lasers may only be permitted if maintenance protocols for the laser devices can be demonstrated [15, 16]. Anesthesiologists and anesthesia nurses need sufficient knowledge and experience because the overall responsibilities of laser device operation and safety during the operation should only be assigned to trained personnel.

6.1.8 Start-Up Operation and Orientation of Laser Equipment

After purchasing a new laser, an orientation session must be held in which all physicians and laser users can participate. Regardless of how often individuals use a laser device, all users must familiarize themselves with the laser equipment. Continuous education regarding the safe use of lasers should be provided every year and when new users are hired. When a hospital purchases a new laser machine or a laser machine with a new wavelength, the hospital must organize a laser surgery orientation session in which all users, including practitioners, anesthesiologists, and operation room nurses, must participate. The orientation treatment must be performed similarly to an actual procedure, employing all equipment, such as surgical microscopes, video equipment, and protective devices. Through orientation, important information and issues with the device are uncovered.

6.1.9 Use in Restricted Zones

Lasers should be used only in controlled locations. Only essential personnel are allowed in these locations, and all protective goggles must be worn. The windows in the area where the laser is used must be blocked by a material that can prevent the laser from being emitted outside the laser chamber. However, no blocks are required when the CO_2 laser is used. When using a laser, users must employ specific signs and pay attention to everyone surrounding them. All entrances must be marked to alert incoming individuals of an ongoing laser procedure. Protective goggles must match the wavelengths indicated in the room entrance to be used by incoming people [17]. A sign can be placed around the door to indicate that the laser is in use (Fig. 6.4). Moreover, if the practitioner is not using the laser, it is safe to change to "standby" mode in the "ready" mode. The following checklist is recommended while preparing for laser surgery.

6.1.10 Inspection and Maintenance

Pre-use inspections must be performed by laser safety personnel. These include inspection of laser fiber calibration and fiber, handpiece, and waveguide defects; ensuring beam and therapeutic beam matching; and inspection of the laser working environment. More detailed inspections must be performed regularly, and the inspection personnel must be specially trained by the manufacturer.

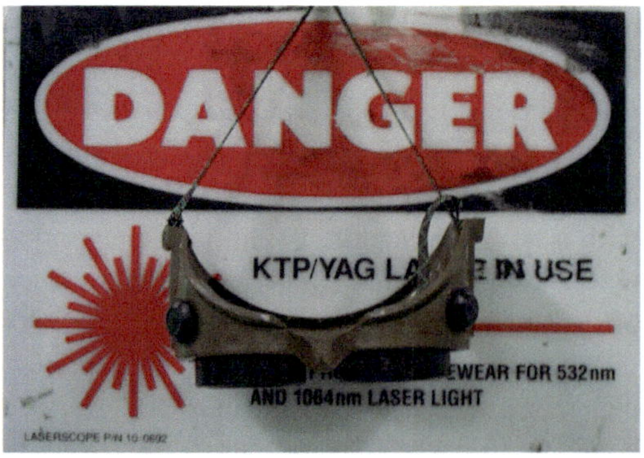

Fig. 6.4 A sign may be placed around the door to indicate the ongoing use of laser

The American Organization of Registered Nurses (AORN) has adopted the following guidelines for the safe use of laser equipment during surgery [18].

1. All healthcare professionals must be warned of areas where the laser is in use through appropriate labeling.
2. Adequate eye protection must be provided to both patients and healthcare professionals.
3. Patients and healthcare professionals must be provided with adequate skin protection against accidentally emitted or incorrectly reflected laser beams.
4. Patients and healthcare professionals must be protected from inhaling smoke emitted from lasers.
5. Patients and healthcare professionals must be protected against laser-related fire hazards.
6. Patients and healthcare professionals must be protected from laser-related electrical hazards.
7. For the safe use of lasers, safety policies and procedures should be adopted.

In 2004, the AORN installed a laser safety program in private clinics and general hospitals, which mandates that individuals who utilize lasers must acquaint themselves with and adhere to these safety regulations. Among others, it recommends that the areas where the laser is in use require additional precautionary measures, such as protection from flammable and explosive hazards associated with the laser [19].

Medical lasers are useful for the diagnosis and treatment of illnesses. However, they can cause serious damage to patients undergoing laser treatment and the medical personnel involved. To prevent these risks, healthcare professionals require sufficient training in the use of lasers. Medical institutions have established appropriate guidelines and precautions for the safe use of lasers, which should be implemented and practiced to prevent laser-related accidents [20].

6.2 KQ 6.2 How to Manage Postoperative Oral Bleeding Following Transoral Laser or Robotic Surgery?

Hyun Jun Hong

6.2.1 Incidence

Transoral robotic surgery (TORS) has become a widely used minimally invasive approach for the treatment of oropharyngeal cancers. Since the Food and Drug Administration (FDA) approved TORS for T1 and T2 oropharyngeal cancer (OPC) in 2009, its use has increased, leading to careful evaluation of oncologic outcomes and the associated morbidity and mortality of robot-assisted surgery.

Postoperative hemorrhage is a common complication of TORS, with bleeding rates ranging from 3.1% to 13.2% [21, 22]. The overall incidence of post-TORS hemorrhage is relatively low at 5.78%. However, it is higher than that of other common oropharyngeal surgeries such as tonsillectomy, which has a postoperative bleeding rate of 4.8% in adults [21, 23, 24].

Even a moderate postoperative oral hemorrhage can lead to airway compromise, aspiration, asphyxiation, and potential cardiopulmonary arrest. The severity of post-TORS hemorrhage ranges from minor bleeding managed with observation to severe cases resulting in death (Table 6.1) [25].

A large survey of self-reported complications following TORS in 2015 patients revealed a catastrophic bleeding rate of 3.5% and a mortality rate of 0.3%.

The incidence of major hemorrhage requiring emergent embolization, transcervical artery ligation (TAL), or tracheotomy to control the hemorrhage was even lower, at 2.90% (Fig. 6.5) [21, 26, 27].

The external carotid artery (ECA) or its branches, such as the lingual or facial arteries, can be ligated to prevent postoperative bleeding following TORS [21].

6.2.2 Risk Factors

Large primary tumors, perioperative anticoagulation or antiplatelet therapy, prior radiation therapy, and insufficient surgical experience are associated with significantly increased post-TORS hemorrhage rates.

6.2.3 Prevention

Reconstruction of oropharyngeal defects, when possible, can be technically challenging and is typically reserved for specific situations such as

Table 6.1 Classification of postoperative bleeding after TORS

Classification	Description
Minor	Any description of visualized bright red blood or blood clots resolved without operative management Spontaneous resolved bleeding with conservative management
Intermediate	Diffuse venous oozing or small arterial source bleeding resulting in operating room evaluation or intervention Managed with monopolar or bipolar cautery
Major	Massive bleeding requiring operative intervention Managed with transoral or transcervical vessel ligation or intervention embolization
Severe	Bleeding resulting in life-threatening medical complications: Airway compromise, hypoxia, requiring tracheotomy, cardiopulmonary arrest, hemodynamic instability requiring transfusion

TORS transoral robotic surgery

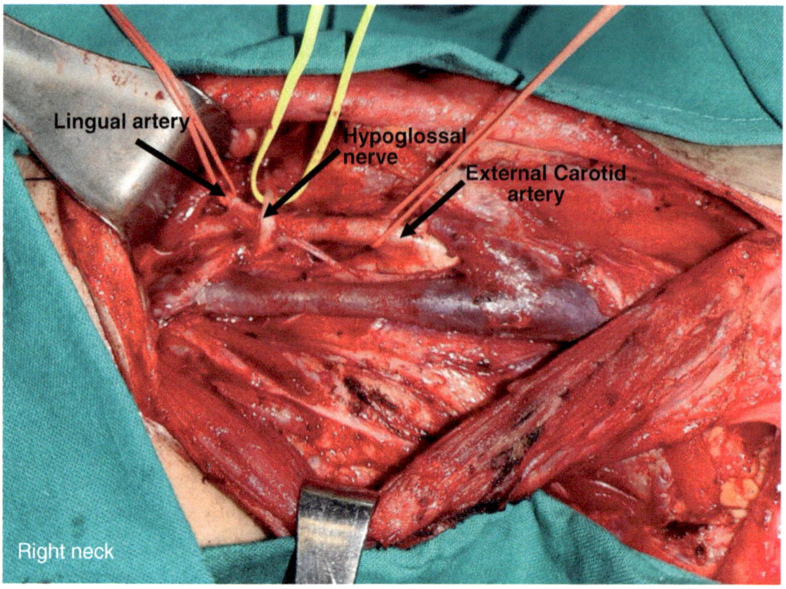

Fig. 6.5 Surgical anatomy for transcervical artery ligation

large palatal defects, significant loss of tongue base volume, fistulas, or exposure of the carotid artery [28]. This reconstruction may help reduce secondary bleeding by covering the defect and preventing the formation of granulation tissue. To prevent catastrophic bleeding, some groups have suggested transcervical arterial ligation (TAL) of either the ECA or its branches to diminish the arterial blood flow to the surgical site [21, 23, 26, 28, 29]. Studies have indicated that TAL is associated with a reduction in severe bleeding rates according to the Mayo Postoperative Bleeding Severity Classification (Table 6.1), although an overall decrease in post-TORS bleeding rates has not been observed [25]. TAL is considered an important adjunct for preventing postoperative hemorrhage during neck dissection (ND) concurrent with TORS, such as transoral oropharyngectomy. Concurrent ND offers the advantage of controlling the ECA and its branches with relatively low morbidity associated with pharyngocutaneous fistula rates (4%). Although TAL does not lower the overall incidence of post-TORS hemorrhage, it may reduce the incidence of major bleeding [28]. Previous reports have suggested that prophylactic TAL results in a significant but statistically insignificant decrease in the relative risk of major post-TORS bleeding (RR = 0.40, 95% CI = 0.15–1.07) [21]. In this study, 45 NDs with TAL were required to prevent major post-TORS hemorrhages necessitating operative control, emergent tracheostomy, TAL, embolization, cardiac arrest, or death [21].

Expert Opinion

To prevent postoperative hemorrhage, the facial or lingual arteries are sometimes ligated. Additionally, to control bleeding, a medium-sized TachoSil (Takeda Pharmaceutical Company Limited, Tokyo, Japan) sheet is cut into nine equal pieces and evenly applied to the oropharyngeal surgical bed (Jun-Ook Park).

Patients with a history of radiation exposure and advanced tumors are at a higher risk of postoperative hemorrhage. In these patients, prophylactic TAL may reduce the incidence of severe bleeding after TORS. Post-TORS patients who are unable to protect their airways should be strongly considered for prophylactic tracheostomy to assist with airway protection.

Management Protocols

Managing postoperative oral bleeding following transoral laser or robotic surgery is crucial for ensuring patient comfort and preventing complications. The following steps and guidelines should be followed:

1. **Assess the Bleeding:** Evaluate the severity of the bleeding. Minor bleeding can often be managed conservatively, while severe bleeding requires immediate medical attention.
2. **Position the Patient:** Position the patient comfortably and upright to minimize the risk of aspiration and reduce blood flow to the head and neck regions.
3. **Monitor Vital Signs:** Continuously monitor vital signs, including blood pressure and heart rate, especially if bleeding is severe. Rapid changes may indicate the need for more intensive interventions.
4. **Clear the Airway:** Ensure that the patient's airway is clear, and they are breathing normally. If severe bleeding obstructs the airway, suctioning or other emergency measures should be employed.
5. **Apply Direct Pressure:** Apply direct pressure to the bleeding site using sterile gauze or a clean cloth. Instruct the patient to bite down gently on the gauze to help control bleeding, maintaining constant pressure for at least 20–30 min.
6. **Avoid Aggravating Factors:** Advise the patient to avoid activities that could increase bleeding, such as vigorous rinsing, spitting, or drinking through a straw.
7. **Transfusion:** Blood transfusions may be necessary to restore hemoglobin levels in cases of significant blood loss.
8. **Medications:** If bleeding persists, the surgeon or healthcare provider may prescribe medications such as tranexamic acid or topical hemostatic agents to control the bleeding.
9. **Surgical Intervention:** If bleeding cannot be controlled using the aforementioned measures, the surgical team should be consulted immediately for further assessment and intervention. They may need to return to the operating room for further exploration and repair.

Prevention is preferable to treatment; thus, the surgical team must take precautions during the procedure to minimize the risk of postoperative bleeding. Additionally, patients should be informed about potential risks and provided with clear postoperative care instructions to reduce the likelihood of complications.

Expert Opinion

To prepare for potential massive postoperative hemorrhage, a tracheotomy is performed in most cases. In such events, the tracheotomy tube is ballooned, and the oral cavity is packed with gauze as a temporary hemostatic measure until the patient can be transported to the operating room (Jun-Ook Park).

6.3 KQ 6.3. How to Manage Supraglottic Stenosis Following Transoral Laser or Robotic Supraglottic Laryngectomy

Young Ho Jung

6.3.1 Supraglottic Stenosis Following Transoral Laser or Robotic Supraglottic Laryngectomy

Following the removal of the tumor and surrounding tissue in the supraglottis or hypopharynx with the help of a laser or robot, tissue defects may lead to aspiration. When these defects are reconstructed using a flap, stenosis can occur if the flap is excessively large. This problem can be resolved by excising the enlarged tissue [30–34].

In contrast, when supraglottic and hypopharyngeal resections are performed using a laser or robot, a CO_2 laser or monopolar Bovie is used. In this case, the temperature of the tissue can increase to 150 °C–200 °C, causing significant thermal damage to the surrounding tissue. Consequently, unexpected supraglottic stenosis may develop, and if resection extends to the vocal or false vocal cords, glottic stenosis may also ensue [23, 35, 36].

6.3.2 How to Prevent Postoperative Supraglottic Stenosis

Prevention of postoperative supraglottic stenosis begins with patient selection. Failure to select appropriate patients can lead to unavoidable postoperative supraglottic stenosis or can make proper management challenging [37, 38].

Patient age is the most important factor for consideration. The risk of aspiration pneumonia due to defects in the supraglottic region after surgery is high in older patients. Therefore, supraglottic, supracricoid partial, and vertical partial laryngectomies are limited in older patients. Even if the decision to operate is made because the older patient's pulmonary function or physical strength is good relative to the patient's age, if the structure that should normally be resected is deliberately left during surgery, adhesion between the remaining structures can cause supraglottic stenosis. Leaving at least half of the epiglottis is beneficial to prevent aspiration pneumonia; however, the remaining tissue can adhere to the opposite defect site and can cause stenosis [35, 39].

In case postoperative radiation therapy is performed, the adhesion between the tissues can worsen due to continuous local mucosal inflammation in addition to heat damage by a laser or monopolar Bovie. Unless concerns regarding oncological safety exist, radiation therapy is best avoided.

Expert Opinion

Adding radiation therapy after partial laryngectomy increases the risk of stenosis, aspiration, and dysphagia, with higher radiation doses leading to more severe complications. A postoperative radiation dose of 60 Gy is associated with greater risks than a dose of 50 Gy; thus, avoiding radiation or using the lowest effective dose may help reduce the risk of laryngeal stenosis (Jung Je Park).

Moreover, preserving the perichondrium of the thyroid cartilage as much as possible during surgery is beneficial. If the tumor does not invade the cartilage and is naturally dissected above the perichondrium, it is better to preserve the perichondrium than to remove it completely and expose the cartilage. This can not only reduce stenosis due to adhesions after surgery but can also prevent radiochondronecrosis that can occur after postoperative radiation therapy.

6.3.3 Treatment

The patient (Fig. 6.6) had a remaining epiglottis that obstructed the airway during inhalation. Although the epiglottis plays a protective role, it can also cause airway obstruction. The patient could walk and run without difficulty and did not exhibit any signs of inspiratory stridor. Therefore, no special treatments were required. However, surgical treatment may be necessary if the patient experiences respiratory distress or stridor during physical activity. Laser surgery can be used to remove portions that fold inwards; however, supraglottoplasty is generally recommended. Supraglottoplasty is a technique commonly used for pediatric laryngomalacia, in which the epiglottis folds into the supraglottic airway. By using a laser to burn the mucosa on the ventral side of the epiglottis carefully, the tendency for inward collapse of the epiglottis is reduced.

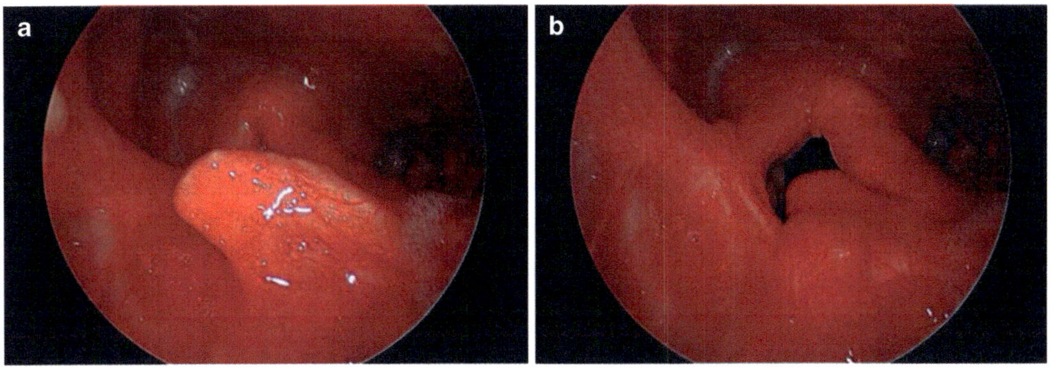

Fig. 6.6 Remaining epiglottis that partially obstructs the airway. (**a**) Resting, remaining left epiglottis after supraglottic laryngectomy. (**b**) During inspiration, the epiglottis is pulled down and partially obstructs the glottis

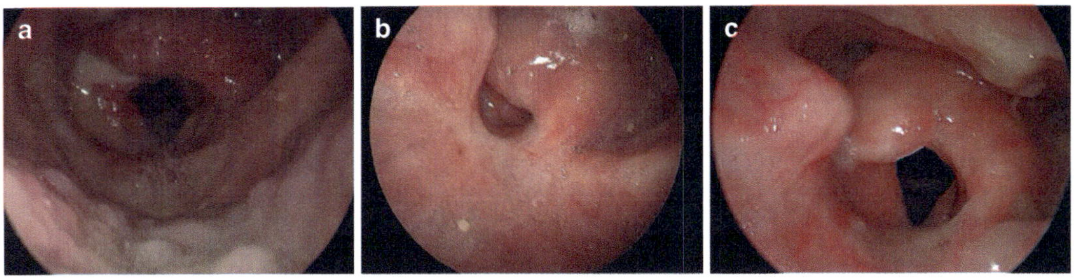

Fig. 6.7 Postoperative post-radiotherapy supraglottic stenosisPostoperative post-radiotherapy supraglottic stenosis. (**a**) Four weeks after supraglottic laryngectomy with robot, the patient has mobile and visible bilateral vocal cords. (**b**) Two months after radiotherapy, the vocal cords are invisible and covered by supraglottic synechiae. (**c**) After incising and excising the narrowed area using a KTP (potassium-titanyl-phosphate) laser and local triamcinolone injection, the patient has visible and mobile vocal cords

Suturing the epiglottis to the vallecula may also be considered; however, caution is required to avoid complications [36, 40].

In some cases, after supraglottic robotic laryngectomy, significant adhesions in the larynx can occur before the wounds heal completely. To address this, bougination and balloon dilation can be used as initial methods. When performing these procedures under general anesthesia, ventilation can be administered if a tracheostomy is performed. Otherwise, a temporary apnea technique should be used to monitor oxygen saturation. Another option is to use a Coblator to dissect or excise a narrow area. Using a CO_2 laser to incise the stenotic area may result in less bleeding, but the stenosis may worsen after 1 or 2 months. While incising the stenotic area using a cold instrument poses the disadvantage of difficulty in controlling bleeding, the Coblator offers the advantage of minimal tissue damage and reduced restenosis. This is because it is used under irrigation with normal saline at approximately 75 °C. If a laser is used, a potassium-titanyl-phosphate (KTP) laser is recommended because of its excellent hemostatic effect and minimal damage to the surrounding tissue. After incising or excising the narrowed area, local injection of corticosteroids such as triamcinolone or local injection of anticancer antibiotics, such as mitomycin C, can help to prevent adhesion recurrence. In cases of severe laryngotracheal stenosis, laryngotracheal reconstruction surgery is performed. The use of a tracheostomy tube or stoma retainer can help prevent recurrent stenosis by preventing negative pressure. Systemic steroids may also be used for 1 or 2 weeks; however, their efficacy is limited. The patient shown in Fig. 6.7 had laryngotracheal stenosis, which was treated using a KTP laser to excise the narrowed area and with local triamcinolone injection to resolve the stenosis [32, 41, 42].

Supraglottic stenosis is generally easier to resolve than subglottic or glottic stenosis. Cases requiring radical surgical treatments, such as laryngeal stenting, laryngotracheal reconstruction, partial cricotracheal reconstruction, or total laryngectomy, are uncommon.

6.4 KQ 6.4. How to Manage Persistent Dysphagia Following Transoral Laser or Robotic Supraglottic Laryngectomy

Young Ho Jung

6.4.1 Persistent Dysphagia

Esophageal phase problems may arise from the failure of the cricopharyngeus muscle to relax or impaired peristaltic movement within the esophagus. However, these are rarely observed following laser or robotic surgery. Most cases of dysphagia stem from complications in tongue movement during the oral phase or issues concerning cricopharyngeus muscle relaxation, which can result from problems with laryngeal elevation during the pharyngeal phase [30, 31, 39, 41, 43].

Aspiration and aspiration pneumonia occur due to several factors, including the removal of protective structures, such as the epiglottis and false and true vocal cords, which are involved in laryngeal protection, or due to complications from impaired vocal cord movement caused by thermal damage to the recurrent laryngeal nerve or adhesions in the vocal cord area, leading to unilateral or bilateral vocal cord paralysis [23, 30, 31, 37, 39–44].

6.4.2 How to Prevent Persistent Dysphagia

Patient selection plays a crucial role in preventing aspiration and aspiration pneumonia. In cases where cancer has invaded the arytenoid cartilage or if the patient is affected by vocal cord paralysis, partial or complete removal of the arytenoid cartilage during surgery becomes necessary. Postoperative vocal cord paralysis becomes inevitable, rendering glottic closure difficult due to tissue loss, thereby increasing the risk of aspiration. In such cases, it is advisable to consider concurrent chemoradiation therapy without surgery or neoadjuvant chemotherapy followed by surgical intervention. Effective neoadjuvant chemotherapy can lead to favorable tumor responses, enabling reduction of the resection range and minimizing tissue loss [41, 45].

Expert Opinion
Postoperative dysphagia patients might initially have asymptomatic dysphagia that is only identified through objective examinations. After surgery, dysphagia and difficulty with oral intake may become apparent. Clinicians should perform objective examinations preoperatively, such as videofluoroscopic swallow study (VFSS), using the Penetration-Aspiration scale. (Jung Je Park)

For performing supraglottic laryngectomy, complete removal of the epiglottis is visually appealing; however, for effective laryngeal protection, it is beneficial to retain the contralateral epiglottis, or at least part of it, while ensuring oncological safety (Fig. 6.8, Video 6.1). When using a CO_2 laser for supraglottic laryngectomy, achieving a transverse cut can be challenging, particularly for separating the false from the true

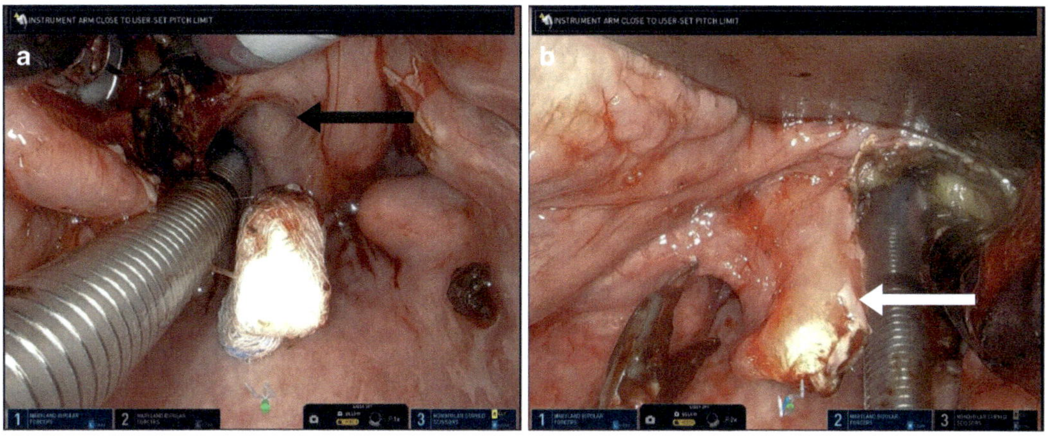

Fig. 6.8 Preserving the contralateral epiglottis, or a portion thereof, to ensure oncologic safety. (**a**) Right supraglottic cancer (black arrow) is being removed using transoral robotic surgery. (**b**) Left epiglottis (white arrow) is saved to prevent aspiration

vocal cord at the ventricle. Therefore, utilizing robotic assistance is preferable. Even with robotic assistance, the surgery should be performed in a low-power cutting mode to prevent vocal cord adhesion or recurrent laryngeal nerve palsy caused by thermal damage to the surrounding tissues [34, 44].

6.4.3 Treatment of Persistent Dysphagia

The key difference between transoral laser or robotic and conventional supraglottic laryngectomy is the preservation of the upper half of the thyroid cartilage during the transoral surgery. In conventional supraglottic laryngectomy, approximation of the hyoid bone and lower half of the thyroid cartilage facilitates laryngeal elevation and reduces the incidence of aspiration by posterior tilting of the larynx [23, 44].

Therefore, more aggressive postoperative swallowing rehabilitation is required in the case of transoral surgery. Swallowing rehabilitation exercises, such as the Mendelsohn maneuver as well as effortful and supraglottic swallowing, should be performed vigorously. For transoral surgery, aspiration may decrease, and swallowing may become more natural after 1 or 2 months, when the scar contracture of the lesion is formed. During this period, attention should be paid to lung toileting, and a tracheostomy should be performed, if necessary, to prevent pulmonary complications while continuing swallowing training.

In cases of unilateral vocal cord adhesion or recurrent laryngeal nerve palsy caused by thermal damage to the surrounding tissues, injection laryngoplasty can be performed, if necessary, to relieve symptoms. For vocal cord adhesion caused by thermal damage, the movement of the vocal cords is limited, but atrophy of the vocal cord muscles is not observed; therefore, dysphonia and aspiration are often not severe.

Problems related to the esophageal phase, such as failure to relax the cricopharyngeal muscle or impaired peristaltic movement of the esophagus, are rare. If the cricopharyngeal muscle spasm is confirmed by videofluoroscopy, a Botox injection can be considered. When considering Botox injection for cricopharyngeal muscle relaxation failure, administration can be performed both via intraoral and percutaneous approaches. In the transoral approach, the injection is targeted at the ring-shaped cricopharyngeal muscle, identified by elevating the cricoid cartilage under general anesthesia. The injection is delivered into the muscles in the central area of the posterior part of the cricopharyngeal muscle and in the left and right anterior 120° areas of the muscle, with 20 IU administered to each area of the muscle, totaling 60 IU. The percutaneous approach is performed under local anesthesia and electromyographic guidance. Localization can be challenging due to the poor function of the cricopharyngeal muscle. However, such instances are rare following transoral supraglottic laryngectomy. Therefore, cricopharyngeal muscle relaxation failure may be a secondary manifestation resulting from impaired laryngeal elevation rather than an isolated issue. Therefore, emphasis should be placed on prioritizing rehabilitation exercises covered in the previous discussion.

References

1. Rhee CK, Chung PS, Jeong PS. Laser safety in laryngeal microsurgery using CO_2 laser. Korean J Bronchoesophagol. 1998;4:159–64.
2. Moseley H. Operator error is the key factor contributing to medical laser accidents. Lasers Med Sci. 2004;19:105–11.
3. Beyea SC. Preventing fires in the OR. AORN J. 2003;78:664–6.
4. Wolf GL, Sidebotham GW, Lazard JL, Charchaflieh JG. Laser ignition of surgical drape materials in air, 50% oxygen, and 95% oxygen. Anesthesiology. 2004;100:1167–71.
5. Hermens JM, Bennett MJ, Hirshman CA. Anesthesia for laser surgery. Anesth Analg. 1983;62:218–29.
6. Norton ML, Strong MS, Vaughan CW, Snow JC, Kripke BJ. Endotracheal intubation and Venturi (jet) ventilation for laser microsurgery of the larynx. Ann Otol Rhinol Laryngol. 1976;85(5 Pt 1):656–63.
7. Talmage EA. Endotracheal tube is not necessary for laryngeal microsurgery. Anesthesiology. 1981;55:332.
8. Hirshman CA, Leon D, Porch D, Everts E, Smith JD. Improved metal endotracheal tube for laser surgery of the airway. Anesth Analg. 1980;59:789–91.
9. Spiess BD, Ivankovich AD. Anesthetic management of laser airway surgery. Semin Surg Oncol. 1990;6:189–93.
10. Wolf GL, Simpson JI. Flammability of endotracheal tubes in oxygen and nitrous oxide enriched atmosphere. Anesthesiology. 1987;67:236–9.
11. Geffin B, Shapshay SM, Bellack GS, Hobin K, Setzer SE. Flammability of endotracheal tubes during Nd-YAG laser application in the airway. Anesthesiology. 1986;65:511–5.
12. Kim DH, Jung PS, Kim JS. The effects of blood and normal saline on laser-resistant endotracheal tube combustion. Korean J Anesthesiol. 1995;29:798–805.
13. Sesterhenn AM, Dünne AA, Braulke D, Lippert BM, Folz BJ, Werner JA. Value of endotracheal tube safety in laryngeal laser surgery. Lasers Surg Med. 2003;32:384–90.
14. American National Standards Institute. Safe use of lasers in health care facilities. ANSI Z136.3–1988. New York: American National Standards Institute; 1988.
15. Dorsey JH. Education and credentialing of the gynecologic laser surgeon. Obstet Gynecol Clin N Am. 1991;18:661–5.
16. Ossoff RH. Implementing the ANSI Z 136.3 laser safety standard in the medical environment. Otolaryngol Head Neck Surg. 1986;94:525–8.
17. Wamsley CE, Hoopman J, Kenkel JM. Safety guidelines concerning the use of protective eyewear and gauze during laser procedures. Aesthet Surg J. 2020;41:1179.
18. Association of Operating Room Nurses. Recommended practices. Laser safety in the practice setting. AORN J. 1989;50:1015–20.
19. Association of perioperative Registered Nurses Recommended Practices Committee. Recommended practices for laser safety in practice settings. AORN J. 2004;79(836–8):841–4.
20. Woo SH, Chung P-S, Lee SJ. Safe use of medical lasers. Med Lasers. 2021;10(2):68–75.
21. Stokes W, Ramadan J, Lawson G, Ferris FRL, Holsinger FC, Turner MT. Bleeding complications after Transoral robotic surgery: a meta-analysis and systematic review. Laryngoscope. 2021;131(1):95–105.
22. Zenga J, Suko J, Kallogjeri D, Pipkorn P, Nussenbaum B, Jackson RS. Postoperative hemorrhage and hospital revisit after transoral robotic surgery. Laryngoscope. 2017;127(10):2287–92.
23. Sethi RKV, Chen MM, Malloy KM. Complications of Transoral robotic surgery. Otolaryngol Clin N Am. 2020;53(6):1109–15.
24. Asher SA, White HN, Kejner AE, Rosenthal EL, Carroll WR, Magnuson JS. Hemorrhage after transoral robotic-assisted surgery. Otolaryngol Head Neck Surg. 2013;149(1):112–7.
25. Hockstein NG, Weinstein GS, O'Malley BW Jr. Maintenance of hemostasis in transoral robotic surgery. ORL J Otorhinolaryngol Relat Spec. 2005;67(4):220–4.
26. Sharbel DD, Abkemeier M, Sullivan J, Zimmerman Z, Albergotti WG, Duvvuri U, et al. Transcervical arterial ligation for prevention of postoperative hemorrhage in transoral oropharyngectomy: systematic review and meta-analysis. Head Neck. 2021;43(1):334–44.
27. Crawford JA, Bahgat AY, White HN, Magnuson JS. Hemostatic options for Transoral robotic surgery of the pharynx and base of tongue. Otolaryngol Clin N Am. 2016;49(3):715–25.

28. Gabrysz-Forget F, Mur T, Dolan R, Yarlagadda B. Perioperative safety, feasibility, and oncologic utility of transoral robotic surgery with da Vinci xi platform. J Robot Surg. 2020;14(1):85–9.
29. Bollig CA, Gilley DR, Ahmad J, Jorgensen JB. Prophylactic arterial ligation following transoral robotic surgery: a systematic review and meta-analysis. Head Neck. 2020;42(4):739–46.
30. Dziegielewski PT, Kang SY, Ozer E. Transoral robotic surgery (TORS) for laryngeal and hypopharyngeal cancers. J Surg Oncol. 2015;112(7):702–6.
31. Hamilton D, Paleri V. Role of transoral robotic surgery in current head & neck practice. Surgeon. 2017;15(3):147–54.
32. Lucioni M, Bertolin A, Lionello M, Giacomelli L, Ghirardo G, Rizzotto G, et al. Transoral laser microsurgery for managing laryngeal stenosis after reconstructive partial laryngectomies. Laryngoscope. 2017;127(2):359–65.
33. Lucioni M, Marioni G, Mangialaio M, Rizzotto G. CO(2) laser treatment of laryngeal stenoses after reconstructive laryngectomies with cricohyoidopexy, cricohyoidoepiglottopexy or tracheohyoidoepiglottopexy. Eur Arch Otorrinolaringol. 2007;264(2):175–80.
34. Razafindranaly V, Lallemant B, Aubry K, Moriniere S, Vergez S, Mones ED, et al. Clinical outcomes with transoral robotic surgery for supraglottic squamous cell carcinoma: experience of a French evaluation cooperative subgroup of GETTEC. Head Neck. 2016;38(Suppl 1):E1097–101.
35. Canzi P, Maiorano E, Sovardi F, Nardo M, Occhini A, Benazzo M. A rare presentation of recalcitrant oropharyngeal stenosis in a 54-year-old male patient following Transoral robotic surgery for obstructive sleep apnea. Am J Case Rep. 2022;23:e937123.
36. Misiolek M, Orecka B, Czecior E, Namyslowski G. CO_2 laser treatment of laryngeal stenoses after supracricoid laryngectomies: comment on: Lucioni M, Marioni G, Mangialaio M, Rizzotto G (2007) CO_2 laser treatment of laryngeal stenoses after reconstructive laryngectomies with cricohyoidopexy, cricohyoidoepiglottopexy or tracheohyoidoepiglottopexy. Eur arch Otorhinolaryngol 264: 175-180. Eur Arch Otorrinolaringol. 2007;264(8):981–2.
37. van der Woerd B, Patel KB, Nichols AC, Fung K, Yoo J, MacNeil SD. Functional outcomes in early (T1/T2) supraglottic cancer: a systematic review. J Otolaryngol Head Neck Surg. 2018;47(1):76.
38. Vilaseca I, Bernal-Sprekelsen M. Transoral laser microsurgery for locally advanced laryngeal cancer. Acta Otorrinolaringol Esp. 2013;64(2):140–9.
39. Hans S, Chekkoury-Idrissi Y, Circiu MP, Distinguin L, Crevier-Buchman L, Lechien JR. Surgical, oncological, and functional outcomes of Transoral robotic Supraglottic laryngectomy. Laryngoscope. 2021;131(5):1060–5.
40. Shapshay SM, Wang Z, Rebeiz EE, Perrault DF Jr, Pankratov MM. "Window" laryngoplasty: a new combined laser endoscopic and open technique for conservation surgery. Ann Otol Rhinol Laryngol. 1994;103(9):679–85.
41. Hassid S, Krug B, Deheneffe S, Daisne JF, Delahaut G, Lawson G, et al. Treatment of supraglottic squamous cell carcinoma with advanced technologies: observational prospective evaluation of oncological outcomes, functional outcomes, quality of life and cost-effectiveness (SUPRA-QoL). BMC Cancer. 2023;23(1):493.
42. Burgess LP. Laryngeal reconstruction following vertical partial laryngectomy. Laryngoscope. 1993;103(2):109–32.
43. Dabas S, Gupta K, Ranjan R, Sharma AK, Shukla H. Oncological outcome following TORS in HPV negative supraglottic carcinoma. Indian J Cancer. 2019;56(1):9–14.
44. Scott SI, Madsen A, Rubek N, Charabi BW, Wessel I, Jensen CV, et al. Dysphagia and QoL 3 years after treatment of oropharyngeal cancer with TORS or radiotherapy. Laryngoscope. 2023;133(8):1893–8.
45. Peretti G, Piazza C, Mora F, Garofolo S, Guastini L. Reasonable limits for transoral laser microsurgery in laryngeal cancer. Curr Opin Otolaryngol Head Neck Surg. 2016;24(2):135–9.

7 Conventional Partial Laryngectomy with/Without Pharyngectomy

Young-Hoon Joo

7.1 KQ 7.1. How to Manage Airway Narrowing and Failure of Weaning Tracheostomy Following Conventional Partial Laryngectomy

Young-Hoon Joo

Current treatment options for laryngeal cancer include radical surgery, such as total laryngectomy. Organ preservation surgery, such as partial laryngectomy, radiotherapy, and chemotherapy, may be administered as a standalone treatment or in various combinations, depending on the site and stage of the laryngeal cancer. Although total laryngectomy (TL) represents a curative approach for locally advanced laryngeal cancer (stages III and IV), patients often refuse it due to the considerable impact on their quality of life, which includes the loss of a normal voice and the need for a permanent tracheostomy. Over the last few decades, organ preservation has become one of the most studied issues in head and neck oncology [1].

Organ-preservation surgery includes the following options: (1) Extended cordectomy for small lesions of the third anterior section of the vocal cords; (2) Frontolateral partial laryngectomy for vocal cord lesions extending to the anterior commissure; (3) Vertical hemilaryngectomy, which allows the removal of vocal cord lesions that, although still limited, extend into the supraglottic and/or subglottic region; (4) Partial horizontal laryngectomy for lesions of the supraglottic larynx (which is often complicated by the postoperative onset of difficulty in swallowing, with a tendency to aspirate ingested material into the airways, causing severe complications, particularly in older adults); (5) Supracricoid partial laryngectomy (SCPL), which is used for lesions of the supraglottis that extend to one or both vocal cords and which allows sparing of the cricoarytenoid unit and enables physiological phonation and deglutination without a permanent tracheostomy; and (6) Vertical hemipharyngolaryngectomy (VHPL) for hypopharyngeal lesions extending to the larynx. VHPL combines the resection of laterally localized extended pharyngolaryngeal tumors with immediate microsurgical reconstruction using a radial forearm fasciocutaneous free flap, including the palmaris longus tendon, for glottis reconstruction.

Supplementary Information The online version contains supplementary material available at https://doi.org/10.1007/978-981-96-1860-6_7.

Y.-H. Joo (✉)
Department of Otolaryngology—HNS, Bucheon St. Mary's Hospital, The Catholic University of Korea, Bucheon, Kyounggi-do, South Korea
e-mail: joodoct@catholic.ac.kr

K.-J. Cho, J.-O. Park (eds.), *Management of Head and Neck Surgery Complications*,
https://doi.org/10.1007/978-981-96-1860-6_7

7.1.1 Aspiration Following Conventional Partial Laryngectomy

Aspiration is the most life-threatening complication associated with treatment for head and neck cancer. Malnutrition, compromised pulmonary function, anxiety, and depression are well-known sequelae of aspiration. Postoperative pulmonary complications contribute significantly to the morbidity, mortality, and length of hospitalization following this procedure.

Wide resection of the tumor, along with a margin of normal tissue, can result in damage to the muscles that are critical for deglutition. Postoperative aspiration is related to the site and size of the tumor, the type of surgery performed, and the reconstruction technique. Patients with cancer often have impaired immunity due to malnutrition and cancer therapies, such as chemotherapy. Aspiration pneumonia can be fatal. However, due to the occurrence of aspiration in virtually all patients undergoing partial laryngectomy, preoperative assessment of the pulmonary status and prevention of postoperative pulmonary complications is necessary. Pulmonary complications frequently occur after partial laryngectomy procedures, leading to significant morbidity. In some cases, these complications necessitate a transition to complete laryngectomy. The incidence of pulmonary complications after supraglottic laryngectomy is 6–47% and 0–13%, respectively [2]. SCPL results in a complete and bilateral resection of the paraglottic space, including, when required, one arytenoid cartilage on the tumor-bearing side (Video 7.1). Compared to conventional vertical partial and supraglottic laryngectomies, SCPL is considered a conservative laryngeal procedure that mostly interferes with the sphincteric function of the larynx [3]. Lewin et al. reported that the postoperative complication rate, including pneumonia and subcutaneous emphysema, after SCPL was 26% [4]. The authors also reported that the postoperative overall complication rate was 32.4%, which was slightly higher than that of conventional supraglottic and vertical partial laryngectomies reported in the literature [5].

Pulmonary function tests (PFTs) help to assess patients' suitability for partial laryngectomy. Although PFTs can diagnose obstructive lung disease, the results do not translate into effective risk prediction for individual patients. Chow et al. reported that PFTs of patients who undergo partial laryngectomy could not help to predict postoperative complications reliably [2]. In our previous study, the forced expiratory volume in 1 s/forced vital capacity ratio was a statistically significant independent predictor of postoperative pulmonary complications [5]. We concluded that PFTs might not be needed unless a significant ventilation impairment is detected in the patient's medical history or physical examination.

Park et al. reported that the decannulation time was significantly delayed in patients with one arytenoid (extended SCPL) [6]. Even when considering the compensatory function of the remaining epiglottis (which functions as a laryngeal sphincter) in patients who have undergone SCPL, the mean decannulation and nasogastric tube removal times differed significantly according to the extended procedure of unilateral arytenoidectomy. Because arytenoids are the only remaining structures of the laryngeal sphincter in patients with SCPL, additional resection of one arytenoid naturally affects function negatively. Closure of the neoglottis can be achieved because of the posterior movement of the base of the tongue and epiglottis and the forward and inward rotational movement of the residual arytenoid. It follows that the conservation of both arytenoids, which collaborate with each other, allows better closure of the neoglottis.

Expert Opinion

During a horizontal partial laryngectomy, preserving at least one side of the superior laryngeal nerve is a priority for preventing postoperative aspiration and dysphagia. (Kwang Jae Cho).

7.1.2 Airway Narrowing Following Conventional Partial Laryngectomy

Nontumoral symptomatic laryngeal stenosis appears to be a rare complication of SCPL, occurring in only 14 patients (3.7%) in a cohort of 376 consecutive patients who underwent SCPL at a single institution over 20 years [7]. Laryngeal stenosis after SCPL can be divided into two groups [7]. Group I consists of patients with immediate laryngeal stenosis in whom decannulation could not be performed after surgery because of insufficient restoration of the laryngeal airway. This complication results from inadequate placement of the impaction sutures. SCPL disrupts the lateral support of the epiglottis by dividing the pharyngoepiglottic folds. Therefore, if the impaction sutures fail to support the epiglottic cartilage in this fashion, the entire epiglottis prolapses backward over the airway. Group 2 includes patients with delayed symptomatic laryngeal stenosis. Various factors contribute to airway narrowing at the impaction level, such as misalignment between the hyoid bone and cricoid cartilage or a smaller female larynx, as well as factors leading to a more aggressive cicatricial formation, such as the use of preoperative or postoperative radiotherapy, diabetes mellitus, or gastroesophageal reflux, which may predispose the patient to postoperative airway narrowing.

> Patients complaining of dyspnea due to postoperative persistent stenosis of the neolaryngeal lumen can be discharged with a tracheostomal cannula, and a transoral laryngeal microsurgery revision of the neoglottis should be scheduled at the second through third postoperative month in the absence of spontaneous recovery.

Recurrent and persistent laryngeal cancer after radiotherapy is associated with more aggressive growth patterns (infiltrative with multiple foci), has a higher tendency for extralaryngeal spread and subglottic extension, is more often undifferentiated, and more frequently presents with intravascular and perineural invasion than do the primary tumors. Therefore, TL is the most commonly performed salvage procedure in patients with recurrent or persistent laryngeal cancer after radiotherapy. Nevertheless, salvage TL is associated with an increased risk of wound formation and other systemic complications. SCPL is a valuable alternative treatment for selected recurrent laryngeal cancers. A systematic review revealed that the pooled mean larynx preservation rate after SCPL for radiorecurrent laryngeal cancer was 85.2% (95% CI 0.78–0.90%, 228 patients) [8]. The pooled mean decannulation rate was 92.1% (95% CI 0.86–0.95%), based on data reported for 213 patients. The time from surgery to decannulation could not be extracted reliably from the articles because of variable reporting methods and because some studies excluded patients with delayed decannulation. The incidence of laryngeal stenosis, which requires further surgery to enhance airway patency and facilitate tracheostomy decannulation, ranges from 0% to 8%. The pooled mean rate of laryngeal stenosis was 3.9% (95% CI 0.01–0.08%) based on a study of 144 patients. In a multicentric study, Bertolin et al. reported that 7% of 70 patients who underwent salvage SCPL suffered decannulation failure because of postoperative laryngeal stenosis [9]. The reported rate of TL for functional failure ranged from 0% to 10%.

VHPL allows the resection of advanced lateralized hypopharyngeal cancer extending to the laryngeal wall of the pyriform sinus, even with arytenoid fixation or extension to the thyroid cartilage in selected cases [10]. It enables a broader resection for hypopharyngeal cancer that has invaded the larynx, which encompasses removing a vertical section of the thyroid cartilage through the anterior commissure to the upper border of the cricoid cartilage. Additional resections, including supraglottic laryngectomy and/or partial cricoid cartilage resection, can be performed in patients with supraglottic or subglottic extension.

Acknowledging the potential for chronic or life-threatening aspiration after open conservation surgery is crucial because the function may be better preserved after VHPL, allowing aspiration-free swallowing and better prosthetic speech restoration. The main reason for aspiration after partial laryngectomy is glottic insufficiency, resulting from the partial or subtotal removal of the laryngeal sphincter. To recreate the glottic plane and sphincter function successfully during VHPL, we follow several principles: [1] Ensuring adequate support for the glottic chink with a tendon of sufficient tension; [2] Making a chink of the appropriate size on the neoglottis to allow complete closure and prevent aspiration; [3] Preserving a patent airway with a neoglottic chink of the appropriate size (approximately 5–6 mm); and [4] Attempting the creation of an anterior commissure in the neoglottis, not only to achieve good shape but also to attain better functional results. Another critical aspect of laryngeal reconstruction is maintaining the height of the posterior buttress at the level of the arytenoid cartilage on the normal side (Fig. 7.1).

Some patients with laryngopharyngeal cancer who are treated with VHPL may develop pharyngoesophageal strictures. Z-plasty can be performed at the pharyngoesophageal anastomotic site to prevent strictures and may help reduce the stricture rate in such cases. Despite the lack of statistical significance, we found elevated rates of pharyngoesophageal stricture in patients treated with concurrent chemoradiation as compared to those treated with surgery or radiation alone.

Expert Opinion

In supraglottic partial laryngectomy, the following technique is crucial for preventing postoperative laryngeal stenosis: The endolaryngeal incision should extend down into the ventricle, immediately above the TVC, while maintaining the same level on both sides. (Kwang Jae Cho).

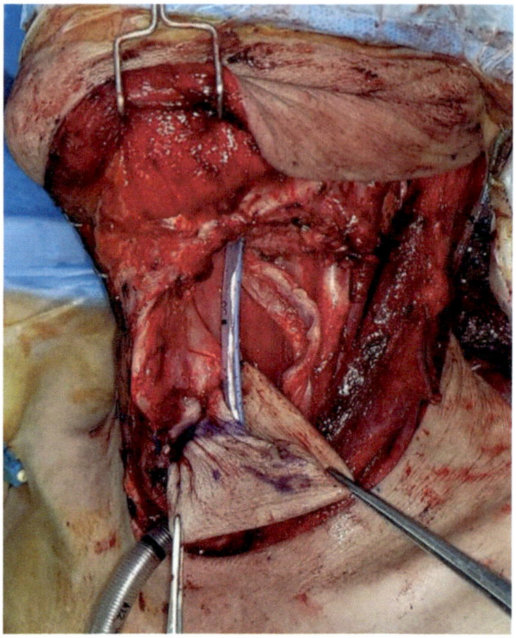

Fig. 7.1 The glottic reconstruction. The palmaris longus tendon has been passed through the hole in the thyroid-cricoid cartilage

7.2 KQ 7.2. How to Manage Pexy Rupture Following Horizontal Partial Laryngectomy

Young-Hoon Joo

Disorders of the pexy line are infrequent complications after partial laryngectomy. The reported incidence of pexy rupture ranges from 0.8% to 4.9%. In a large series, Rizzotto et al. detected pexy rupture in 4 of 469 cases [11]. According to the literature, the early postoperative period is the most common period for the development of this complication. Diagnosis is supported by the presence of splitting at the hyoid–cricoid or thyroid cartilage junction and elevation of the neck flap with subcutaneous emphysema. Some authors have identified several predisposing factors for pexy detachment, including transection of the cricoid arch by sutures, partial resection, or a non-ossified cricoid, and the need to relocate a

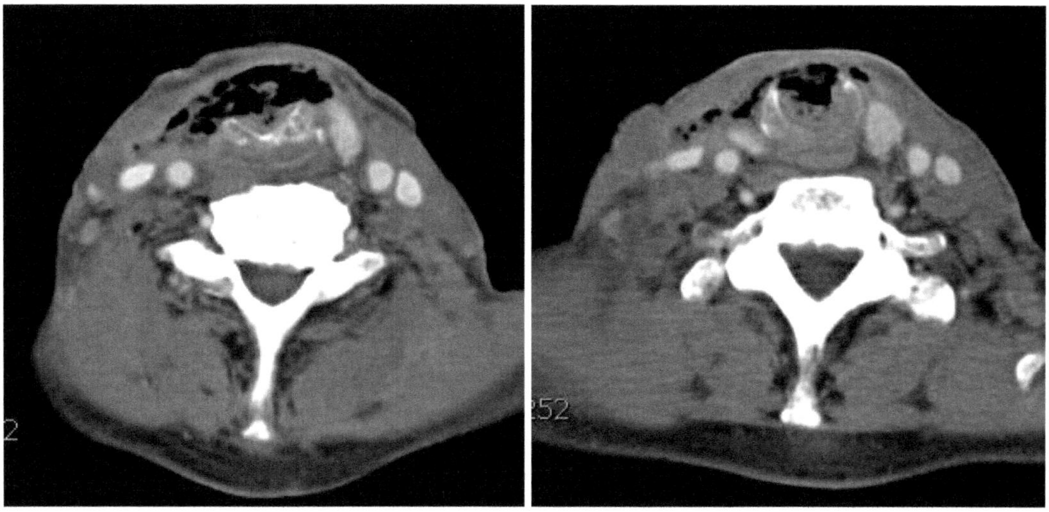

Fig. 7.2 Computed tomography findings in a patient with pexy rupture following supracricoid partial laryngectomy. Subcutaneous emphysema appears as an air accumulation with the elevation of the neck flap

tracheal cannula in an emergency [12]. Other authors have suggested that previous laryngeal irradiation is one of the most critical risk factors for pexy rupture, due to osteitis induced in the hyoid bone [13].

Diagnosis of Pexy Rupture
A pexy line rupture is confirmed when a gap exceeding 30 mm is present between the lower border of the hyoid bone and the cricoid cartilage on CT in a patient who has difficulty in swallowing (Fig. 7.2).

To avoid this complication, before performing a pexy, Naudo et al. suggested a mediastinal dissection of the anterior tracheal wall to reduce the tension at the level of the suture line and inclusion of the first two tracheal rings in the pexy, when feasible [14]. Tension-free sutures are made 1 cm away from the midline at the time of pexy in the initial surgery to avoid pexy rupture. Suturing may be preceded by gently flexing the patient's head.

Pexy line rupture is a rare complication that may occur in patients with a normal postoperative course after partial laryngectomy. Signs and symptoms of detachment of the pexy appear in the first few days after wound healing (8–tenth postoperative day) in nearly all patients (9/10). Dysphagia is the most frequently reported symptom. When pexy detachment occurs, the residual portion of the larynx cannot move upward to allow for satisfactory swallowing. Bleeding from the cervical wound occurs early, suddenly, and dramatically, which is sufficient to necessitate emergency revision surgery in the operating room. Bleeding also suggests an unexpected failure of ligation of a vessel, possibly following increased intrathoracic pressure exerted by the patient during effort. The absence or reduction in the sensitivity of the hypopharyngeal–laryngeal structures may be related to intraoperative surgical errors when the superior laryngeal nerve is not spared. Wound infection, characterized by fever onset and diastasis of the cervical wound, may be observed. Aspiration pneumonia, dyspnea, and dysphonia may also occur.

Treatment of Pexy Rupture
Pexy rupture is commonly treated using revision surgery of the pexy line. In the revision surgery, the patient undergoes a second operation in which the region of the pexy is identified, and a re-suturing of the pexy is performed.

TL is seldom necessary. Open revision surgery is most suitable for significant detachment of the pexy when it is diagnosed early during the patient's hospitalization, in cases where marked alteration of the neoglottis impedes swallowing, and in patients with infection or bleeding. Prompt diagnosis of pexy rupture is crucial. Early intervention prevents respiratory or infectious complications and severe bleeding, safeguarding the overall health of the patient.

Expert Opinion

Pexy rupture is a significant risk when performing a supracricoid partial laryngectomy as a salvage procedure after radiation therapy failure. In the presence of cricoid transection, procedures such as tracheo-crico-hyoido-epiglottopexy or tracheo-crico-hyoidopexy may be required, and salvage total laryngectomy may need to be considered for safety. (Kwang Jae Cho)

References

1. Lefebvre JL, Calais G. Larynx preservation, state of the art. Cancer Radiother. 2005;9:37–41.
2. Chow JM, Block RM, Friedman M. Preoperative evaluation for partial laryngectomy. Head Neck Surg. 1988;10(5):319–23.
3. Laccourreye O, Brasnu D, Périé S, Muscatello L, Ménard M, Weinstein G. Supracricoid partial laryngectomies in the elderly: mortality, complications, and functional outcome. Laryngoscope. 1998;108(2):237–42.
4. Lewin JS, Hutcheson KA, Barringer DA, May AH, Roberts DB, Holsinger FC, et al. Functional analysis of swallowing outcomes after supracricoid partial laryngectomy. Head Neck. 2008;30(5):559–66.
5. Joo YH, Sun DI, Cho JH, Cho KJ, Kim MS. Factors that predict postoperative pulmonary complications after supracricoid partial laryngectomy. Arch Otolaryngol Head Neck Surg. 2009;135(11):1154–7.
6. Park JO, Joo YH, Cho KJ, Kim NG, Kim MS. Functional and oncologic results of extended supracricoid partial laryngectomy. Arch Otolaryngol Head Neck Surg. 2011;137(11):1124–9.
7. Diaz EM Jr, Laccourreye L, Veivers D, Garcia D, Brasnu D, Laccourreye O. Laryngeal stenosis after supracricoid partial laryngectomy. Ann Otol Rhinol Laryngol. 2000;109(11):1077–81.
8. De Virgilio A, Pellini R, Mercante G, Cristalli G, Manciocco V, Giannarelli D, Spriano G. Supracricoid partial laryngectomy for radiorecurrent laryngeal cancer: a systematic review of the literature and meta-analysis. Eur Arch Otorrinolaringol. 2018;275(7):1671–80.
9. Bertolin A, Lionello M, Ghizzo M, Cena I, Leone F, Valerini S, et al. Salvage open partial horizontal laryngectomy after failed radiotherapy: a multicentric study. Laryngoscope. 2020 Feb;130(2):431–6.
10. Kim MS, Joo YH, Cho KJ, Park JO, Sun DI. A classification system for the reconstruction of vertical hemipharyngolaryngectomy for hypopharyngeal squamous cell carcinoma. Arch Otolaryngol Head Neck Surg. 2011;137(1):88–94.
11. Rizzotto G, Crosetti E, Lucioni M, Succo G. Subtotal laryngectomy: outcomes of 469 patients and proposal of a comprehensive and simplified classification of surgical procedures. Eur Arch Otorrinolaringol. 2012;269:1635–46.
12. Laccourreye O, Brasnu D, Laccourreye L, Weinstein G. Ruptured pexis after supracricoid partial laryngectomy. Ann Otol Rhinol Laryngol. 1997;106:159–62.
13. Decotte A, Serrano E, Woisard V, Rose X, Percodani J, Pessey JJ, et al. Ruptured pexis after supracricoid partial laryngectomy: a series of 5 cases. Rev Laryngol Otol Rhinol (Bord). 2009;130:225–9.
14. Naudo P, Laccourreye O, Weinstein G, Jouffre V, Laccourreye H, Brasnu D. Complications and functional outcome after supracricoid partial laryngectomy with cricohyoidoepiglottopexy. Otolaryngol Head Neck Surg. 1998;118:124–9.

Total Laryngectomy with/Without Pharyngectomy

8

Jae Hong Park, Wonjae Cha, Jeong-Yeon Ji,
and Jung-Hae Cho

8.1 KQ 8.1. How to Manage Pharyngocutaneous Fistula Following Total Laryngectomy

Jae Hong Park

Early detection is crucial in the treatment of pharyngocutaneous fistulas. Symptoms of pharyngocutaneous fistulas typically emerge approximately 7–11 days postsurgery and subsequently progress to a fistula. It is vital to identify the fistula promptly and implement appropriate treatment to prevent severe complications, such as carotid artery rupture. In the initial stages, the leaked saliva accumulates in the subcutaneous layer. However, external signs, such as redness or swelling, might not be readily observable, limiting surface assessments. Typically, a drainage tube is placed postoperatively in a location vulnerable to fistulas. Diagnosis can be made by observing the color and presence of foamy bubbles in the drained fluid or, in cases of a significant fistula, by noting the inflation of a vacuum-sealed hemobag. Moreover, measuring amylase levels in the drained fluid, which would sharply increase in the presence of a fistula, or having the patient swallow a colored substance, such as methylene blue or a colored beverage, and then observing the color of the drained fluid (Fig. 8.1a), can provide a direct indication of a fistula. Barium swallow radiography is the most basic and definitive test for detecting a fistula and is usually performed 1–2 weeks after surgery. If complications, such as mediastinitis or pulmonary issues due to the fistula, are suspected, a non-ionic hydrosoluble contrast medium is used. Given that the false-negative rate of barium swallow is approximately 14%, thorough observation of the aforementioned clinical symptoms is necessary. Once a fistula is confirmed using the barium swallow test, an immediate CT scan can delineate the extent of inflammation and salivary accumulation caused by the fistula (Fig. 8.1b) [1–4].

Supplementary Information The online version contains supplementary material available at https://doi.org/10.1007/978-981-96-1860-6_8.

J. H. Park (✉)
Department of Otolaryngology—Head and Neck Surgery, Soonchunhyang University Cheonan Hospital,
Cheonan-si, Chungcheongnam-do, Republic of Korea

W. Cha (✉) · J.-Y. Ji
Department of Otorhinolaryngology—Head & Neck Surgery, Seoul National University Bundang Hospital, College of Medicine, Seoul National University,
Seongnam-si, Gyeonggi-do, Republic of Korea

J.-H. Cho (✉)
St. Vincent's Hospital,
Suwon-si, Gyeonggi-do, Republic of Korea
e-mail: jhchomd@catholic.ac.kr

K.-J. Cho, J.-O. Park (eds.), *Management of Head and Neck Surgery Complications*,
https://doi.org/10.1007/978-981-96-1860-6_8

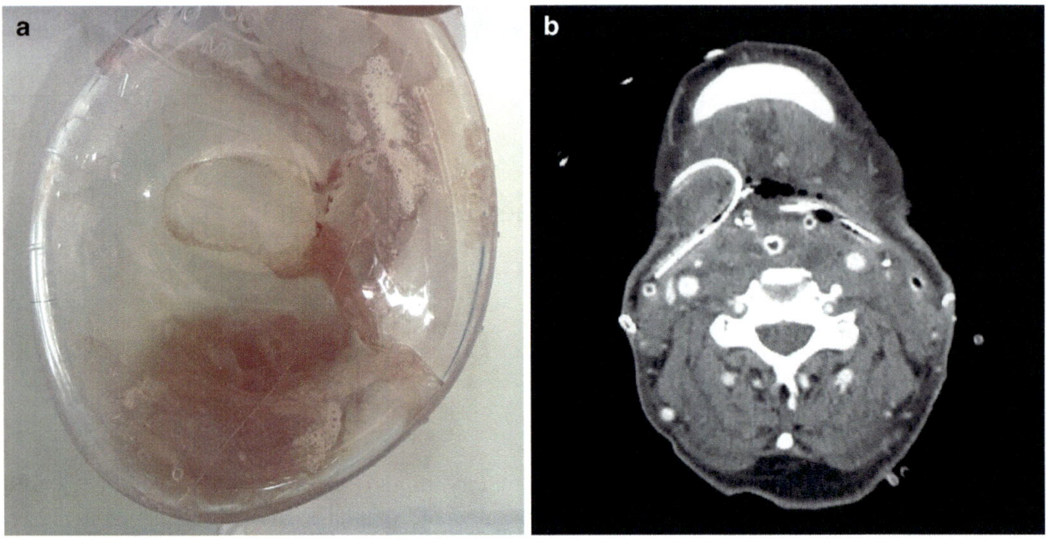

Fig. 8.1 Signs suggestive of pharyngocutaneous fistulas. (**a**) Discharge color in a patient with a pharyngocutaneous fistula. (**b**) Computed tomography findings in a patient with a pharyngocutaneous fistula

Early detection of fistulas can prevent complications. Therefore, it is essential to monitor for fistulas closely in the early postoperative phase by observing drainage and measuring amylase levels. If amylase levels increase significantly as compared to the immediate postoperative period, the presence of a fistula can be preliminarily confirmed by having the patient swallow a colored fluid. If a fistula is suspected, it is vital to verify its location and extent using a barium swallow test and CT scan.

8.1.1 Treatment of Pharyngocutaneous Fistula

After identifying a fistula, unless there is an imminent threat of life-threatening complications, such as carotid artery rupture, conservative treatment should be initiated. However, for patients who have undergone radiation therapy, conservative treatment alone often proves challenging, necessitating early consideration for surgical intervention [5–7].

8.1.2 Conservative Treatment

Expert Opinion
When percutaneous endoscopic gastrostomy is not feasible for a patient with a pharyngocutaneous fistula, a surgical gastrostomy or feeding jejunostomy should be performed. (Joon Kyoo Lee)

1. **Oral Intake Restriction**
   Upon detecting a pharyngocutaneous fistula, oral intake must immediately be restricted. Depending on the patient's condition, a nasogastric tube may be inserted for short-term use, whereas long-term solutions could involve the insertion of a gastrostomy tube via percutaneous endoscopic gastrostomy to bypass the pharynx and esophagus for nutrition. Restricting oral intake often results in decreased salivary production, which may lead to poor oral hygiene and associated complications. Complications can also arise from infections through a fistula. Therefore, maintaining oral hygiene through regular gargling is crucial [7–9].

2. **Appropriate Antibiotics**
   Initial bacterial identification and antibiotic susceptibility testing are necessary to treat the infections caused by fistulas. Retesting during treatment is essential to check for the presence of additional bacterial or fungal infections. Before the bacterial identification results are available, aggressive antibiotic treatment comparable to that used for deep infections or necrotizing fasciitis is needed. Empirically, broad-spectrum antibiotics, including metronidazole, should be administered, particularly those that are effective against anaerobic bacteria [10, 11].
3. **Compression Dressing**
   Wet-to-dry dressing is a disinfection method that mechanically removes exudates and wound debris, thereby aiding wound healing. A clean gauze is moistened with isotonic solutions, such as saline or diluted (1/4 or 1/2) povidone-iodine. The wet gauze is wrung out, applied to the wound, and topped with dry gauze. The dressing should be changed at least twice daily. When applying pressure, strong focal pressure directly to the fistula area reduces fluid leakage and prevents the spread of leaked fluid into the neck space. The areas adjacent to the fistula are also secondarily compressed [10, 12].
4. **Negative-pressure dressing.**
   Applying negative pressure with a sponge suction tip and using local compression dressing helps to divert the leaking saliva away from the neck space, preventing its spread [13, 14].
5. **Stimulation of the Wound and Granulation Tissue Formation**
   If the pharyngocutaneous fistula is small and considerably distant from the vital structure, stimulating the growth of granulation around the opening of the fistula can assist in its closure. Common stimulation methods include repeatedly scraping the inner side of the fistula with a curette or using 30% trichloroacetic acid (TCA) for chemical stimulation. Recently, the author had experience in treating fistulas using an electrocautery device to simulate granulation tissue growth along the inner mucosal edge of a fistula, successfully sealing it [7, 10, 15].

Expert Opinion

A controlled pharyngocutaneous fistula typically takes more than 1 week to heal. Closing the controlled fistula often presents challenges, particularly as these fistulas frequently occur after salvage surgery following radiation therapy, which impedes granulation formation around the controlled fistula. In the author's experience, curettage and negative pressure dressing (CuraVac) need to be used for about a week. Once the controlled fistula defect size reduces, the closure is completed by suturing the inner mucosa and the external skin layer separately. (Dong-Il Sun).

In the conservative treatment of pharyngocutaneous fistulas, protecting the vital structures from saliva and inflammation and stimulating the granulation of the fistula to ensure that it fills with granulation tissue and narrows is important. Various methods, such as physical stimulation using a curette or chemical or electrical stimulation, have been introduced. To divert saliva effectively, a method using continuous negative pressure is recommended.

8.1.3 Surgical Treatment Exteriorization (Formation of Controlled Pharyngocutaneous Fistula)

If the saliva flow into the neck space cannot be prevented by conservative treatment, a controlled pharyngocutaneous fistula must be formed by suturing the pharyngeal mucosa and nearest skin to divert saliva externally, protecting the carotid artery (Fig. 8.2a). A flexible endoscope can be introduced into the pharynx to identify the pharyngeal opening of the fistula. Transparent endoscopic light, which is seen from the outside, can be helpful in determining the outside opening of the controlled fistula tract, which should be away from the tracheostoma. The fistula can be managed more efficiently using the previously described negative-pressure dressing. When creating a saliva diversion, care should be taken to direct the saliva away from blood vessels with a high risk of bleeding. During suturing around the fistula (stoma) and skin, it should be ensured that saliva does not flow into other parts of the neck. Continuous negative-pressure tubes or sponge tips can be placed in the fistula to ensure that saliva is only discharged to the outside (Fig. 8.2b). If oral intake is restricted for a long period, a gastrostomy may be more helpful than maintaining a nasogastric tube [7, 10, 15].

8.1.4 Pedicled Flap

If a pharyngocutaneous fistula is detected early and is small, in patients without a history of radiation therapy, favorable results can be achieved with conservative treatment alone. However, if the fistula is large or if the patient has a history of radiation exposure, the fistula tends to progress. As previously mentioned, additional risks must be prevented. Physical barriers should be created between vital structures, including the carotid artery, and saliva from the fistula. For this procedure, a flap with a high survival rate and rich blood flow is required. This allows antibiotics to reach the wound adequately, and the muscular and fatty layers can absorb exudates and fill the empty space in the neck. The donor site should be selected from a range outside the previous radiation fields. The pectoralis major myocutaneous (PMMC) flap is the most suitable and reliable. Another commonly used pedicled flap is the latissimus dorsi flap.

If the pharyngocutaneous fistula does not close completely after conservative treatment or pedicled flap surgery, additional flap transplantation may be required. The choice of flap depends on the patient's condition and the surgeon's preference, and the options include free and local flaps. Small and minor artificial pharyngocutaneous fistulas can be sutured using surrounding advancement flaps. However, if the internal mucosal entrance of the fistula remains wider than the skin outlet, suturing the skin alone is not an efficient method. In such cases, curettage or electrocoagulation can be performed to narrow the mucosa. Suturing and advancement flap techniques can be attempted once the flaps are determined to be sufficiently narrow. Fistulas that do not close using this method require a local rotational flap, for which the author prefers the deltopectoral flap, which can be folded because it is thin. After using the PMMC flap to close the pha-

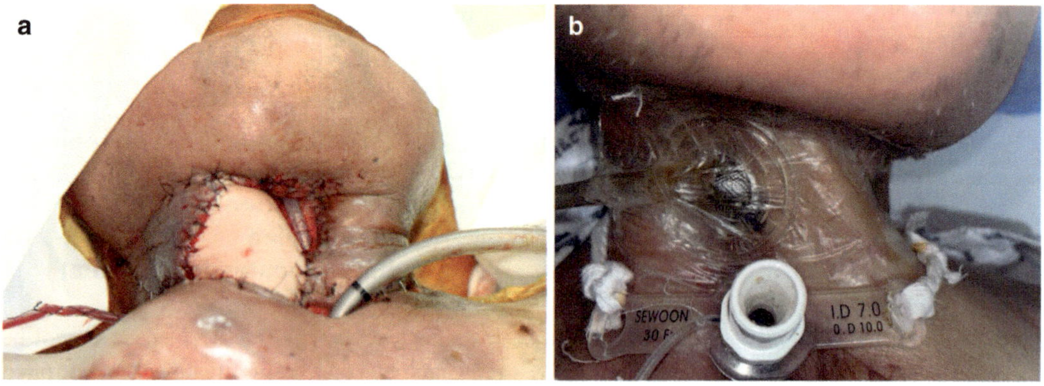

Fig. 8.2 Controlled pharyngocutaneous fistulas. To design a pathway for salivary bypass that avoids the carotid artery. (**a**) The skin is incised, and the pharyngeal mucosa is sutured to the skin. (**b**) A continuous negative pressure sponge tip is placed in the fistula

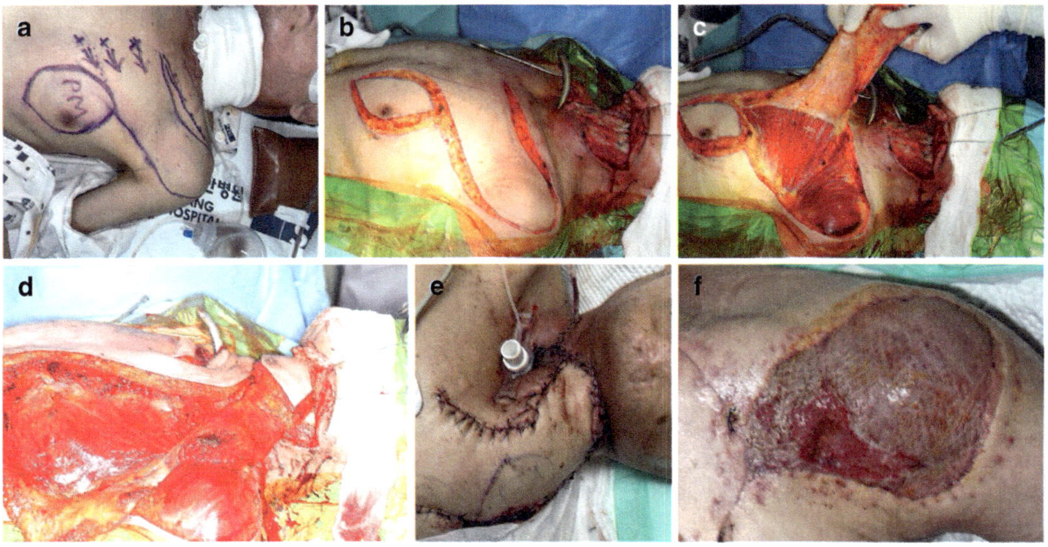

Fig. 8.3 (**a**) Reconstruction of the pharyngeal wall using the pectoralis major myocutaneous (PMMC) flap and the deltopectoral (DP) flap. Due to the thickness of the PMMC flap, skin closure was difficult, and thus a DP flap from the same side was designed. (**b**) A skin incision of the DP and PMMC flaps was made (**c**), the DP flap was elevated first (**d**), and the pectoralis major muscle flap was elevated. (**e**) Elevated PMMC and DP flaps were transplanted into the defect area. The pharynx and skin are completely covered with these flaps. (**f**) The skin defect at the donor site of the DP flap on the shoulder is covered with a split-thickness skin graft

ryngeal defect, if the primary closure of the neck skin is challenging due to its volume, a deltopectoral flap can be simultaneously designed on the same or opposite side (Fig. 8.3). However, the deltopectoral flap has a limited range of rotation; therefore, it is preferable to design it on the same side to cover a wider range [7, 10, 15–18].

For patients with a history of radiation treatment or those with a large pharyngocutaneous fistula, it is recommended to consider early closure using a free or pedicled flap. If surgery is delayed and inflammation progresses to the carotid artery wall, serious complications, such as carotid artery blowout, can occur. In cases where the skin has become thick due to inflammation or where a significant skin defect occurs, using the PMMC flap may make closing of the wound challenging due to its volume. Thus, simultaneous application of another pedicled flap, such as the deltopectoral flap, may be necessary.

Expert Opinion

EndoVAC Summary

Endoluminal vacuum-assisted closure therapy (EndoVAC) can be applied using vacuum pressure within the cavity. The general method is as follows: It can be applied under general anesthesia or with local anesthesia using lidocaine solution for the oropharynx and nasal cavity. A 14-Fr. Levin tube is passed through one nostril and out through the mouth, then cut to the perforated area (Fig. 8.4a). A hydrophilic foam dressing (V.A.C.® Granufoam™) Dressing; KCI Manufacturing, Athlone, Ireland), used to protect wounds with heavy exudate for secondary healing, is designed to fill the pharyngeal tube adequately (Fig. 8.4b). A hole large enough for the Levin tube is cut in the middle of one end of the sponge, using scissors, and a clamp is used to extend the hole to the other end without completely penetrating it (Fig. 8.4c). The Levin tube and sponge are fixed in place with sutures at

(continued)

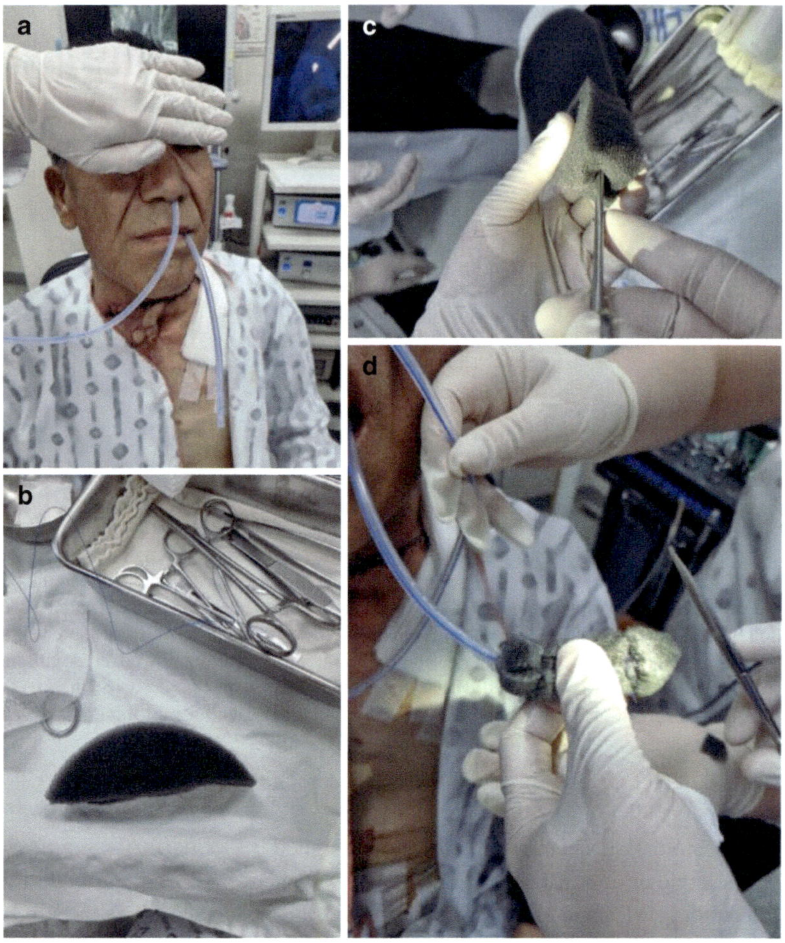

Fig. 8.4 (**a**) Levin tube (14 French-size) is passed out of the mouth through the one nasal cavity and cut at the end of any hole. (**b**) A hydrophilic sponge for secondary wound healing (V.A.C.® Granufoam™ Dressing, KCI Manufacturing, Westmeath, Ireland) is prepared and designed to be fitted into the intraluminal space of the pharynx. (**c**) A hole is made into the middle of one side of the sponge and advanced using clamps until the very end of the other side. (**d**) The Levin tube and the sponge are anchored together with two stitches

two locations (Fig. 8.4d). When inserting the tube under local anesthesia, the fixed sponge is grabbed with a clamp under the guidance of a flexible laryngoscope and positioned in the pharynx through the mouth to ensure proper insertion (Fig. 8.5). The end of the Levin tube exiting through the nasal passage is maintained in a vacuum state by applying a negative-pressure wound dressing (KCI Medical Products Ltd., Wimborne Dorset, UK). The pressure is maintained at 125 mmHg in continuous mode, and the setup is made portable for easy patient movement. Occasionally, if the pressure shifts to positive momentarily when the patient opens their mouth and does not revert back to negative pressure, it can be connected to a wall suction in the hospital room to revert to negative pressure quickly. If the patient needs to move, it should be reconnected immediately upon returning to the hospital room to ensure that negative pressure is applied.

This EndoVAC therapy has the advantage of being directly applicable to the pharyngeal sites causing pharyngocutaneous fistulas. By applying negative pressure, it prevents the retention of additional oral contents, such as saliva, in the deep neck space and blocks contents refluxed from

(continued)

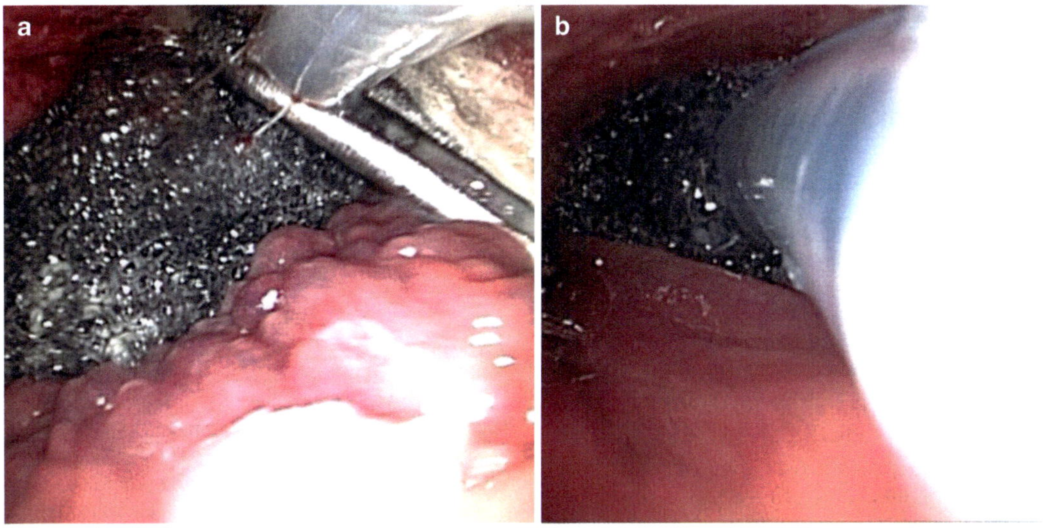

Fig. 8.5 The sponge is grasped and inserted into the oropharynx at the point of dehiscence endoluminally under the guide of flexible laryngoscopy (**a**). The final position is confirmed by flexible laryngoscopy (**b**)

the stomach from re-entering the neck. Even in patients who cannot undergo general anesthesia, application can be performed under mild sedation, depending on the situation, and it can be an alternative to resolve pharyngocutaneous fistulas in patients requiring large and prolonged reconstructive surgery. EndoVAC can also be preemptively inserted during initial pharyngeal reconstruction in patients where postoperative pharyngocutaneous fistula is expected and can prevent issues when reconstructing the pharynx using a flap. Through one nostril, the EndoVAC can be inserted, and through the other, a nasogastric tube can be inserted to provide enteral nutrition simultaneously. Even doctors who cannot perform advanced reconstructive surgery, such as flap reconstruction, perform this procedure relatively easily after some training. However, it has a few disadvantages; it is not recommended when the perforation site is near a large vessel or when the vessel is exposed. The Levin tube can cause nasal irritation and pain, or the sponge lodged in the oropharynx for an extended period can cause discomfort in the pharynx. Due to limited space for insertion, the site of the perforation must be carefully identified beforehand. The sponge, which adheres to the surrounding tissues due to the negative pressure, may not easily detach with mild traction or may cause minor bleeding after separation, which can be removed after dripping saline. The sponge cannot be left in place for long periods, and exudate can clog the system; thus, replacing the sponge approximately every 5 days is recommended. Although not common, subsequent stenosis of the lumen may occur with the use of EndoVAC, which can then be treated with dilatation or stent insertion. (Joon Kyoo Lee).

(continued)

8.2 KQ 8.2. How to Prevent and Manage Tracheostomal Stenosis Following Total Laryngectomy?

Jae Hong Park

Tracheostomal stenosis is a common complication of laryngectomy, with a reported incidence ranging from 4% to 55%. Factors that increase the risk of tracheostomal stenosis include closure methods, lack of mucosal approximation, excessive tension, fistula formation, tracheal infection, and a history of radiotherapy [19–21].

Tracheostomal stenosis can be categorized into various types based on appearance and potential causes [19].

1. Vertical slit—typically a linear or slit-like narrowing.
2. Concentric—a uniform narrowing around the entire circumference of the tracheostoma.
3. Inferior shelf—this could result from compression by the sternal heads of the sternocleidomastoid muscle, scar contraction, or redundant skin folds.

Tracheostomal stenosis can lead to inadequate secretion clearance, intermittent airway obstruction, as well as insufficient space for tracheoesophageal puncture and voice prosthesis placement [22]. Various tracheostomaplasty methods, such as Z-plasty, tracheal splits, and advanced flaps, have been introduced in the literature. However, all these techniques fundamentally share the principle of widening the section of the excised organ and preventing it from narrowing again by using a skin flap [19, 22, 23].

Tracheostomal stenosis is a potentially serious complication that can occur after the creation of a tracheostomy, and accurate knowledge of its prevention and treatment is crucial. In this chapter, we share our experiences in preventing and treating tracheostomy stenosis during tracheostomy creation.

Tracheal Incision Method: The manner in which the trachea is incised plays a pivotal role in preventing tracheostomy stenosis. We particularly favor a technique that preserves part of the posterior tracheal wall, aiming to resect four or more tracheal rings in an oblique pattern. This method enlarges the tracheal cross-section, reducing the risk of tracheostoma stenosis (Fig. 8.6).

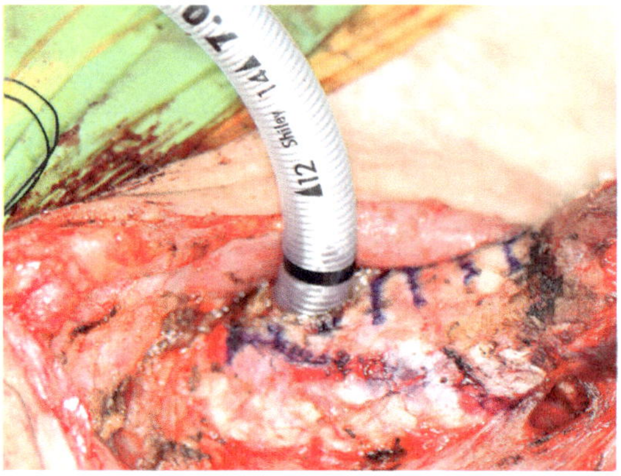

Fig. 8.6 Pattern of tracheal resection. The oblique pattern of tracheal resection is designed to include at least four or more tracheal rings. During this procedure, a portion of the posterior wall is preserved. This allows it to be spread out posteriorly and anchored when sutured to the skin

> **Expert Opinion**
> There is an opinion that performing tracheal resection in an oblique pattern destroys more of the cartilage framework, compromising the structural integrity. Therefore, some advocate for transverse resection to preserve the intact cartilage rings. (Joon Kyoo Lee).

Suturing Technique: Before suturing the anterior wall of the trachea to the skin, it is advisable to anchor the anterior trachea wall to the periosteum of the sternum or the bilateral clavicular heads. This helps prevent the tracheostomy from sagging downward toward the mediastinum. Moreover, the upper skin flap should be properly designed to spread over the posterolateral walls of the trachea and sutured for effective anchoring of the posterolateral tracheal wall in the superolateral direction, which can spread the posterolateral wall bilaterally. Care should be taken as inadequate excision of the upper skin

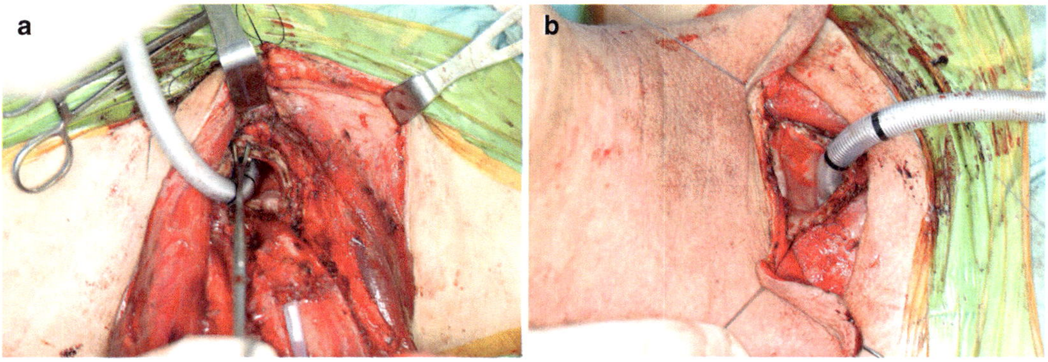

Fig. 8.7 Tracheostoma formation. (**a**) The anterior wall of the resected trachea is anchored to the sternum or the clavicle head's periosteum to prevent it from sagging downward. (**b**) The posterior-lateral wall is spread out and fixed to the upper skin flap to prevent the tracheostoma from constricting and curling inward

flap can lead to sagging, causing the posterolateral wall of the trachea to shrink inward [24–28] (Fig. 8.7).

Expert Opinion
When suturing the trachea to the skin, the entire tracheal cartilaginous portion should be included in the lower flap and the upper flap should be connected to the membranous portion. (Joon Kyoo Lee).

Expert Opinion
When tracheostomal stenosis occurs, it often recurs even after surgical correction. Therefore, preventing the development of such stenosis is crucial during the initial surgery. The most important factor is to ensure that no tension is created when suturing the stoma. To achieve this, sufficient cervicomediastinal dissection along the pretracheal fascia layer must be performed to ensure the mobility of the trachea. Additionally, rather than stitching the stoma to the skin in a 1:1 ratio, a more open and wide-spread shape should be created by sewing with a bit more extension. (Dong-Il Sun).

If tracheostomal stenosis occurs postoperatively and requires surgical intervention, the following steps should be undertaken [28] (Fig. 8.8, Video 8.1):

- Dissect and separate the skin and trachea. Following the excision of the surrounding soft tissues, aim to expose as much of the trachea as possible while considering the positioning of nearby vessels, with the goal of exposing four or more tracheal rings.
- Based on the cross-section of the tracheostoma, incisions should be made at the 3, 6, and 9 o'clock positions, vertically cutting through the tracheal wall. The vertical incision should encompass approximately four tracheal rings or more; however, if this is not possible, the incision should be made as long as feasible.
- Ensure that the strips from the vertically incised anterior tracheal wall are pulled inferolaterally and sutured securely to the periosteum of the bilateral clavicular heads.
- Subsequently, the anterior and lateral defects of the tracheal wall should be covered using an advanced skin flap.
- The posterior wall of the trachea should be securely sutured to the skin on both the upper sides to prevent downward sagging.

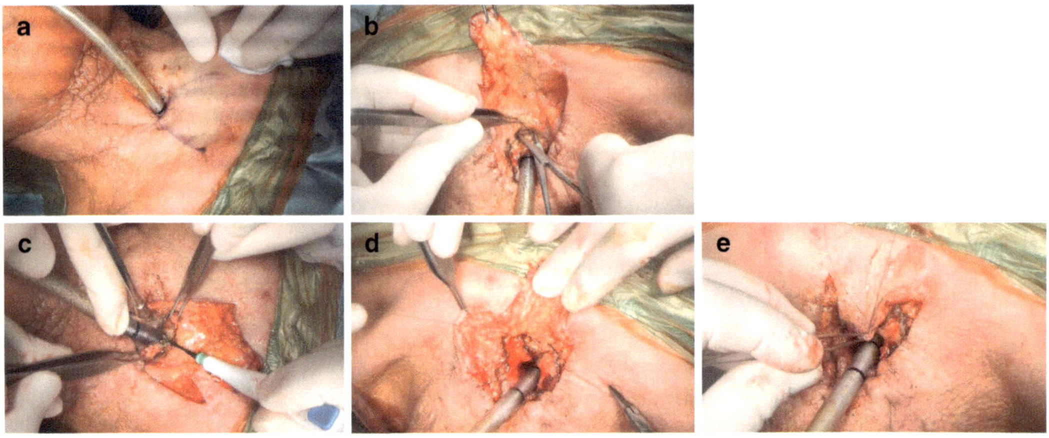

Fig. 8.8 Tracheal split and anterior advanced skin flap. (**a**) The incision was designed for the anterior advanced flap. (**b**) The skin and trachea are separated, surrounding muscle and connective tissues are excised, and, considering the position of surrounding vessels, if possible, at least four segments of the trachea are fully exposed. (**c**) Based on the cross-section of the tracheostoma, incisions are made in the 3, 6, and 9 o'clock directions to vertically split the tracheal wall. (**d**) The left and right strips of the vertically split anterior tracheal wall are pulled laterally and sutured securely to the periosteum of both clavicle heads. (**e**) Subsequently, the anterior and lateral defect of the tracheal wall is covered with an advanced skin flap

Expert Opinion

Before considering surgical stomaplasty, administering multiple steroid (triamcinolone) injections into the fibrous portion can help alleviate stenosis to some extent. Additionally, if surgery is later required, the procedure can be performed with less tension, providing an advantage. (Joon Kyoo Lee)

◆ When initially creating the tracheostoma, to prevent it from sagging downward, the anterior wall should be fixed to the periosteum of the sternum or bilateral clavicular heads, while the posterolateral walls should be pulled up and secured to the upper skin flap with appropriate tension on both sides. In the case of a narrowed tracheostoma, it should be revised and resected in a manner that creates an oblique cross-section to enlarge the tracheostoma. Subsequently, the tracheal wall should be split, pulled inferolaterally, and fixed to both sides downward to bilateral clavicular heads.

8.3 KQ 8.3. How to Prevent and Manage Pharyngoesophageal Stenosis Following Total Laryngectomy

Wonjae Cha and Jeong-Yeon Ji

Pharyngoesophageal stenosis (or stricture) is a late complication that can occur due to an inadequate pharyngeal circumference following total laryngectomy or laryngopharyngectomy, often stemming from a pharyngoesophageal fistula. This condition is particularly concerning as it impacts swallowing quality and nutritional intake [29].

8.3.1 Prevention

Techniques to prevent pharyngoesophageal stenosis include choosing appropriate primary closure techniques, such as types of closure, cricopharyngeal myotomy, and considerations of mucosa availability to guide flap reconstruction choices.

To understand and prevent pharyngoesophageal stenosis, the incidence and risk factors should be considered. A comparison between salvage and primary laryngectomy cases revealed a higher incidence rate in salvage cases (33% vs. 8%) [30]. Exploration of flap reconstruction versus primary closure revealed that flap reconstruction exhibited a lower incidence (5% vs. 21%) [30]. However, salvage cases involving tubed flap reconstruction increased the likelihood of pharyngoesophageal stenosis formation as compared to primary closure [31]. Interestingly, in primary cases, the incidence of stenosis did not correlate with flap reconstruction or adjuvant radiation therapy [31].

Primary closure techniques, including types of closure and cricopharyngeal myotomy, are important for preventing stenosis. Closing both the mucosal and muscle layers yielded superior swallowing function as compared with mucosa-only closure, which resulted in a larger mean pharyngeal diameter and reduced tonicity [32]. T-type and vertical closures were the most frequently performed for pharyngeal reconstruction (Fig. 8.9) and yielded similar outcomes [33]. Cricopharyngeal myotomy, which lowers peak pharyngeal pressure as compared to a procedure without myotomy, has been advocated due to its potential to decrease the chances of fistulas and to prevent dysphagia due to cricopharyngeal muscle spasm [34]. Some surgeons have proposed that a short myotomy of the upper esophageal sphincter and inferior constrictors should be a routine procedure during total laryngectomy, whereas others have suggested a long myotomy involving all the pharyngeal constrictor muscles [32]. However, previous studies have demonstrated no significant differences in the use of cricopharyngeal myotomies [33]. Nevertheless, this result may be biased because the decision to perform cricopharyngeal myotomy was made at the time of pharyngeal reconstruction, particularly when dealing with a narrow pharyngeal lumen [32]..

The decision regarding flap reconstruction and the choice of flap are contingent on the available mucosal tissue. A radial forearm free flap (RFFF) is an option, although it has a stenosis rate of 13–36% after reconstruction [30, 35]. Patched RFFF with a minimum 2-cm mucosa strip is preferred over tubed RFFF, particularly due to its lower stricture rate. Recently, many surgeons have preferred the anterolateral thigh free flap (ALT FF) because of its reduced donor site morbidity and suitability for dilation due to its ample tissue volume [29].

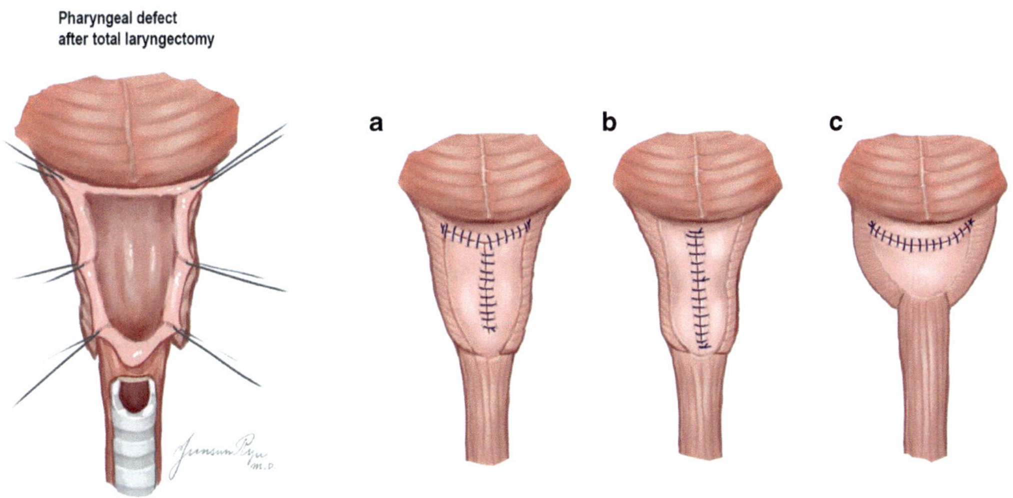

Fig. 8.9 Closure method for reconstruction of pharynx. (**a**) T-type closure. (**b**) Vertical closure. (**c**) Transverse closure

Expert Opinion
Pharyngoesophageal stenosis frequently fails to resolve despite repeated bougination. In such cases, an esophageal stent can be a useful treatment option. During reconstructive surgery using a flap, the author recommends making a vertical incision at the esophageal junction where stenosis occurs and inserting the flap into the split esophageal mucosa with suturing. This technique helps to extend the luminal circumference, thereby preventing stenosis. (Dong-Il Sun).

8.3.2 Diagnosis

Differentiating pharyngoesophageal stenosis from possible tumor recurrence is crucial, and endoscopy and biopsy should precede the start of management.

Diagnosis of pharyngoesophageal stenosis requires vigilance to distinguish it from potential tumor recurrence. Endoscopy and biopsy are vital tools for confirming or ruling out tumor involvement [36]. The presence and extent of pharyngoesophageal stenosis are evaluated using endoscopy or modified barium swallow studies [37]..

8.3.3 Management

The management of pharyngoesophageal stenosis involves various methods, of which dilation is the primary approach. For failed cases, esophageal stent or flap reconstruction may be an option.

The management of pharyngoesophageal stenosis involves several strategies. Dilation is the primary treatment approach and can be performed as an outpatient procedure. In some cases of primary closure, a single dilation only may be sufficient; however, many cases require repeated dilation treatments for effective management [31]. Maintaining an adequate lumen size (36 Fr) is essential for efficient swallowing and tracheoesophageal speech production. A bougie or balloon can be used for dilation, widening the stenotic segment and extending the lumen circumferentially [38]. (Fig. 8.10) The clinical efficacy did not differ significantly between bougie and balloon dilation [39]. In some instances, mitomycin C injection can be employed to augment dilation effects [40].

Esophageal stents are an option for treating dilation failures. Most commonly, stents should be considered in patients with recurrent stenosis and a poor prognosis for long-term survival. Flap reconstruction is considered when other methods do not yield desired outcomes. The selection of the tissue for reconstruction depends on various factors. The available options include gastric pull-up, jejunal free flap, RFFF, ALT FF, and pectoralis major free flap.

Expert Opinion
Inserting an esophageal stent carries a risk of migration; thus, careful monitoring is required. (Joon Kyoo Lee).

In conclusion, the prevention and management of pharyngoesophageal stenosis after total laryngectomy is a complex endeavor, requiring a multidisciplinary approach. Understanding the incidence, risk factors, techniques, and interventions involved is crucial for optimizing patient outcomes and preserving the swallowing function.

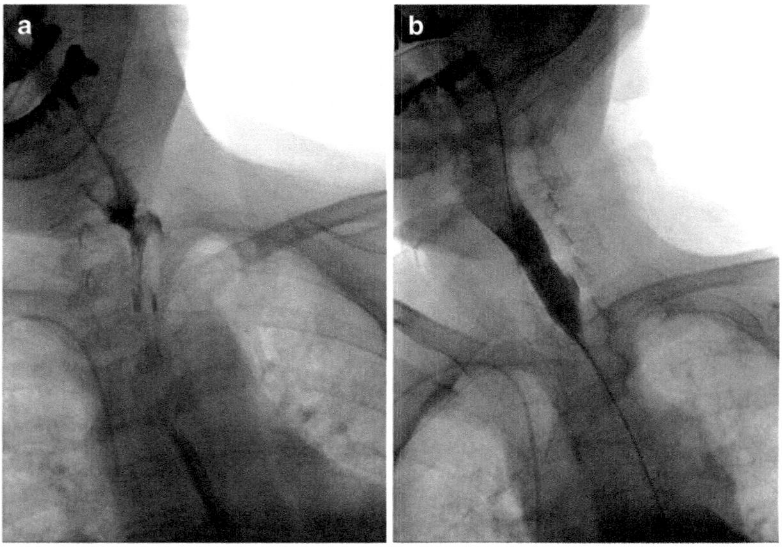

Fig. 8.10 Lateral projections of balloon dilation for pharyngoesophageal stenosis. (**a**) Before dilation, the stenotic portion is noted by fluoroscopy. (**b**) The stenotic portion is widened using balloon dilation

8.4 KQ 8.4. How to Resolve Voice Prosthesis (Provox®)-Related Problems?

Jung-Hae Cho

Although many patients who have undergone total laryngectomy achieve successful voice rehabilitation through tracheoesophageal speech, certain issues can arise with the use of a voice prosthesis (VP; Provox®; Atos Medical AB, Hörby, Sweden). As a VP is not a permanent implant, it requires periodic replacement and management. The status of the VP should be verified at each clinic visit, and the exact nature of any problem that arises should be established. This can easily be checked by requesting the patient to drink water. The adverse events associated with VPs include biofilm formation, leakage, and granulation tissue formation. Biofilm formation on a VP can lead to fungal colonization, which can cause infection and VP failure. Leakage through or around the VP can cause cough or aspiration pneumonia. Granulation tissue formation around the VP can make it difficult to produce a voice or may cause VP extrusion. Problems or adverse events related to the VP should be identified early and should be managed to prevent complications and improve the quality of life.

Expert Opinion

Shunt surgery for a voice prosthesis can be performed either during the initial surgery or secondarily after the completion of adjuvant therapies, such as radiation treatment. The author prefers to perform shunt formation during the initial surgery. This preference is due to the increased risk of complications, such as fistula formation and difficulties in healing, when shunt surgery is performed secondary to radiation therapy, which can impair circulation at the shunt site. (Dong-Il Sun).

8.4.1 Biofilm Formation or *Candida* Overgrowth

Biofilm formation and *Candida* overgrowth are common complications associated with voice prostheses (Fig. 8.11). A silicone VP is easily colonized by microorganisms, particularly *Candida albicans*, which form biofilms that can lead to VP dysfunction [41]. The most common indication for VP replacement is valve incompetence caused by *Candida* overgrowth, which causes fluid leakage through the valve. Antifungal

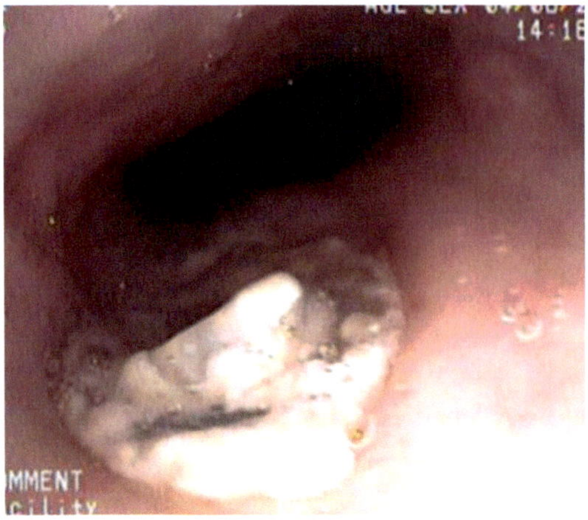

Fig. 8.11 Voice prosthesis in situ with colonization of candidiasis

agents, such as Nystatin or Diflucan, can be applied topically, directly to the VP, with a cleaning brush [42]. Dietary changes, such as the consumption of probiotic dietary products, can decrease the *Candida* burden in the pharynx and esophagus. If VP obstruction occurs, cleaning the prosthesis with suction can be attempted before replacement.

8.4.2 Leakage

The primary reason for prosthesis replacement is leakage through and around the prosthesis (transprosthetic or periprosthetic). Fistula tract enlargement occurs in approximately 7% of patients [43]. In addition, the thickness of the tracheoesophageal (TE) wall (the length of the tracheoesophageal fistula) is known to decrease over time [44]. Reflux has been identified as a major comorbidity causing atrophy of the TE party wall [45]. The prescription of proton pump inhibitors (PPIs) might be a long-term treatment for comorbidities, such as reflux and pharyngeal stenosis, to prevent the recurrence of tracheoesophageal puncture (TEP) tract issues. Both enlargement of the fistula tract and atrophy of the TE party wall cause VP pistoning during swallowing, as well as peripheral leakage, leading to aspiration and coughing. This issue can be resolved by simply inserting a shorter VP. It is best to downsize the length of the VP by only one size (2 mm) because a constricted fit of the VP may cause swelling and edema.

> In the natural course of healing after surgery, the swelling and inflammation of the tissues typically subside. Therefore, a shorter prosthesis is often sufficient to address peripheral leakage during follow-up.

The use of a double-flange VP (Provox XtraSeal®, Atos Medical®, Hörby, Sweden) can be effective in preventing periprosthetic leakage and lengthening the time between replacements [46]. Insertion of Provox XtraSeal® is advisable to use the overshoot mechanism to ensure complete unfolding of the esophageal flange in the lumen of the esophagus (Video 8.2).

TEP site injections with silicone, purse-string sutures around the TEP, and temporary VP removal are strategies for addressing recurrent periprosthetic leakages [47]. The application of a purse-string suture around the TEP tract using an atraumatic absorbable Vicryl 3.0 or non-absorbable suture can be used.

> **Overshooting Method**
> The VP can be overshot into the esophageal lumen and then repositioned correctly using a hemostat. This ensures proper placement of the esophageal flange within the esophagus and ensures that excess tissue is encompassed between the flanges.

If peripheral leakage cannot be resolved with conservative surgical measures, surgical closure of the TEP tract and subsequent repuncture may be necessary. The fistula may need to be closed with primary closure or a vascularized flap (sternocleidomastoid fascia and muscle, pectoralis major, deltopectoral, or radial forearm) [48]. Failure to address tracheoesophageal fistulae can lead to severe aspiration or death.

Transprosthetic leakage is caused by fungal growth on the flapper valve of the prosthesis itself, pressure changes (under pressure) in the neopharynx during swallowing, and stricture of the pharyngoesophageal segment. Using a Provox plug® can manage the central leakage during eating. Another method involves integrating magnets within the VP (Provox ActiValve®, Atos Medical, Hörby, Sweden), which counteracts this issue by facilitating active closure of the valve. A magnet-based valve system to achieve active closure of the valve provides resistance against the inadvertent opening of the valve caused by under pressure during swallowing and/or deep inhalation [49].

> Under pressure is often the cause of early or frequent leakage, in which case the application of a Provox ActiValve® should be considered.

The therapeutic algorithm for VP-related leakage is summarized in Fig. 8.12.

8.4.3 Granulation Tissue (Contact Granuloma)

Careful attention should be paid to any granulomatous changes observed during the examination. Granulation tissue around a tracheoesophageal fistula (TEF) can be caused by local infections or reflux. If it is caused by reflux, treating the reflux with PPIs is important. In addition, cauterization of granulation tissue using a potassium-titanyl-phosphate (KTP) laser may be necessary (Fig. 8.13). Granulation tissue around the VP can also lengthen the TEF, causing the VP to move out of place. This can occur in two ways: inward displacement under the tracheal mucosa (Fig. 8.14) or outward displacement due to esophageal mucosal overgrowth. If the VP is displaced inwards into the tracheal lumen, device removal is mandatory to prevent dislodgment into the trachea. Occasionally, the VP falls out of place and is inhaled into the trachea or bronchial tree. This requires bronchoscopic removal. Overgrowth of the esophageal mucosa around the VP can be verified by performing a transnasal esophagoscope or neck CT (Fig. 8.15). It is rec-

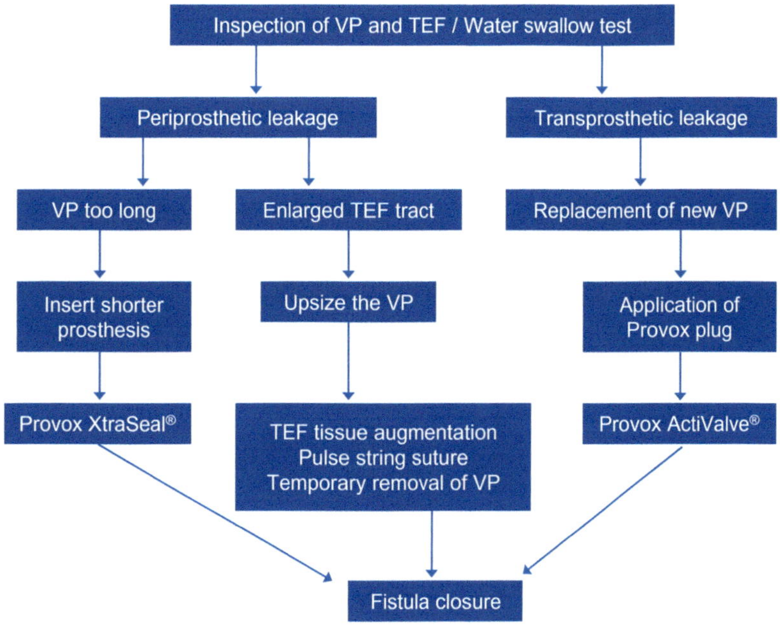

Fig. 8.12 The therapeutic algorithm for the voice prosthesis-related leakage. *VP* voice prosthesis, *TEF* tracheoesophageal fistula

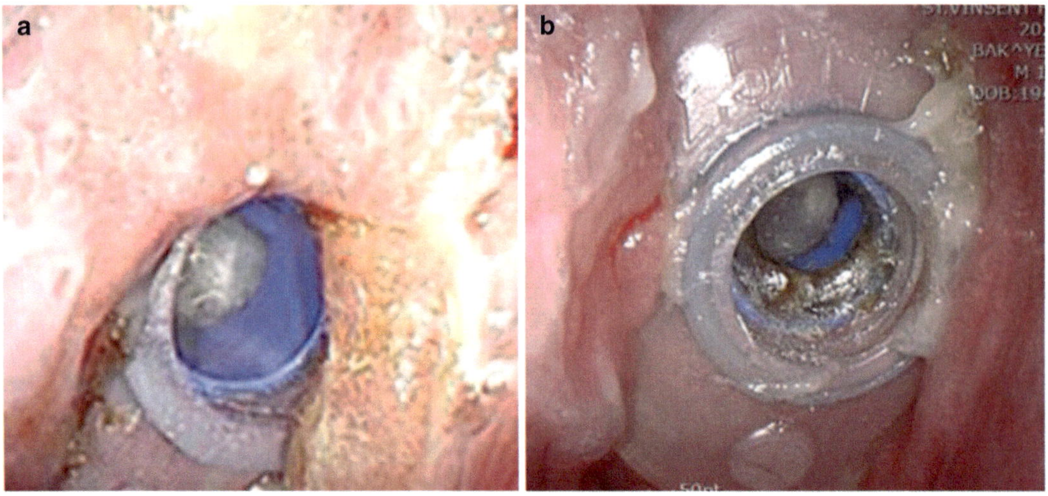

Fig. 8.13 Granulation tissue formation around prosthesis. (**a**) The panel shows granuloma on the voice prosthesis, causing vocal failure, whereas. (**b**) The panel shows the successful removal of granuloma after ablation using KTP (potassium-titanyl-phosphate) laser

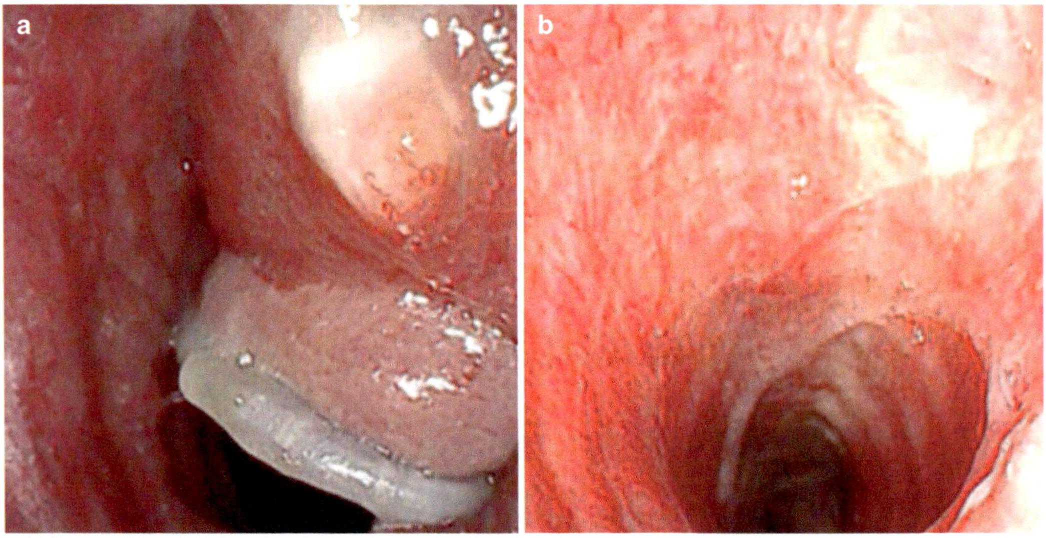

Fig. 8.14 Dislodgement of voice prosthesis (VP) into trachea. (**a**) The panel shows the extrusion of VP into the trachea, causing airway obstruction. (**b**) The panel shows the tracheal lumen and healed tracheoesophageal fistula after the removal of VP

ommended to dilate the full TEF tract because the distal part of the TEF is often narrower than the proximal part. After dilatation, a longer VP is inserted by the overshooting method. If the VP falls out and the patient does not realize it, the TEF may close completely, and the patient will require another tracheoesophageal puncture procedure.

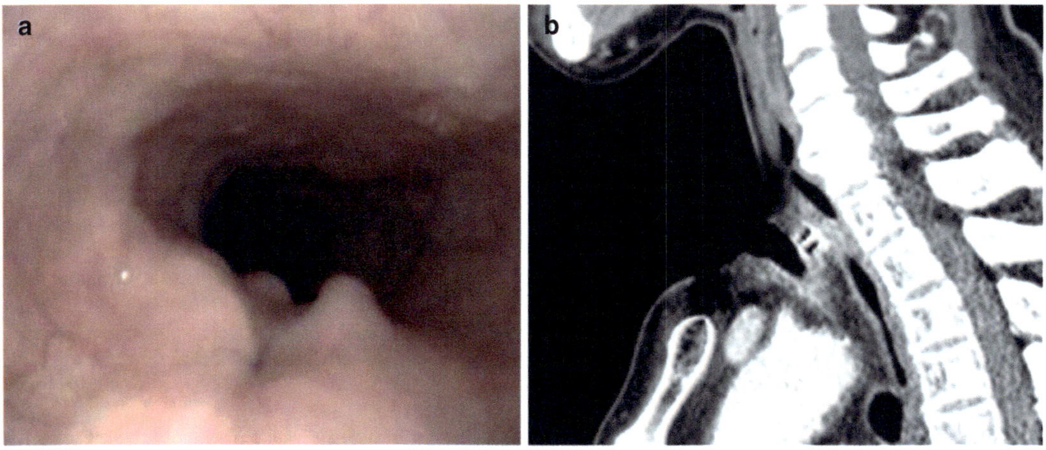

Fig. 8.15 The impacted and hidden voice prosthesis (VP). (**a**) The panel shows the esophageal lumen using a transnasal esophagoscope; the VP is not visible. (**b**) The panel shows the impacted VP in the tracheoesophageal party wall on the neck computed tomography

References

1. Hier M, Black MJ, Lafond G. Pharyngo-cutaneous fistulas after total laryngectomy: incidence, etiology and outcome analysis. J Otolaryngol. 1993;22:164–6.
2. Ikiz AO, Uca M, Guneri EA, Erdag TK, Sutay S. Pharyngocutaneous fistula and total laryngectomy: possible predisposing factors, with emphasis on pharyngeal myotomy. J Laryngol Otol. 2000;114(10):768–71.
3. Friedman M, Venkatesan TK, Yakovlev A, Lim JW, Tanyeri HM, Caldarelli DD. Early detection and treatment of postoperative pharyngocutaneous fistula. Otolaryngol Head Neck Surg. 1999;121:378–80.
4. Moses BL, Eisele DW, Jones B. Radiologic assessment of the early postoperative total-laryngectomy patient. Laryngoscope. 1993;103:1157–60.
5. Makitie AA, Irish J, Gullane PJ. Pharyngocutaneous fistula. Curr Opin Otolaryngol Head Neck Surg. 2003;11(2):78–84.
6. Natvig K, Boysen M, Tausjo J. Fistulae following laryngectomy in patients treated with irradiation. J Laryngol Otol. 1993;107:1136–9.
7. Redaelli de Zinis LO, Ferrari L, Tomenzoli D, Premoli G, Parrinello G, Nicolai P. Postlaryngectomy pharyngocutaneous fistula: incidence, predisposing factors, and therapy. Head Neck. 1999;21:131–8.
8. Cavalot AL, Gervasio CF, Nazionale G, Albera R, Bussi M, Staffieri A, Ferrero V, Cortesina G. Pharyngocutaneous fistula as a complication of total laryngectomy: review of the literature and analysis of case records. Otolaryngol Head Neck Surg. 2000;123:587–92.
9. Boyce SE, Meyers AD. Oral feeding after total laryngectomy. Head Neck. 1989;11:269–73.
10. Myers EN. The management of pharyngocutaneous fistula. Arch Otolaryngol. 1972;95:10–7.
11. Wang SG. Metronidazole effect in prevention of pharyngocutaneous fistula complicating surgery for malignant tumor of the larynx and pharynx. Korean J Otorhinolaryngol-Head Neck Surg. 1989;32:328–34.
12. Nadine BS. Taking care of wounds. In: Practical plastic surgery for nonsurgeons. 2nd ed. Hanley & Belfus; 2007. p. 5.
13. Andrews BT, Smith RB, Hoffman HT, et al. Orocutaneous and pharyngocutaneous fistula closure using a vacuum-assisted closure system. Ann Otol Rhinol Laryngol. 2008;117:298–302.
14. Rosenthal EL, Blackwell KE, McGrew B, et al. Use of negative-pressure dressings in head and neck reconstruction. Head Neck. 2005;27:970–5.
15. Bresson K, Rasmussen H, Rasmussen PA. Pharyngocutaneous fistulae in totally laryngectomized patients. J Laryngol Otol. 1974;88:835–42.
16. Rees R, Cary A, Shack RB, et al. Pharyngocutaneous fistulas in advanced cancer: closure with musculocutaneous or muscle flaps. Am J Surg. 1987;154:381–3.
17. Theogaraj SD, Merritt WH, Acharya G, et al. The pectoralis major musculocutaneous Island flap in single-stage reconstruction of the pharyngoesophageal region. Plast Reconstr Surg. 1980;65:267–76.
18. Kimura Y, Tojima H, Nakamura T, et al. Deltopectral flap for one-stage reconstruction of pharyngocutaneous fistulae following total laryngectomy. Acta Otolaryngol Suppl. 1994;511:175–8.
19. Capper R, Bradley PJ. Etiology and management of tracheostomal stenosis. Curr Opin Otolaryngol Head Neck Surg. 2002;10(2):123–8.

20. Kuo M, Ho CM, Wei WI, Lam KH. Tracheostomal stenosis after total laryngectomy: an analysis of predisposing clinical factors. Laryngoscope. 1994;104(1 Pt 1):59–63.
21. Wax MK, Touma BJ, Ramadan HH. Tracheostomal stenosis after laryngectomy: incidence and predisposing factors. Otolaryngol Head Neck Surg. 1995;113(3):242–7.
22. Montgomery WW. Stenosis of tracheostoma. Arch Otolaryngol. 1962;75:62–5.
23. Kim YH, Kim NH, Seong SY, Hyun DW, Choi HS. Double reversing Z-plasty with inferiorly widening stomaplasty for the management of tracheostomal stenosis. Auris Nasus Larynx. 2010;37(3):361–4.
24. Lam KH, Wei WI, Wong J, Ong GB. Tracheostome construction during laryngectomy—a method to prevent stenosis. Laryngoscope. 1983;93(2):212–5.
25. Suzuki M, Tsunoda A, Shirakura S, Sumi T, Nishijima W, Kishimoto S. A novel permanent tracheostomy technique for prevention of stomal stenosis (triangular tracheostomy). Auris Nasus Larynx. 2010;37(4):465–8.
26. Karonidis A, Tsoutsos D. The inverted V-shaped fasciocutaneous advancement flap effectively solves the complication of tracheostomal stenosis. Ann Plast Surg. 2021;86(3):298–301.
27. Seo GT, Wein LE, Dowling EM, Khorsandi AS, Urken ML. A novel technique for management of stenosis of the postlaryngectomy stoma with preservation of a functional tracheoesophageal puncture following tracheal resection. Head Neck. 2022;44(7):1737–41.
28. Trivedi NP, Patel D, Thankappan K, Iyer S, Kuriakose MA. Stomaplasty—anterior advancement flap and lateral splaying of trachea, a simple and effective technique. J Postgrad Med. 2008;54(1):21–4.
29. Myers EN, Snyderman CH. Operative otolaryngology: head and neck surgery. 3rd ed. Philadelphia, PA: Elsevier; 2017.
30. Tsou YA, Lin MH, Hua CH, Tseng HC, Bau DT, Tsai MH. Comparison of pharyngeal stenosis between hypopharyngeal patients undergoing primary versus salvage laryngopharyngectomy. Otolaryngol Head Neck Surg. 2010;143(4):538–43.
31. Sweeny L, Golden JB, White HN, Magnuson JS, Carroll WR, Rosenthal EL. Incidence and outcomes of stricture formation postlaryngectomy. Otolaryngol Head Neck Surg. 2012;146(3):395–402.
32. Maclean J, Szczesniak M, Cotton S, Cook I, Perry A. Impact of a laryngectomy and surgical closure technique on swallow biomechanics and dysphagia severity. Otolaryngol Head Neck Surg. 2011;144(1):21–8.
33. Walton B, Vellucci J, Patel PB, Jennings K, McCammon S, Underbrink MP. Post-laryngectomy stricture and pharyngocutaneous fistula: review of techniques in primary pharyngeal reconstruction in laryngectomy. Clin Otolaryngol. 2018;43(1):109–16.
34. Horowitz JB, Sasaki CT. Effect of cricopharyngeus myotomy on postlaryngectomy pharyngeal contraction pressures. Laryngoscope. 1993;103(2):138–40.
35. Scharpf J, Esclamado RM. Reconstruction with radial forearm flaps after ablative surgery for hypopharyngeal cancer. Head Neck. 2003;25(4):261–6.
36. Flint PW, Francis HW, Haughey BH, Lesperance MM, Lund VJ, Robbins KT, et al. Cummings otolaryngology : head and neck surgery. 7th ed. Philadelphia, PA: Elsevier; 2020.
37. Spaulding SL, Ansari E, Xing MH, Sandler ML, O'Malley QF, Ho R, et al. Diagnosis and management of pharyngoesophageal stenosis: a comprehensive approach to prophylactic, endoscopic, and reconstructive treatment options. Am J Otolaryngol. 2021;42(5):103003.
38. Ferguson DD. Evaluation and management of benign esophageal strictures. Dis Esophagus. 2005;18(6):359–64.
39. Josino IR, Madruga-Neto AC, Ribeiro IB, Guedes HG, Brunaldi VO, de Moura DTH, et al. Endoscopic dilation with bougies versus balloon dilation in esophageal benign strictures: systematic review and meta-analysis. Gastroenterol Res Pract. 2018;2018:5874870.
40. Gusmon-Oliveira CC, Kuboki YM, de Paulo GA, de Lima MS, Uemura RS, Martins BC, et al. Endoscopic injection of mitomycin C for the treatment of pharyngoesophageal stenosis refractory to endoscopic treatment with dilatation in patients treated for head and neck cancer. Gastroenterol Res Pract. 2018;2018:5428157.
41. Talpaert MJ, Balfour A, Stevens S, Baker M, Muhlschlegel FA, Gourlay CW. *Candida* biofilm formation on voice prostheses. J Med Microbiol. 2015;64(Pt 3):199–208.
42. Pentland DR, Stevens S, Williams L, Baker M, McCall C, Makarovaite V, et al. Precision antifungal treatment significantly extends voice prosthesis lifespan in patients following total laryngectomy. Front Microbiol. 2020;11:975.
43. Hutcheson KA, Lewin JS, Sturgis EM, Kapadia A, Risser J. Enlarged tracheoesophageal puncture after total laryngectomy: a systematic review and meta-analysis. Head Neck. 2011;33(1):20–30.
44. Jiang N, Kearney A, Damrose EJ. Tracheoesophageal fistula length decreases over time. Eur Arch Otorrinolaringol. 2016;273(7):1819–24.
45. Lorenz KJ, Kraft K, Graf F, Pröpper C, Steinestel K. Role of reflux-induced epithelial-mesenchymal transition in periprosthetic leakage after prosthetic voice rehabilitation. Head Neck. 2015;37(4):530–6.
46. Mayo-Yáñez M, Cabo-Varela I, Suanzes-Hernández J, Calvo-Henríquez C, Chiesa-Estomba C, Herranz G-BJ. Use of double flange voice prosthesis for periprosthetic leakage in laryngectomised patients: a

prospective case-crossover study. Clin Otolaryngol. 2020;45(3):389–93.
47. Parrilla C, Longobardi Y, Galli J, Rigante M, Paludetti G, Bussu F, et al. Periprosthetic leakage in tracheoesophageal prosthesis: proposal of a standardized therapeutic algorithm. Otolaryngol Head Neck Surg. 2021;165(3):446–54.
48. Lane C, Wright M, Linton J, Goyal N. Surgical closure of enlarged tracheoesophageal fistula after laryngectomy: a systematic review of techniques. Am J Otolaryngol. 2023;45(1):104023.
49. Mayo-Yáñez M, Chiesa-Estomba C, Lechien JR, Calvo-Henríquez C, Vaira LA, Cabo-Varela I. Long-term outcomes and cost-effectiveness of a magnet-based valve voice prosthesis for endoprosthesis leakage treatment. Eur Arch Otorrinolaringol. 2022;279(8):4167–72.

Part IV

Trachea and Bronchus

9 Tracheostomy

Kyoung Ho Oh, Changmyeon Song, and Inn-Chul Nam

9.1 KQ 9.1. How Do We Prevent Possible Complications in Conventional Tracheostomy?

Kyoung Ho Oh

Tracheotomy is a relatively common procedure performed to provide a safe and less damaging airway in cases of upper airway obstruction or when intubation is expected to be maintained for more than 2 weeks. It is generally performed as a planned operation, but sometimes as an emergency procedure, which requires a precise understanding of the technique and anatomy, as it must be performed within a short period. Additionally, the intricate physiological and anatomical complexities of the patient are often not fully understood in such expedited procedures; therefore, greater vigilance is required to prevent complications. Tracheotomy is a relatively safe procedure. However, as with any surgery, unexpected complications may occur. Most complications are reversible with proper care; however, severe complications or lack of proper care can lead to irreversible sequelae, such as brain damage due to hypoxia. Consequently, the surgeon performing tracheostomy should have a thorough knowledge of the complications of tracheotomy, should be able to predict them in advance, and must take appropriate and prompt action when they occur. This chapter discusses complications that can occur during and after surgery.

9.1.1 Intraoperative Complications

9.1.1.1 Bleeding

Anatomically, no major arteries pass through the area of the neck where a tracheostomy is performed, reducing the risk of significant bleeding. If bleeding occurs, it is generally limited, involves the external jugular vein, or may happen during thyroidotomy. Therefore, locating the bleeding site and performing electrocautery or compression for hemostasis is often sufficient. Furthermore, during tracheotomy under local anesthesia, the patient's blood pressure often rises during the surgery; therefore,

K. H. Oh (✉)
Department of Otolaryngology-Head and Neck Surgery, Korea University Ansan Hospital, College of Medicine, Korea University, Ansan-si, Republic of Korea
e-mail: ohkyoungho@korea.ac.kr

C. Song (✉)
Department of Otolaryngology-Head and Neck Surgery, College of Medicine, Hanyang University, Seoul, Republic of Korea

I.-C. Nam (✉)
Department of Otolaryngology—Head and Neck Surgery, Incheon St. Mary's Hospital, College of Medicine, The Catholic University of Korea, Incheon, Republic of Korea
e-mail: entnam@catholic.ac.kr

K.-J. Cho, J.-O. Park (eds.), *Management of Head and Neck Surgery Complications*, https://doi.org/10.1007/978-981-96-1860-6_9

controlling blood pressure and stabilizing the patient's condition often helps to control bleeding. In addition, it is recommended that patients with coagulation disorders are prepared and treated in advance, such as by administering platelets before surgery [1]. Intermittent thyroid ima artery may also be present in a few patients. If bleeding in this area is confirmed, electrocautery may be adequate for hemostasis (Fig. 9.1). If bleeding is excessive, rupture of the left innominate vein should be checked. Compression can achieve temporary hemostasis, followed by two steps to determine the focus of bleeding. If a tear in the innominate vein is confirmed, the area is typically compressed using a gauze-type hemostatic agent and sutured in consultation with a vascular surgeon. As the innominate artery lies below the vein, it rarely sustains any damage. However, in some cases, rupture of the innominate artery may occur because of dissection of a false lumen, such as in patients who are short-necked or those with obesity. The treatment for rupture of this artery is the same as that for vein rupture; however, the incidence of side effects is higher; therefore, close observation is required following surgery. Such damage to this major vessel can cause a cerebrovascular or cardiovascular accident due to the formation of a thrombus; therefore, it is recommended that the patient's condition be closely monitored for several days, preferably in an intensive care unit.

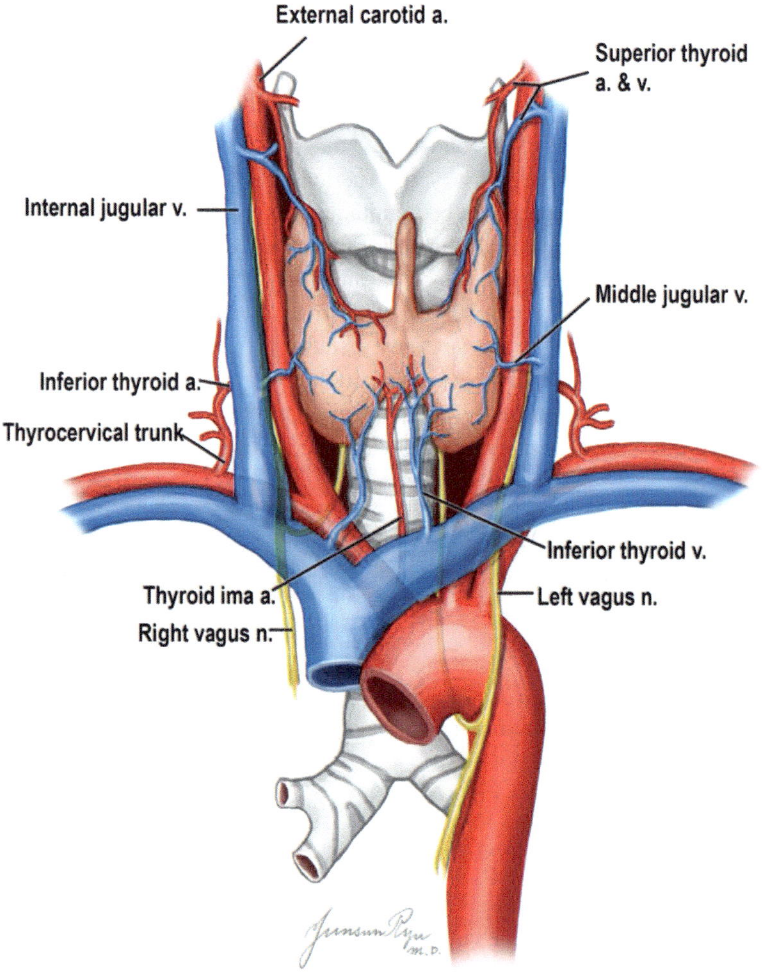

Fig. 9.1 Anatomy of tracheotomy. The thyroid ima artery is found in 1%–4% of cases and branches from either the aorta or innominate artery to course toward the isthmus of the thyroid gland. *a* artery; *v* vein, *n* nerve

If excessive bleeding occurs during tracheotomy, the procedure should be stopped immediately. Subsequently, the exact site of bleeding should be located, and the corresponding blood vessel should be sutured. Additionally, it should be noted that excessive dissection of the surgical area to find the bleeding site may tear more blood vessels and make suture challenging. Therefore, surgeons should apply pressure to the bleeding site and call for help from a more experienced surgeon.

Expert Opinion

Pin-point puncture of the innominate artery can cause continuous pumping of a small amount of blood, which cannot be easily controlled by compression or any hemostatic agents. If pumping of blood continues, a special suture technique performed by a vascular surgeon may be needed. In the case of large amount of intraoperative bleeding, incision for tracheotomy is usually not sufficient for searching or exposing the bleeding focus. Thus, extension of the incision is the first and most important step. (Si-Youn Song).

9.1.1.2 Emphysema

Although emphysema occurs unexpectedly after surgery, it is sometimes caused by excessive bagging after inserting a tube into a false lumen at the time of surgery. If the true lumen is found and the tube is inserted, prophylactic antibiotics are administered, and the affected area should be properly compressed. It disappears within a few weeks thereafter.

Expert Opinion

Subcutaneous emphysema that occurs after a tracheotomy is caused by strong pressure being applied to the tracheotomy site, often due to actions such as coughing. Therefore, use of a cuffed tracheotomy tube and maintaining cuff inflation for an appropriate duration after the surgery is important to prevent pressure from being exerted on the tracheotomy site. Additionally, to prevent pressure within the trachea from dispersing into the subcutaneous tissue, it is effective to create a tracheotomy site that is sufficiently larger than the tube and to suture the skin and trachea together. (Tack Kyun Kwon).

Too much packing around the tracheotomy tube to prevent post-operative bleeding or too tight suturing of the incision may cause emphysema. (Si-Youn Song).

9.1.1.3 Bronchospasm

Bronchospasm during tracheotomy rarely occurs in adults but occasionally affects infants. Bronchospasm may be suspected if the partial pressure of oxygen decreases and the partial pressure of carbon dioxide increases despite correct tube placement. If bronchospasm is suspected, inhaled agents, such as epinephrine, isoproterenol, or β_2 agonists, should be administered immediately in collaboration with the anesthetist or attending physician. If there is any possibility that the tracheostomy tube is not appropriately inserted, endotracheal intubation should be performed.

9.1.1.4 Laceration of Tracheal Posterior Wall

> **Expert Opinion**
> Posterior tracheal wall injury can occur with tracheotomy, particularly in pediatric patients, even when making a vertical incision in an urgent tracheotomy. After performing an urgent vertical incision tracheotomy, the posterior wall of the trachea must be inspected and repair performed if any injury is identified. (Tack Kyun Kwon).

During intubation, the tube should be inserted using rotation to align the angle of the tube so as to prevent potential laceration of the posterior wall of the trachea. The posterior wall is closely spaced with the vertebrae; therefore, it usually heals spontaneously, even if lacerated, without further treatment. Nevertheless, in such cases, subcutaneous emphysema and pneumothorax are more likely to occur postoperatively, and active surveillance is necessary.

9.1.1.5 Injury to Adjacent Structures

> **Expert Opinion**
> If proper neck extension is not achieved, the tracheotomy site may be positioned deeper, increasing the risk of complications. (Il-Seok Park).
>
> In cases of tracheal deviation caused by a tumor, a neck CT scan is useful not only for identifying the lateral deviation of the trachea, but also for assessing the depth and its relationship with surrounding major vessels. (Jin Ho Sohn).

If the trachea is challenging to locate due to the patient's obesity or short neck, or if the trachea deviates due to a thyroid tumor, damage to adjacent organs, such as the esophagus or recurrent laryngeal nerve, may occur due to incorrect dissection. Consequently, chest radiography should be performed before surgery to check for tracheal deviations. Damaged organs should be appropriately treated, such as using primary suturing of the esophagus and neurorrhaphy of the nerve.

9.1.2 Postoperative Complications

9.1.2.1 Subcutaneous Emphysema, Pneumomediastinum

Emphysema may occur in approximately 9% of cases despite proper tracheotomy, particularly if a false lumen is inadvertently created or if a tear is present in the posterior wall of the trachea [2]. Emphysema usually resolves within a few weeks with compression of the affected area and administration of prophylactic antibiotics to prevent infection at the affected site.

9.1.2.2 Pneumothorax

Pneumothorax after tracheotomy occurs in approximately 1% of cases and is generally caused by a misplaced tracheostomy tube and subsequent injury to the pleura [3]. It is rarely caused by a tear in the posterior mucosal wall of the trachea or a preexisting alveolar sac that ruptures during surgery [3]. When a pneumothorax occurs, the patient complains of pleuritic pain and dyspnea, which can be diagnosed using auscultation and chest radiography. In the event of pneumothorax, consultation with cardiothoracic surgery and respiratory medicine specialists is crucial to initiating treatment, which may involve chest tube insertion.

9.1.2.3 Delayed Bleeding

In rare cases, if the innominate artery is traumatized at the time of surgery, a pseudoaneurysm may rupture, causing massive bleeding several days after the surgery (Fig. 9.2). Consequently, in the event of trauma to the innominate artery, a postoperative enhanced neck CT should be performed.

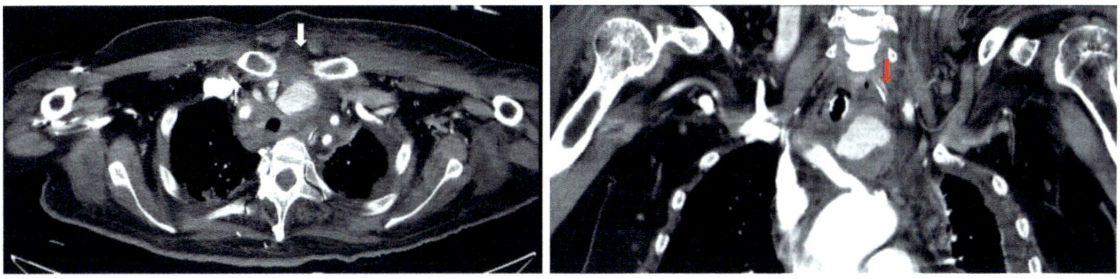

Fig. 9.2 Computed tomography finding of pseudoaneurysm following tracheotomy. Irregularly shaped contrast enhancement in the upper mediastinum (white and red arrows)

> **Expert Opinion**
> In cases where the neck is short or the tracheostomy site is positioned too low, delayed bleeding may occur weeks or even months later. (Il-Seok Park).

9.1.2.4 Wound Infection

Tracheotomy wound infection occurs in approximately 2–4% of cases [4]. The tracheotomy stoma is considered a clean-contaminated wound, making it challenging to keep the wound clean after surgery. Thus, administering perioperative antibiotics can help to reduce the incidence of postoperative wound infections [5]. Following the onset of an infection, daily dressings should be applied with antibiotics that target skin flora, such as coagulase-negative staphylococci (e.g., *Staphylococcus epidermidis* or *Staphylococcus aureus*).

> **Expert Opinion**
> To prevent wound infection, keeping the tracheostoma clean is important. Thus, frequent removal of discharge around the tracheostoma and frequent change of dressing is needed. (Si-Youn Song).

> **Expert Opinion**
> The unexpected dislodgement of a tracheostomy cannula can lead to a serious situation, potentially resulting in patient death. Therefore, in high-risk patients—such as those who are obese, have a short neck, are uncooperative, or in particular, pediatric patients—creating a preventive fenestration, which involves suturing the skin and trachea together, may be necessary. (Tack-Kyun Kwon).
>
> Tracheal stenosis may also occur, and recently, when tracheostomies have been performed during neurosurgery or respiratory medicine (percutaneous dilatational tracheostomy, PDT) procedures, the tracheostomy site may be created laterally, or in the case of PDT, the trachea may be pushed inward. This can narrow the tracheal lumen, cause tracheal chondritis, and make the removal of the tracheostomy tube difficult. (Il-Seok Park).
>
> When reinserting the tracheal cannula, it is safe to illuminate the tracheostomy tract with a headlight and, if necessary, use retractors or other instruments to secure a clear view during the insertion. (Jin Ho Sohn).
>
> It would be beneficial to consider two more causes of accidental decannulation. The first is when the neck strap of the

(continued)

tracheal cannula is loose or untied; thus, it is necessary to secure the neck strap tightly at an appropriate length. The second cause involves position changes in patients using an artificial ventilator. To prevent this, it is important to disconnect the ventilator tube from the tracheal cannula before changing the patient's position and to apply pressure to ensure that the tracheal cannula does not come out during the position change. (Jin Ho Sohn).

9.1.2.5 Unintended Decannulation

In patients with obesity, the tube is frequently not inserted deep enough into the trachea, which may lead to its dislodgement due to patient movement. Additionally, tube blockage can occur due to inadequate evacuation or removal of mucus from the tube or due to a dry environment, potentially causing the tube to dislodge if the patient coughs heavily. If the tube dislodges, it must be reinserted into the same stoma; however, the stoma may narrow rapidly following dislodgement. No excessive force should be applied while the tube is inserted into the narrowed stoma. When reinsertion of the tube is challenging, an attempt should be made to open the stoma immediately using Kelly forceps or nasal speculum while providing oxygen through a mask, followed by a fresh attempt to insert the tube. If this method proves unsuccessful, assistance should be sought from a trained otolaryngologist, and attempts should be made to provide oxygen through a mask bag. If the patient complains of respiratory distress following tube insertion or if bagging through the tube fails, the tube may have been inserted into a false lumen. In such cases, the tube should be promptly removed. A trained otolaryngologist should attempt tube insertion while providing sufficient oxygen through a mask. If hypoxia occurs during the procedure, a neurological examination should be performed. Generally, if tube dislodgement occurs in a patient who has undergone tracheostomy and has a stable stoma, the ward staff should follow the sequence illustrated in Fig. 9.3.

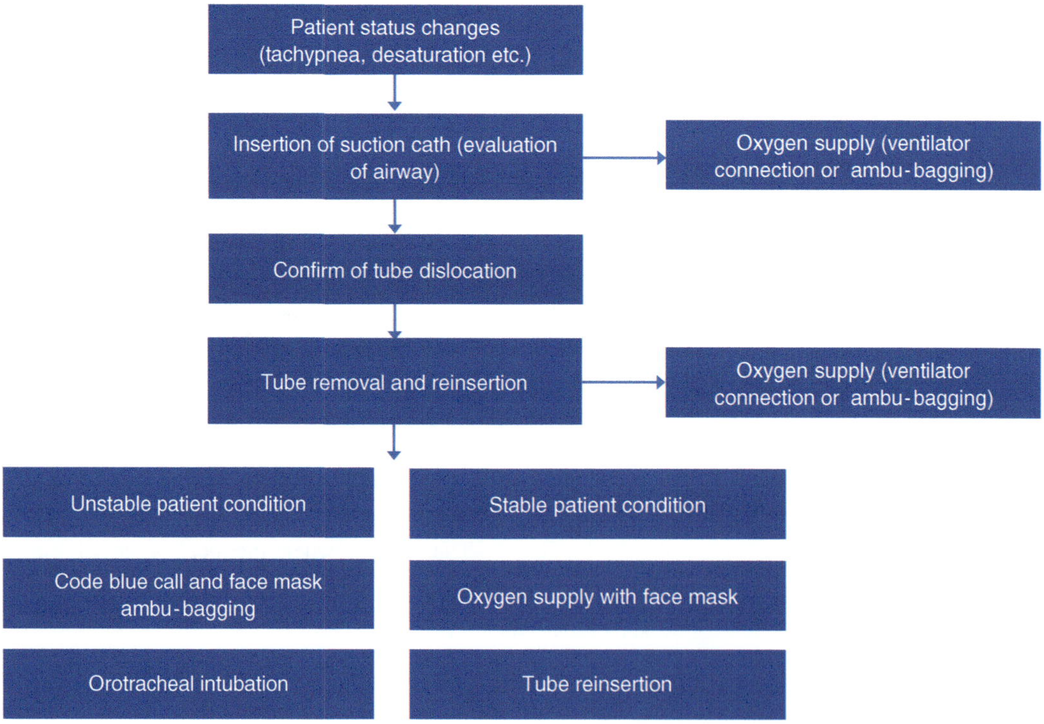

Fig. 9.3 Algorithm for unintended decannulation

9.2 KQ 9.2. How to Manage the Long-Term Complications of Tracheostomy—Peristomal Granulation and Suprastomal Stenosis

Changmyeon Song

9.2.1 Peristomal Granulation

Peristomal granulation is a common complication of prolonged indwelling tracheostomy tubes. In most cases, the granulation tissue around the stoma is self-limiting and does not impede tube replacement. However, a risk of bleeding remains if the granulation tissue becomes irritated, typically during tube changes due to traumatic forces. Occasionally, sizable peristomal granulations may develop, potentially obstructing the stoma and complicating the insertion of a new tube after removing the previous tube.

Expert Opinion
Intralesional or peri-lesional steroid injection may be helpful for managing granuloma. (Si-Youn Song).

Conservative management is recommended for small, non-bleeding granulations that do not interfere with tube replacement. Regular dressing with an antibiotic ointment can help prevent infection and bleeding. In cases of intermittent bleeding, compression with an epinephrine-soaked gauze can be used for adequate control.

Expert Opinion
Using cup forceps designed for nasal endoscopic surgery makes it easy to remove granuloma tissue, and the bleeding is minor and self-limiting; thus, cauterization is rarely needed. (Jin Ho Sohn).

Management of a large and complex peristomal granuloma involves excision using cold-steel instruments, such as knives and scissors, followed by cauterization with bipolar forceps. If a granuloma protrudes externally, excision and cauterization can be performed under local anesthesia. Typically, the pressure exerted by the tube against the stomatal skin and soft tissue acts as a compressive force to arrest bleeding.

General anesthesia may be necessary to manage granulation tissue inside the trachea, either above the stoma (suprastoma) or at and below the stoma (Fig. 9.4). In cases where the patient is conscious with an intact coughing response, bleeding from granuloma excision can lead to severe coughing and irritation. This may create emergent situations that hinder reinsertion of the tracheostomy tube. When surgical procedures are performed under general anesthesia, two options can be considered: converting the airway to orotracheal intubation or intermittently unplugging and inserting the tube through the stoma during surgery. Granulation tissue can be removed using a cold knife, monopolar or bipolar forceps, or a coblator [6].

Small amounts of granulation tissue situated outside the trachea can be monitored conservatively or excised under local anesthesia. Conversely, when a substantial granuloma is positioned within the trachea, causing hindrance to tracheotomy tube changes, or in vases where the granuloma continues to bleed, surgical excision of the granuloma under general anesthesia is advisable. The airway can be converted to orotracheal intubation, or the tube can be intermittently removed and reinserted during the course of the surgery.

Expert Opinion
After removing the granuloma, avoid exposing the wound and close the surgical site by suturing between healthy tissue and skin. This will help to prevent recurrence. (Tack-Kyun Kwon).

(continued)

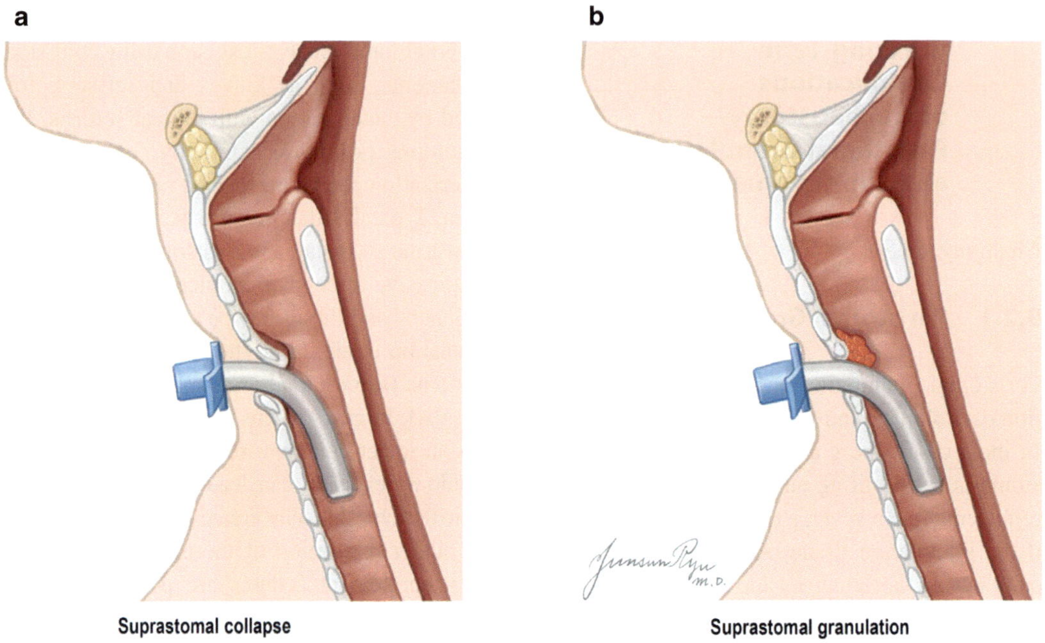

Fig. 9.4 Suprastomal collapse (**a**) and suprastomal granulation (**b**)

> Most granulomas inside the trachea can be removed under local anesthesia using an endoscope and cup forceps designed for nasal endoscopic surgery. (Jin Ho Sohn).

9.2.2 Laryngotracheal Stenosis

Tracheal stenosis is one of the most common long-term complications associated with tracheotomy, with an incidence rate of 2% [7]. Suprastomal and tracheal stenosis arise from irritation of the tracheal mucosa or cartilage rings or the disruption of blood flow caused by the tracheotomy tube or tube balloon. Prior orotracheal intubation may predispose individuals to subglottic and tracheal stenosis. Low-pressure ballooning is preferred to mitigate this complication, and efforts have been made to minimize trauma from the tube. Suprastomal stenosis may result from invagination of the anterior suprastomal trachea, which commonly contributes to decannulation failure [8].

The treatment choice for airway stenosis depends on the length and severity of the condition. Simple stenosis is characterized by a short stricture that is less than 1 cm in length and is limited to the tracheal mucosa. In contrast, complex stenosis involves a longer stricture or stenosis with a lesion extending to the tracheal wall, with or without tracheomalacia [9]. Bronchoscopic assessment should be performed to evaluate the extent and degree of stenosis.

> **Expert Opinion**
> Three-dimensional reconstruction chest computed tomography is very helpful for evaluating tracheal stenosis. (Si-Youn Song).

A less invasive approach for treating simple stenosis involves bougienage or balloon dilatation. Additionally, simple stenosis can be managed through steroid injection, endoscopic excision with or without a laser, and topical application of mitomycin C to reduce the risk of restenosis following these procedures. Tracheal resection with end-to-end anastomosis may be warranted in cases of severe, complex, and recurrent stenosis that hinders respiration when using a tracheotomy tube. However, interventional bronchoscopic treatments, including stent insertion, may be considered when surgical intervention is impractical due to comorbidities or when the stenosis exceeds 5–6 cm in length [10].

Treatment Options for Subglottic and Tracheal Stenosis (Fig. 9.5)

- Steroid injection
- Endoscopic bougienage/dilatation
- Endoscopic excision with or without laser
- Spray cryotherapy
- Topical application of mitomycin C
- Tracheal (cricoid) resection with end-to-end anastomosis
- Bronchoscopy interventions, including stent insertion

Expert Opinion

The efficacy of mitomycin C is controversial. Some reports suggest that, while it may delay the wound healing process, it does not have a significant effect on reducing stenosis. Therefore, it should be used with caution. (Tack-Kyun Kwon).

In cases of mild suprastomal stenosis, simple excision of the inwardly deviated tissue may suffice. In slightly more severe cases, the trough method, which involves pulling the inwardly deviated tissue outward to expand the tracheal lumen, can be effective. (Jin Ho Sohn).

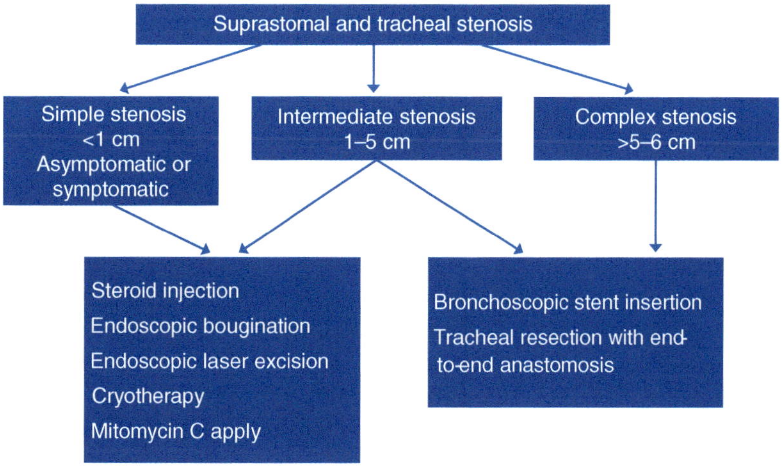

Fig. 9.5 Treatment algorithm for suprastomal and tracheal stenosis

9.3 KQ 9.3. How to Manage the Long-Term Complications of Tracheotomy—Tracheoesophageal Fistula and Tracheomalacia

Changmyeon Song

9.3.1 Tracheoesophageal Fistula

Tracheoesophageal fistula (TEF) is a rare complication that may arise from the prolonged use of a tracheotomy tube. Reports suggest that TEF occurs in less than 1% of patients undergoing tracheotomy [11]. Symptoms of TEF include aspiration of food material, gastric dilatation, recurrent episodes of aspiration pneumonia, and the inability to ventilate the lungs effectively. Factors such as injury, infection, inflammation, and necrosis of the posterior tracheal mucosa caused by the cannula and pressure can contribute to the development of tracheoesophageal fistula. Additionally, simultaneous placement of a nasogastric tube may increase the risk of fistula formation [12].

Expert Opinion

Metal plate and screw used for fixation of C-spine fracture can increase the risk of fistula formation. (Si-Youn Song).

To prevent the occurrence of a TEF, it is crucial to reposition the cuff or alleviate tracheal compression by adjusting the size of the tracheostomy tube or utilizing an elongated tube. The incidence of TEF has significantly decreased with the adoption of high-volume, low-pressure balloon cuffs in tracheotomy tubes [13].

Expert Opinion

Another cause of TEF after a tracheotomy is direct pressure injury to the tracheal posterior wall from the tip of the tracheal cannula. To prevent direct pressure from the tip of the tracheal cannula on the tracheal posterior wall, after inserting the tracheal cannula into the trachea, a flexible endoscope should be inserted through the inside of the tracheal cannula to check if the tip of the cannula is pressing on the tracheal posterior wall. If so, the tip of the cannula can be slightly trimmed or it can be replaced with another cannula with a different curvature. (Jin Ho Sohn).

Assessment of the fistula involves endoscopic examinations of the inner mucosa of the trachea through bronchoscopy and evaluating esophageal lesions through esophagoscopy. Furthermore, imaging examinations, such as computed tomography, magnetic resonance imaging, and esophagograms, provide additional information regarding the severity of the TEF.

Conservative management can be considered for small, asymptomatic TEFs. This procedure involves lowering the cuff of the tracheotomy tube below the fistula and converting the nasogastric tube into a gastrostomy to promote fistula healing. Notably, spontaneous healing of a TEF is uncommon, and most cases require surgical intervention for repair.

During TEF repair, insertion of viable tissue between the trachea and esophagus is crucial [14]. In cases of a small TEF, the membranous tracheal mucosal fistula is addressed by directly suturing the tracheal defect. The esophageal fistula is repaired using a two-layer technique: the inner esophageal mucosal defect is initially repaired, followed by suturing of the outer esophageal muscles using an interrupted technique. To prevent fistula recurrence, a local rotation flap of the strap muscles can be inserted between the repaired tracheal and esophageal sites [12].

For larger defects in the posterior tracheal wall, a more extensive surgical approach involving tracheal resection and end-to-end anastomosis with simultaneous primary closure of the esophageal fistula is necessary. The procedure begins by exposing the anterior wall of the trachea and avoiding injury to the bilateral recurrent laryngeal nerves. Minimizing the exposure of the upper and lower tracheal levels to the fistula site to prevent compromised perfusion of the healthy trachea is important.

The trachea is then resected both above and below the level of the fistula, and ventilation is secured by inserting a tube into the distal trachea. The orotracheal tube is pulled upward to ensure that it remains below the level of the larynx, as it will be reinserted after end-to-end anastomosis. After resection of the tracheal defect, the esophagus is fully exposed, and the defect is repaired using absorbable sutures. Following the removal of the ventilation tube, the remaining orotracheal tube is advanced below the defect level.

End-to-end anastomosis of the healthy upper and lower trachea is achieved with multiple 3–0 Vicryl sutures. While the orotracheal tube is typically extubated later, some surgeons may opt for temporary tracheotomy below the sutured level, facilitating early extubation if deemed preferable.

Treatment Options for Tracheoesophageal Fistula (Fig. 9.6)

- Lower the position of the cuff in the trachea
- Convert to temporary gastrostomy
- Perform primary repair of tracheal and esophageal defects
- Insert a viable tissue (e.g., strap muscle) between the trachea and esophagus
- Perform end-to-end anastomosis of the trachea and repair the esophageal fistula

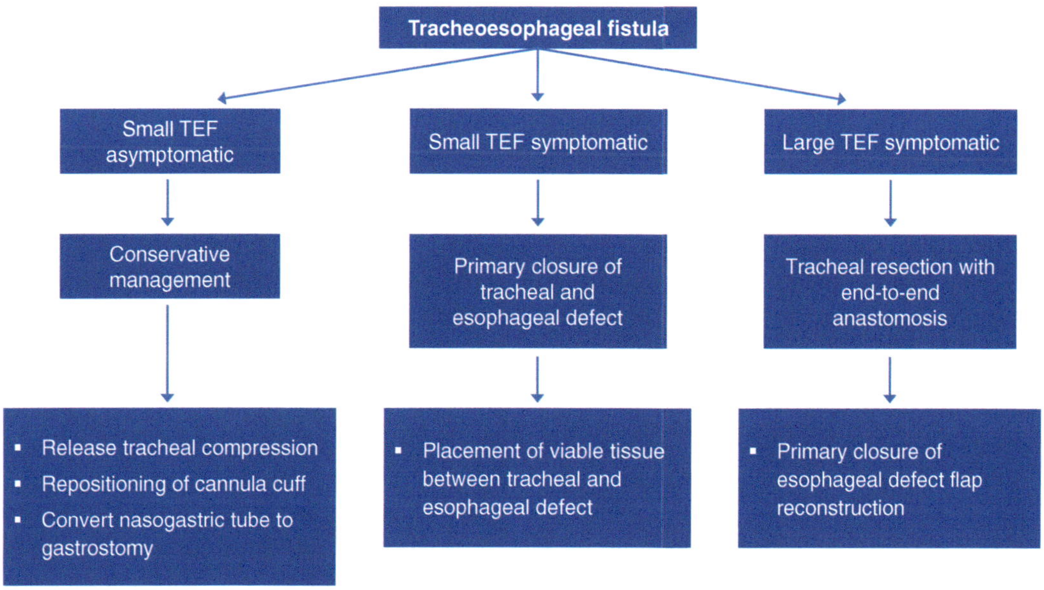

Fig. 9.6 Algorithm for the management of a tracheoesophageal fistula. *TEF* tracheoesophageal fistula

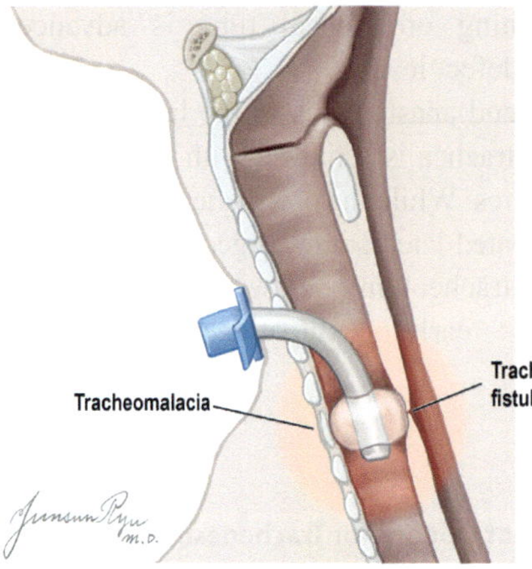

Fig. 9.7 Prevalent location for tracheomalacia and tracheoesophageal fistula

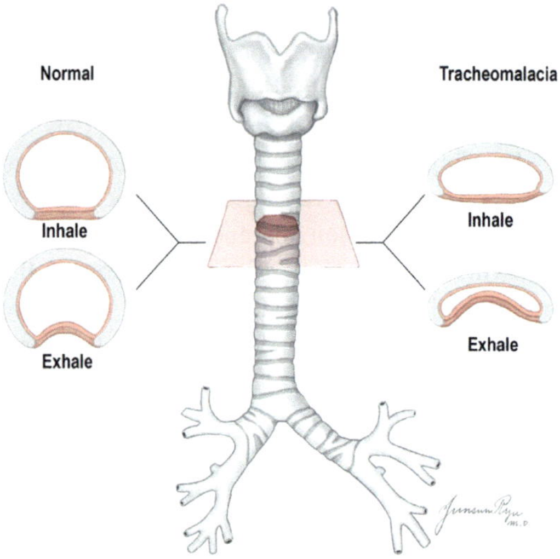

Fig. 9.8 Change of tracheal lumen during respiration in tracheomalacia

9.3.2 Tracheomalacia

Patients requiring a tracheotomy tube with a balloon for ventilation, often due to conditions such as degenerative neuromuscular diseases, may experience widening of the cervical trachea and tracheomalacia (Fig. 9.7). This is primarily attributed to factors such as the pressure exerted by the tube balloon, the use of an oversized cannula, and inflammation in the tracheal region [15]. Tracheal narrowing or collapse typically becomes apparent during exhalation before being observed during inhalation. To prevent tracheomalacia, cuff pressure should be minimized, aiming for a target pressure of <25 mmHg. This approach helps to mitigate the risk of tracheal complications associated with excessive pressure on the tracheotomy tube (Fig. 9.8) [16].

Treating tracheomalacia can be complex, particularly when it is associated with severe tracheal stenosis. In mild cases, continuous positive pressure may provide relief. In cases of small focal tracheomalacia, adjusting the tracheotomy tube to position the cuff distal to the pathological portion can be beneficial. Bronchoscopic stent insertion is often recommended in cases of diffuse tracheomalacia, and these stents are typically left in place for more than 6 months. If the malacia portion is localized, tracheoplasty may be considered as a potential treatment option [13]. Tracheal resection and end-to-end anastomosis are seldom performed; however, a comprehensive evaluation is imperative to assess any coexisting pathology in the upper airway. This meticulous assessment is crucial to determine the most appropriate course of action for addressing tracheal conditions.

9.4 KQ 9.4. How to Manage Massive Arterial Bleeding Following Tracheotomy

Inn-Chul Nam

Any peristomal bleeding in a patient undergoing tracheotomy should prompt a full clinical investigation to ascertain the underlying cause. The differential diagnosis of tracheostomy bleeding is determined based on the time interval between the tracheotomy and bleeding onset. Bleeding that occurs within 48 h is classified as "early," and that occurring days or months later is termed "late." Bleeding within 48 h of tracheotomy is typically associated with local factors, such as injury of the anterior jugular or inferior thyroid veins, systemic coagulopathy, erosion secondary to tracheal suction, or bronchopneumonia. Bleeding occurring 3 days to 6 weeks after tracheotomy should be considered an indication of a tracheal innominate artery fistula, unless otherwise proven. Other causes of catastrophic pulmonary hemorrhage include pulmonary artery flotation catheter-induced arterial rupture, thoracic aneurysmal rupture, and, less commonly, vascular fistula (from the carotid artery or inferior thyroid artery). Hemorrhage occurring more than 6 weeks postoperatively is rarely related to tracheal innominate artery fistulas and is more likely to be secondary to granulation tissue, tracheobronchitis, or malignancy.

Massive hemorrhage caused by erosion of the innominate artery is the most common delayed fatal complication of tracheostomy. The most common risk factor for this complication is low tracheostomy [17]. Two possible mechanisms underlie innominate artery erosion. The first mechanism involves erosion of the tip of the tracheostomy tube through the anterior tracheal wall. Anterior angulation of a right-angled tracheostomy tube or incorrect curvature of the tube may cause the end to erode the anterior tracheal wall. The second mechanism is the direct erosion of the innominate artery by the tracheostomy tube outside the trachea (Fig. 9.9). This complication can be prevented by placing the tracheostomy tube through the second and third tracheal rings and using a tracheostomy tube with the correct curvature [18].

Bleeding from the innominate artery after a tracheostomy is usually fatal. Warning signs of impending massive bleeding from the innominate artery include premonitory minimal bleeding (sentinel bleeding) and pulsation of the tracheostomy tube that coincides with the heartbeat. These signs have been reported to be pathognomonic of innominate arterial bleeding [19]. Cuff inflation should be the first procedure to control hemorrhage. Cuff inflation is more likely to be effective if the tracheostomy tube erodes through the anterior wall of the trachea into the innominate artery at the level of the cuff. However, this maneuver may not stop bleeding if the innominate artery is eroded by direct contact with the tracheostomy tube. In this case, the innominate artery should be dissected off the trachea using the index finger and should be occluded against the sternum (Fig. 9.10). The tracheostomy tube should be removed and replaced with a cuffed orotracheal tube. The index finger may be inserted through the tracheostomy wound and advanced posteroinferiorly along the trachea into the mediastinum behind the innominate

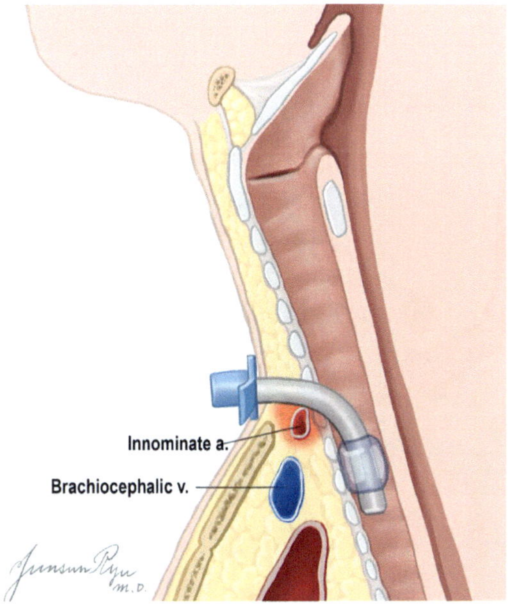

Fig. 9.9 The relationship of the tracheostomy tube to the innominate artery in low tracheostomy. *a* artery, *v* vein

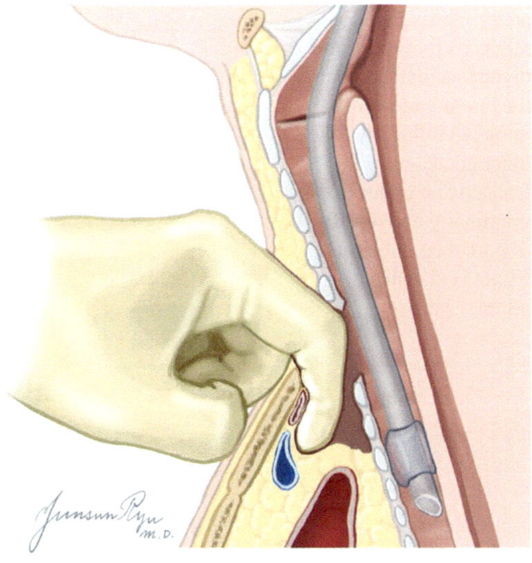

Fig. 9.10 Technique of occlusion of innominate artery by digital pressure against sternum. The procedure requires blunt dissection of the artery from the anterior wall of the trachea

artery with blunt digital dissection. To avoid tearing of the innominate artery, the finger should press against the trachea during dissection. Once the vessel is occluded, the patient should be transported to the operating room, and the innominate artery should be divided and the ends oversewn. The innominate artery is best exposed through median sternotomy.

Expert Opinion
Whether the tip of the tracheostomy tube is pressing on the anterior tracheal wall can be confirmed by inserting a flexible endoscope through the inner diameter of the tracheostomy tube. If the tip of the tracheostomy tube is pressing on the tracheal wall, you can either slightly trim the tip of the tube or replace it with a tracheostomy tube with a different curvature. This method also helps to prevent tracheal stenosis caused by irritation from the tip of the tracheostomy tube. (Jin Ho Sohn).

Newly developed difficulty in passing the suction catheter through the tracheotomy tube may be a sign of tracheotomy tube related complication and must be examined with a fiberscope. (Si-Youn Song).

After sternotomy, the innominate artery is exposed by division of the thymus, with superior retraction of the innominate vein. The artery is encircled on both sides of the tracheal innominate arterial fistula to gain vascular control (Fig. 9.11). The fistula site is usually small and surrounded by an inflamed and indurated arterial wall. Repairing the defect in the innominate artery can fail, with a higher rate of recurrent bleeding and death compared to dividing the artery. The innominate artery should be debrided back to the healthy tissue and should be closed. Management of tracheal defects can be individualized by allowing granulation to occur during resection. Regardless of the method used, vascu-

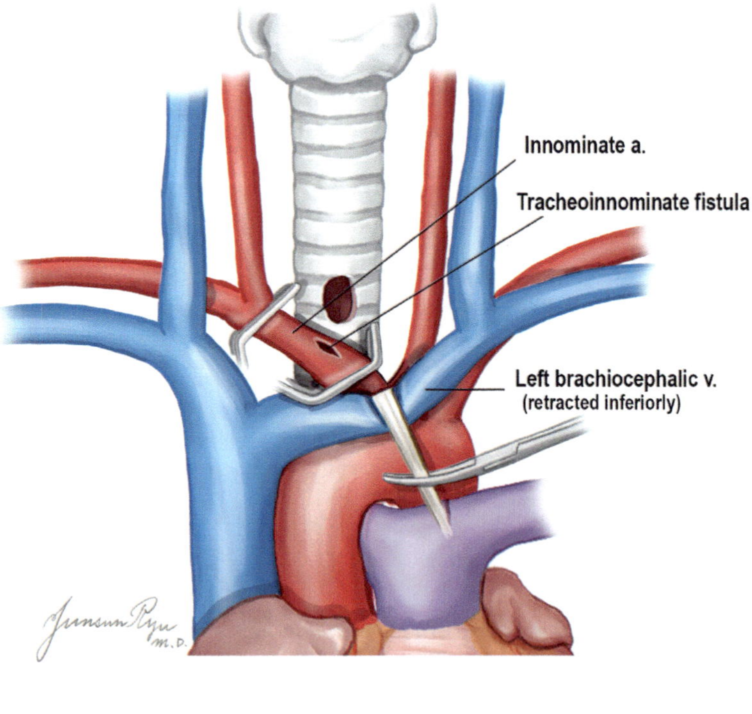

Fig. 9.11 Surgical repair of the innominate artery. Through a median sternotomy, the thymus is divided, and the innominate vein is retracted inferiorly. The innominate artery is isolated and controlled proximally and distally. The tracheoinnominate fistula is visualized. *a* artery, *v* vein

larized tissue needs to be interposed between the tracheal defect and the divided ends of the innominate artery to eliminate dead space, prevent infection, and reduce the risk of rebleeding. The pectoralis major muscle flap is ideal for this purpose. [20].

A recent report highlighted the successful management of tracheal innominate artery fistulas using percutaneous endovascular stenting of the innominate artery, either as a definitive procedure or as a temporary measure [21]. While these non-surgical management strategies may be successful, they are unlikely to be available in an emergency. Therefore, immediate surgery is currently the treatment of choice.

- All tracheostomy bleeding should be considered a sentinel bleed, and the source must be identified, even if the bleeding resolves.
- Low tracheostomy is one of the most common risk factors for innominate artery bleeding.
- When innominate artery bleeding occurs, the first treatment is digital compression using the index finger through the tracheostoma.
- After the initial management, the trachea–innominate artery fistula should be repaired in the operation room.

9.5 KQ 9.5. How to Prevent Possible Complications in Percutaneous Dilatational Tracheostomy

Inn-Chul Nam

The complications of percutaneous dilatational tracheostomy (PDT) are comparable to those following open surgical tracheotomy [22]. Complications of PDT are traditionally divided into early and late complications. Early complications include bleeding, infection, pneumothorax, technical failure, and perioperative hypoxia due to tube obstruction or accidental decannulation. Late complications include the development of granulation tissue resulting in airway stenosis, failure to decannulate or upper airway obstruction with respiratory failure after decannulation, tracheoesophageal fistula, tracheomalacia, tracheal stenosis, and trachea–innominate artery fistula [23]. Since most complications do not differ markedly from those of surgical tracheotomy, they will not be described separately here, and we will focus on complications specific to PDT and determine how they can be prevented.

PDT is a semi-blind technique that relies on surface markings for accurate anatomical identification. Therefore, careful patient selection is important to determine the success of this procedure. Surface landmarks, such as the thyroid or cricoid cartilage, cricothyroid membrane, tracheal rings, and the sternal notch, should be easily identified and marked. Therefore, patients with obesity or those with short and large necks may make the identification of key landmarks more challenging. Although a short, obese neck has been considered to be a relative contraindication for PDT, many studies support the use of PDT in patients with obesity [24].

Previous neck surgery is regarded as a contraindication for PDT [25]. The rationale for this is that it hampers the identification of landmarks and distorts the normal internal anatomy. Prior tracheostomy is considered a relative contraindication for PDT due to the presence of scar tissue and possibly altered anatomy. However, according to a prospective study, repeated PDT had no significant complications, and no cases required conversion to surgical tracheotomy [26]. In addition, a residual tracheostomy scar may help in the identification of landmarks in patients with large necks or ambiguous external anatomy.

Other anatomical considerations should include the ease with which an endotracheal tube can be replaced if it were to be dislodged in the periprocedural period prior to establishing an airway with a tracheostomy tube. Patients with laryngeal edema, vocal cord paralysis, subglottic stenosis, and maxillofacial trauma should be approached with care in this regard, and proper planning, equipment, and staff should be available in the event that the airway is lost and cannot be easily reestablished before the tracheostomy tube is inserted and secured.

Bleeding is the most common complication of both surgical and percutaneous tracheotomies and is estimated to occur in approximately 5% of patients. However, bleeding is more likely to be associated with PDT than with surgical tracheotomy [27]. Early bleeding, within 48 h of the procedure, is usually minor and originates from the superficial veins. A more serious cause of hemorrhage is a trachea–innominate arterial fistula, which usually occurs later. Although the majority of bleeding is minimal, the potential for more severe and catastrophic bleeding is present. In one study of 497 cases, bleeding complicated the procedure in 24 (4.8%) cases, with six of these requiring conversion to an open tracheotomy [25]. Furthermore, PDT was associated with a 0.17% incidence of lethal complications, most of which were due to bleeding (38%), with 31% of the hemorrhagic deaths occurring at the time of tube insertion [28].

Several vessels and structures may sustain damage during PDT, resulting in bleeding. These include the inferior thyroid vein, anterior jugular vein, or thyroid isthmus itself. The thyroid ima artery is an anatomical variant present in 3% of the population. This small artery can arise directly from the brachiocephalic trunk, carotid artery, or even the aortic arch and often lies immediately anterior to the tracheal midline [25]. Once significant bleeding is identified, the initial response should be to place direct digital pressure over the tracheostomy site, which is usually sufficient in cases of small vessel injury. If the guidewire has already been placed, it should be left in situ to allow the insertion of a dilator to tamponade any bleeding and assist with rescuing airway access. In case of failure of digital pressure to achieve bleeding control, the endotracheal tube should be advanced to the normal position, and the tube cuff should be inflated to protect the airway. Then, the tracheotomy incision should be extended, and the bleeding vessel should be located and subsequently ligated. If PDT is deemed difficult to perform, a switch to surgical tracheostomy should be made.

To prevent bleeding during PDT, a thorough assessment should be performed in all patients, including an examination of the neck for identifiable landmarks or obvious vessels. This should be conducted in the position where the procedure will be performed to allow for movement from the neutral position. Previous imaging modalities, particularly computed tomography scans, should be reviewed for the presence of problematic vessels.

Another method for preventing complications, including bleeding during PDT, is ultrasound. With the increasing availability of affordable mobile ultrasound systems, real-time ultrasound guidance is now widely used during routine invasive procedures, such as the insertion of percutaneous drains and vascular access catheters. The role of ultrasound during various airway procedures has also been the focus of attention in recent years. Ultrasound has been reported to improve the safety profile of PDT. The theoretical advantage of preprocedural ultrasound is its ability to identify cervical anatomy and aberrant pretracheal vasculature to avoid immediate vascular complications. Arterial pulsation palpated over the anterior neck prior to PDT has been confirmed by ultrasound, which prevented a potentially serious complication [29]. It also helps in selecting the proper size and length of the tracheostomy tube, particularly in patients with an increased pretracheal soft tissue diameter. Intraprocedural ultrasound may assist not only in revealing potentially aberrant vessels, but also in identifying the preferred puncture location and guiding needle puncture of the trachea. Real-time imaging can be used to identify the desired level of puncture in the sagittal plane in the midline over the trachea, while right-angle rotation of the probe allows for an out-of-plane approach to guide the needle tip toward the midline. In patients with obesity and in those with anatomical deformities due to chronic musculoskeletal pathology, prior injuries, and surgical procedures, palpation of traditionally used anatomical landmarks may be difficult or even impossible. A suboptimal position of the tracheal puncture can subsequently lead to tracheostomy tube malpositioning. Tracheal tube malposition, which results in a tube lying at an angle to the tracheal axis and abutting the lateral or posterior tracheal wall, can cause partial tube lumen obstruction, which has been implicated in failure to wean from ventilation and otherwise unexplained episodes of desaturation. Ultrasound may be even more useful in these patients.

Another tool that can reduce complications during PDT is a (flexible) bronchoscope. Since PDT was first described in 1985, many possible complications have been noted to be primarily caused by the blind nature of the procedure. Incorrect tracheal puncture during PDT can result in malpositioning of the tube and insertion of the tube into a false passage (not into the tracheal lumen, but into the paratracheal space), which can result in hypoxia, subcutaneous emphysema, and hemothorax. This has led to the common practice of passing a fiberoptic bronchoscope down the endotracheal tube before passing a needle into the trachea. This not only allows visualization of the needle and subsequent guidewire passage, but also serves as a safeguard as the tube is pulled back during the procedure. A unique complication of PTD is unexpected extubation while pulling back the endotracheal tube to secure space during tracheal puncture and dilatation. To secure the airway during PDT, the endotracheal tube must be positioned immediately below the vocal cords. Premature extubation can be prevented by using bronchoscopic guidance. The most important advantage of bronchoscopy-guided PDT is that the surgeon can easily and accurately locate the tracheostomy site. This is made possible by trans-illumination of the fiberoptic bronchoscope light inside the trachea and by direct visualization of the puncture needle and dilator with the camera attached to the bronchoscope (Fig. 9.12). Accurate localization of the tracheostomy site provides another advantage, such as preventing repeated puncture attempts with a puncture needle and resulting in a short procedural time [30]. The next important advantage is the prevention of posterior tracheal wall injury by direct visualization during puncture and dilatation. Moreover, bronchoscopy-guided PDT is beneficial for training. However, this technique has several drawbacks, such as carbon dioxide retention, decreased oxygen tension resulting from partial occlusion of the endotracheal tube by bronchoscopy, increased intracranial pressure, and additional costs [31]. However, the benefits of bronchoscopy guidance in terms of safety and precision outweigh the potential drawbacks, particularly when it is performed by an inexperienced surgeon or in patients with unfavorable anatomy. Therefore, individual patient factors and clinical considerations should be considered when using bronchoscopic guidance during PDT.

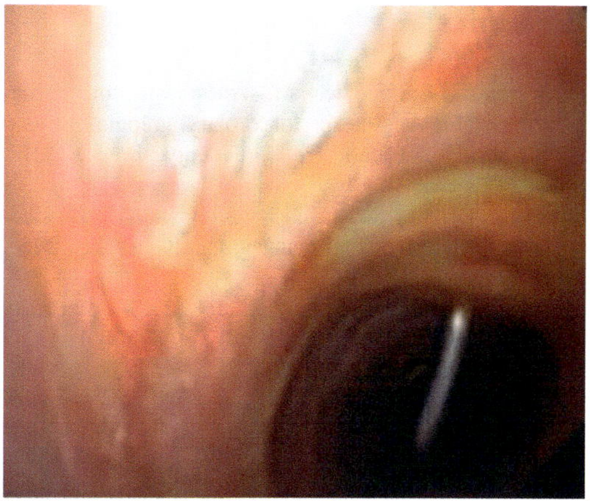

Fig. 9.12 Bronchoscopic view of puncture needle during bronchoscopy-guided percutaneous dilatational tracheostomy

- Complications of PDT are few compared to open surgical tracheostomy.
- Careful patient selection is an important factor in preventing complications of PDT.
- Bleeding is the most common complication of PDT.
- PDT under ultrasound or bronchoscopic guidance can reduce the complication rate of PDT.

Expert Opinion

Although long-term follow-up is necessary, PDT can cause trachea stenosis more frequently than does transcervical invasive tracheotomy. (Il-Seok Park).

References

1. Demirci O, Popovich M. Anesthesia for tracheotomy. In: Anesthesia for otolaryngologic surgery. Cambridge: Cambridge University Press; 2012. p. 255.
2. Myers EN, Carrau RL. Early complications of tracheotomy: incidence and management. Clin Chest Med. 1991;12(3):589–95.
3. Panajaroen P, Tangjaturonrasme N. Pneumothorax after tracheostomy: a prospective study. Otolaryngol Pol. 2015;69(3):26–30.
4. Viau F, Lededente A, Le Tinier J. Complications of tracheotomy. Rev Pneumol Clin. 1988;44(1):24–32.
5. Sittitrai P, Siriwittayakorn C. Perioperative antibiotic prophylaxis in open tracheostomy: a preliminary randomized controlled trial. Int J Surg. 2018;54(Pt A):170–5.
6. Brown CS, Ryan MA, Ramprasad VH, Karas AF, Raynor EM. Coblation of suprastomal granulomas in tracheostomy-dependent children. Int J Pediatr Otorhinolaryngol. 2017;96:55–8. https://doi.org/10.1016/j.ijporl.2017.03.004.
7. Goldenberg D, Ari EG, Golz A, Danino J, Netzer A, Joachims HZ. Tracheotomy complications: a retrospective study of 1130 cases. Otolaryngol Head Neck Surg. 2000;123(4):495–500. https://doi.org/10.1067/mhn.2000.105714.
8. Koitschev A, Graumueller S, Zenner HP, Dommerich S, Simon C. Tracheal stenosis and obliteration above the tracheostoma after percutaneous dilational tracheostomy. Crit Care Med. 2003;31(5):1574–6. https://doi.org/10.1097/01.CCM.0000065189.64560.A8.
9. Zouk AN, Batra H. Managing complications of percutaneous tracheostomy and gastrostomy. J Thorac Dis. 2021;13(8):5314–30. https://doi.org/10.21037/jtd-19-3716.
10. Murgu SD, Egressy K, Laxmanan B, Doblare G, Ortiz-Comino R, Hogarth DK. Central airway obstruction: benign strictures, tracheobronchomalacia, and malignancy-related obstruction. Chest. 2016;150(2):426–41. https://doi.org/10.1016/j.chest.2016.02.001.
11. Epstein SK. Late complications of tracheostomy. Respir Care. 2005;50(4):542–9.
12. De Leyn P, Bedert L, Delcroix M, Depuydt P, Lauwers G, Sokolov Y, et al. Tracheotomy: clinical review and guidelines. Eur J Cardiothorac Surg. 2007;32(3):412–21.
13. Zouk AN, Batra H. Managing complications of percutaneous tracheostomy and gastrostomy. J Thorac Dis. 2021;13(8):5314–30.
14. Macchiarini P, Verhoye JP, Chapelier A, Fadel E, Dartevelle P. Evaluation and outcome of different surgical techniques for postintubation tracheoesophageal fistulas. J Thorac Cardiovasc Surg. 2000;119(2):268–76.
15. Ho EC, Kapila A, Colquhoun-Flannery W. Tracheal ring fracture and early tracheomalacia following percutaneous dilatational tracheostomy. BMC Ear Nose Throat Disord. 2005;5:6.
16. Korean Bronchoesophagological Society Guideline Task F, Nam IC, Shin YS, Jeong WJ, Park MW, Park SY, et al. Guidelines for tracheostomy from the Korean Bronchoesophagological society. Clin Exp Otorhinolaryngol. 2020;13(4):361–75.
17. Mathog RH, Kenan PD, Hudson WR. Delayed massive hemorrhage following tracheostomy. Laryngoscope. 1971;81(1):107–19.
18. Utley JR, Singer MM, Roe BB, Fraser DG, Dedo HH. Definitive management of innominate artery hemorrhage complicating tracheostomy. JAMA. 1972;220(4):577–9.
19. Singh N, Fung A, Cole IE. Innominate artery hemorrhage following tracheostomy. Otolaryngol Head Neck Surg. 2007;136(4 Suppl):S68–72.
20. Roh JL, Na MH, Kim KH. Treating tracheo-innominate artery fistula with interposition of a pectoralis major myocutaneous flap. Eur Arch Otorrinolaringol. 2006;263(2):180–2.
21. Wall LP, Gasparis A, Criado E. Endovascular therapy for tracheoinnominate artery fistula: a temporizing measure. Ann Vasc Surg. 2005;19(1):99–102.
22. Higgins KM, Punthakee X. Meta-analysis comparison of open versus percutaneous tracheostomy. Laryngoscope. 2007;117(3):447–54.
23. Ciaglia P, Graniero KD. Percutaneous dilatational tracheostomy. Results and long-term follow-up. Chest. 1992;101(2):464–7.
24. Romero CM, Cornejo RA, Ruiz MH, Galvez LR, Llanos OP, Tobar EA, et al. Fiberoptic bronchoscopy-assisted percutaneous tracheostomy is safe in obese critically ill patients: a prospective and comparative study. J Crit Care. 2009;24(4):494–500.
25. Muhammad JK, Major E, Wood A, Patton DW. Percutaneous dilatational tracheostomy: haemorrhagic complications and the vascular anatomy of the anterior neck. A review based on 497 cases. Int J Oral Maxillofac Surg. 2000;29(3):217–22.
26. Yilmaz M, Dosemeci L, Cengiz M, Sanli S, Gajic O, Ramazanoglu A. Repeat percutaneous tracheostomy in the neurocritically ill patient. Neurocrit Care. 2006;5(2):120–3.
27. Patel A, Swan P, Dunning J. Does a percutaneous tracheostomy have a lower incidence of complications compared to an open surgical technique? Interact Cardiovasc Thorac Surg. 2005;4(6):563–8.
28. Simon M, Metschke M, Braune SA, Puschel K, Kluge S. Death after percutaneous dilatational tracheostomy: a systematic review and analysis of risk factors. Crit Care. 2013;17(5):R258.
29. Rudas M, Seppelt I. Safety and efficacy of ultrasonography before and during percutaneous dilatational tracheostomy in adult patients: a systematic review. Crit Care Resusc. 2012;14(4):297–301.
30. Shen G, Yin H, Cao Y, Zhang M, Wu J, Jiang X, et al. Percutaneous dilatational tracheostomy versus fibre optic bronchoscopy-guided percutaneous dilatational tracheostomy in critically ill patients: a randomised controlled trial. Ir J Med Sci. 2019;188(2):675–81.
31. Al-Ansari MA, Hijazi MH. Clinical review: percutaneous dilatational tracheostomy. Crit Care. 2006;10(1):202.

10 Airway Surgery for Airway Stenosis or Foreign Body

Eui-Suk Sung and Seong Keun Kwon

10.1 KQ 10.1. How to Manage Tracheal and Bronchial Wall Injury During Endoscopic Airway Surgery During Foreign Body Removal?

Eui-Suk Sung

10.1.1 Prevention of Tracheal and Bronchial Wall Injury

A ventilating bronchoscope was used during airway foreign body (FB) surgery. (Fig. 10.1) Specifically, in children, tracheal wall injury can be reduced by using a bronchoscope that is appropriate for the patient's age. Prior to removal, the application of 4% lidocaine gel to the tracheal wall was also found to be beneficial. Since the tracheal wall is oriented posteriorly as it descends, it is important for the assistant to support the patient's back with their hands during the surgery to properly align the trachea. (Fig. 10.2) Additionally, the type of FB is an important factor in preventing injury. In cases of sharp foreign bodies, there is a risk of bronchial wall damage during removal from a narrow bronchial passage. Therefore, the endoscope must be carefully maneuvered to ensure that the sharp part of the FB does not contact or scratch the wall. If organic material remains on the bronchial wall for a long time, it absorbs moisture, causing the FB to grow and adhere to the bronchial wall due to an inflammatory reaction. This increases the risk of damage to the bronchial wall during removal. To minimize such damage, FBs should not be removed blindly. Instead, endoscopy should be used to monitor the movement of the FB and its gradual removal, taking into account its diameter and orientation. A device suitable for FBs, such as peanut forceps, should be used (Fig. 10.3). For larger FBs, the bronchoscope was withdrawn simultaneously along with the FB.

E.-S. Sung (✉)
Department of Otolaryngology—Head and Neck Surgery, Pusan National University Yangsan Hospital, College of Medicine, Pusan National University, Yangsan, Gyeongnam, Republic of Korea
e-mail: sunges@pusan.ac.kr

S. K. Kwon (✉)
Department of Otorhinolaryngology—Head and Neck Surgery, Seoul National University College of Medicine, Seoul, Korea, Seoul, Republic of Korea

K.-J. Cho, J.-O. Park (eds.), *Management of Head and Neck Surgery Complications*,
https://doi.org/10.1007/978-981-96-1860-6_10

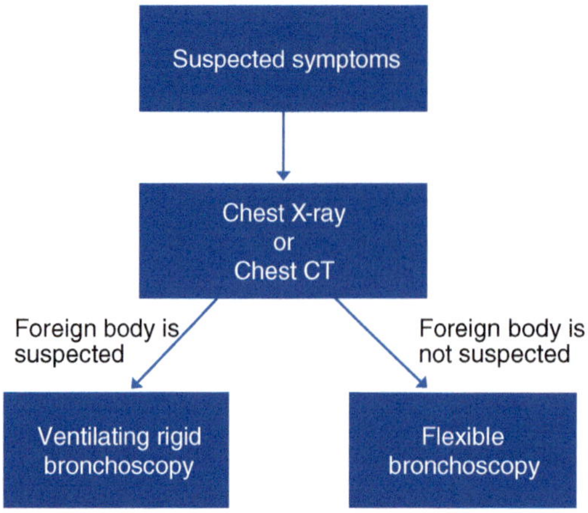

Fig. 10.1 Flow protocol for foreign body suspected symptoms. *CT* computed tomography

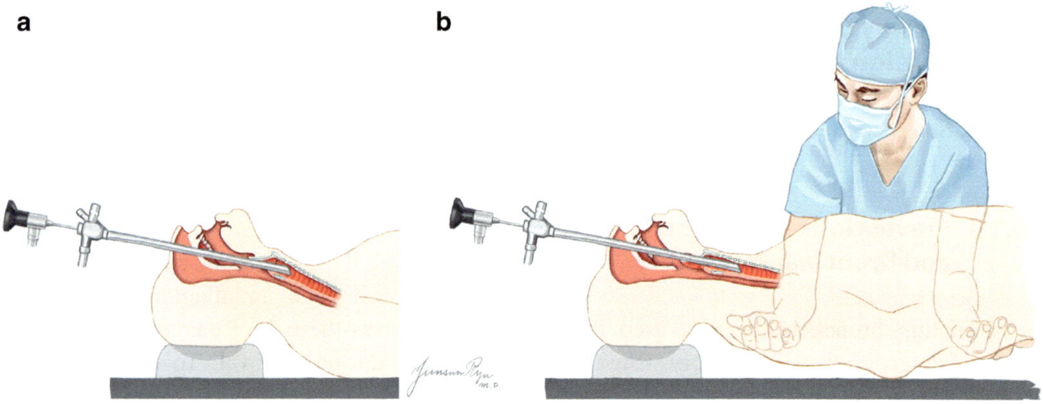

Fig. 10.2 (**a**) Position of the patient in the absence of assistance. (**b**) Position of the patient in the presence of an assistant

Fig. 10.3 Ventilating bronchoscopic instrument. (**a**) Proximal bronchoscope fittings. (**b**) Rigid sucker. (**c**) Rigid ventilating bronchoscope. (**d**) Side-arm forceps. (**e**) Optical forceps

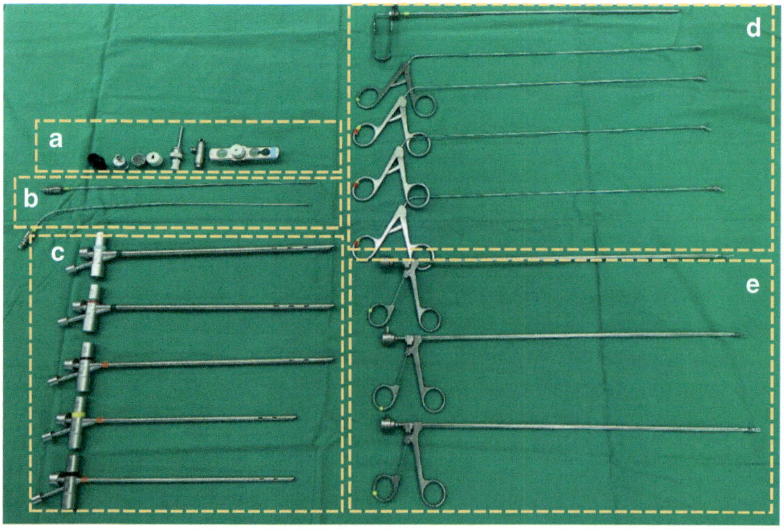

It is essential to prevent damage to the tracheal wall by selecting an endoscope of appropriate size for the patient's age, followed by spraying 4% lidocaine gel to anesthetize the tracheal wall prior to the procedure, adjusting the patient's posture to align with the angle of the endoscope, and using endoscopic instruments that are best suited for the specific foreign body.

Expert Opinion

In smaller pediatric patients, it may be difficult to use forceps attached to the endoscope. If a blind procedure is unavoidable, it is important to stop immediately if resistance is felt when pulling the foreign body with forceps. Repeated endoscopic observation should be performed to confirm the location of the foreign body. (Tack-Kyun Kwon).

Applying 4% lidocaine gel to rigid bronchoscope or spraying 4% lidocaine onto the tracheal wall before removal of foreign body is useful. In cases where the patient is very heavy, the assistant may be unable to continuously support the patient's back with his or her arm. For a lightweight child, it is possible for the assistant to support the back, although this is not the preferred method. This is because if the force used to hold the patient's back is suddenly released, the rigid bronchoscope can cause damage to the mucosa or cartilage ring. The angle of neck flexion is adjusted, and the holder of the suspension laryngoscope is tightened or loosened to advance the rigid bronchoscope tip so that it does not injure the airway mucosa. (Seong Keun Kwon).

It is not possible to prevent the sharp foreign body (FB) from damaging the airway mucosa by just adjusting the endoscope. Hence, the sharp part of the FB must be inserted into the rigid bronchoscope, and then the rigid bronchoscope and FB must be removed together. (Seong Keun Kwon).

The key to removing an FB is to gently suction around the organic FB to remove secretions, carefully check if there is space between the FB and the bronchus and advance the forceps through this space to remove the FB. If there is no space between the FB and the bronchus, the forceps are positioned in front of the FB, the forceps are spread to slightly expand the bronchus, and advanced to sufficiently grasp the FB before removing it. (Seong Keun Kwon).

For very large FBs that do not fit through a bronchoscope, the FB is grasped with forceps and removed with a bronchoscope. If the FB gets caught in the vocal folds and does not pass through, we try removing it by turning the FB and bronchoscope at 90 degrees. (Seong Keun Kwon).

Expert Opinion

To successfully remove an FB without injuring the tracheobronchial wall, selecting an appropriately sized bronchoscope based on the patient's age and growth status is essential. During the insertion of the bronchoscope through the glottis, extending the neck or elevating the chest can facilitate smooth passage through the trachea and bronchus, minimizing the risk of mucosal injury. When removing a sharp FB, it is crucial to ensure that it remains within the bronchoscope. If this is not feasible, at least the sharp end, which poses a risk of injuring the tracheobronchus, should be grasped with forceps or covered by the bronchoscope. (Yoon Se Lee).

Expert Opinion

Performing a flexible bronchoscopy before a ventilating rigid bronchoscopy is recommended, as it provides insight into the location of the foreign body (FB) and helps in planning subsequent steps for its removal if present. (Wei-Chung Hsu).

The CO_2 laser is employed frequently in SGS, while the KTP laser is rarely employed. Alternatively, cold knife incisions are implemented frequently. Similar outcomes are observed in the treatment of SGS with both CO_2 laser and cold knife. (Seong Keun Kwon).

10.1.2 Management of Stenosis Caused by Tracheal and Bronchial Wall Injury

Grades 1 and 2 stenosis can be managed using micro laryngeal bronchoscopy (MLB). The MLB is also used for selected grade 3 stenoses. CO_2 and potassium titanium phosphate lasers are widely used in laryngeal surgery. These lasers are effective in treating early granulation tissue formation, thin webs, and crescentic bands. Risk factors for the failure of subglottic stenosis laser treatment include previous failed outcomes, significant loss of the cartilaginous skeleton, thick circumferential scars greater than 1 cm in length, and posterior commissure involvement. Complications of subglottic stenosis laser treatment include exposure of the perichondrium or cartilage, which can cause chondritis, thermal injury, and tissue scarring. Lasers are also effective for low-grade and noncircumferential stenoses [1].

Traditional methods of managing subglottic stenosis include laser excision and stenting. Although these techniques are effective and still employed by many surgeons, the shearing force exerted on the stenosis during these procedures can cause scarring and may require continuous dilation or extensive open airway surgery. Traditional methods are traumatic to the already formed scars and inflamed tissues. Airway dilation procedures are used to manage airway stenosis.

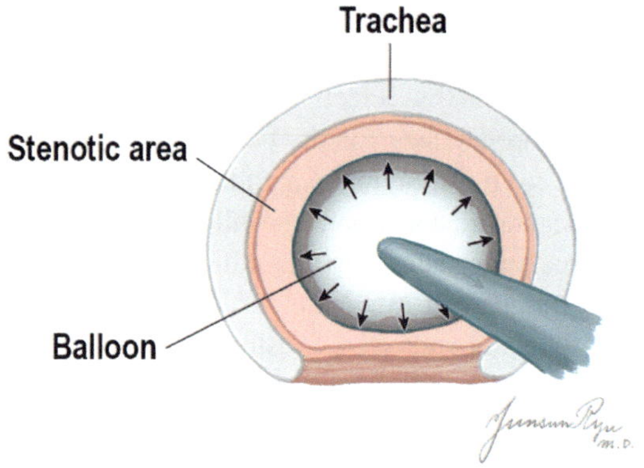

Fig. 10.4 Application of radial pressure of a balloon catheter

Balloon catheters are designed to apply radial pressure to the stenosis [2, 3] (Fig. 10.4), and the diameter is chosen based on the expected age-related size of the airway. Compared with traditional subglottic stenosis treatment, the application of radial pressure to the area of stenosis leads to less scarring and better long-term outcomes, often avoiding the need for airway reconstruction [4]. Gel is applied to the balloon catheter to cushion the stenotic tissue and catheter during balloon laryngoplasty.

10.2 10.2. How to Prevent and Manage Acute Airway Obstruction Following Endoscopic Airway Surgery?

Eui-Suk Sung

Airway obstruction may occur due to tracheal wall spasms during endoscopic airway surgery, often resulting from irritation. Therefore, it is important to avoid direct contact between the tracheal wall and suction devices or forceps. Since, airway obstruction is likely to occur even after surgery, it is necessary to reduce airway edema by administering intravenous steroids during and after surgery. If airway spasms occur after surgery, intubation should be attempted using an endotracheal tube smaller than the appropriate size for the patient's age. In patients with a tracheostomy tube, the cannula may become blocked, necessitating a change to the cannula currently in use or to a smaller cannula. Positive-pressure ventilation using an Ambu bag should be attempted.

Expert Opinion
As the depth of anesthesia decreases and the trachea is stimulated by suction with a metal tip or by bronchoscope friction, laryngospasm and bronchospasm are likely to occur, resulting in hypoxia, dyspnea, and other symptoms. Post-extubation laryngeal edema may be observed after traumatic and multiple attempts of intubation. In patients receiving prolonged periods of intubation, where high cuff pressures may cause edema of laryngeal mucosa. Local trauma following foreign body ingestion can cause significant airway compromise in some cases. Upper airway stimulation in the presence of secretions or inhalation of foreign material may cause laryngeal spasm with adduction of the vocal cords, preventing passage of air to the lungs, leading to hypoxemia. If the patient experiences an airway spasm subsequent to surgery, the physician must employ their hand to elevate the mandible (jaw thrust). The lateral position pushes the tongue and jaw forward due to gravity, hence improving the airway. Before definitive control of the airway is possible, 100% oxygen should be provided with a tightly fitting mask to optimize body oxygen stores. Concurrently, dexamethasone 5 mg is administered intravenously, a smaller endotracheal tube is used to intubate orally, and an endotracheal spray containing salbutamol is used. The patient should be extubated after they have fully recovered from their respiratory distress. (Seong Keun Kwon).

After surgery, the patient was moved to the intensive care unit or general ward for continued monitoring and frequent tracheostomies. The primary reasons for acute airway obstruction after MLB are accidental decannulation of the cannula and blockage of the tracheostomy tube by sputum.

Expert Opinion
During surgery, steroid injections into the stenosis area followed by balloon dilation are employed to prevent recurrent laryngotracheal stenosis after endoscopic procedures. Repeated consecutive endoscopic procedures to remove granulation tissue can further reduce the risk of restenosis post-surgery. (Yoon Se Lee).

The head of the bed was elevated by 30° to reduce the risk of gastric reflux and improve ventilation. Humidified air was administered through the face or through a tracheostomy mask. Immediately after surgery, a large amount of mucus in the larynx was found. Therefore, a humidifying nebulizer was used, and suction was applied to prevent the tubes from becoming blocked with mucus.

Expert Opinion
A nebulizer with mucolytics and a proton pump inhibitor is utilized. When bacterial cultures identify specific microbes, targeted antibiotics can help heal mucosal injuries without leading to secondary infections. (Yoon Se Lee).

The tracheostomy tube was downsized or changed to a cuffless tube at least 72 h post-surgery. This allowed for the formation of a tract, making insertion of the second tube easier. The tracheostomy tube should not be removed until a patent and adequate airway is established. In other words, patients should be able to breathe, and their airways should be protected from aspiration before tube removal. Clinical signs such as the ability to tolerate an obstructed tube and the absence of bronchorrhea, choking, or other signs of aspiration suggest that the patient is ready for decannulation. Flexible laryngoscopy is an excellent tool to confirm airway patency. Patients requiring long-term tracheostomy tube placement should be trained to manage these artificial airways. Caregivers should be familiar with potential complications and skilled in emergency procedures such as removal and reinsertion of the tracheostomy tube.

- Prevention:
  - It is important to be careful not to directly contact the tracheal wall with suction devices or forceps.
  - It is necessary to reduce airway edema by administering intravenous steroids pre- and post-surgery.
  - If airway spasm occurs post-surgery, intubation should be attempted with an endotracheal tube smaller than the size appropriate for the patient's age.
- Management:
  - The head of the bed is elevated by 30° to reduce the chance of gastric reflux and improve ventilation.
  - Humidified air is administered through a face or tracheostomy mask.
  - The tracheostomy tube can be downsized or changed to a cuffless tube at least 72 h post-surgery.

Expert Opinion
If the cannula is obstructed and causing respiratory distress the T-cannula should be replaced promptly, even immediately after tracheostomy. It is important to ensure that the T-cannula can be exchanged promptly following the tracheostomy in children, especially when fenestration sutures are consistently employed. (Seong Keun Kwon).

10.3 KQ 10.3. How to Prevent Recurrent Laryngeal Nerve Damage, Tracheal Ischemia, and Anastomotic Dehiscence after Partial Cricotracheal Resection

Seong Keun Kwon

10.3.1 Preconditioning and Patient Selection Before Open-Airway Surgery

The initial requirement for intubation should be met in cases of acquired stenosis, and mature scar tissue must be formed. Careful waiting is advised if the larynx is reactive and swollen in combination with cardiac disease or aspiration. Tracheal culture must be performed before open airway surgery to select the appropriate antibiotics. If the culture results show methicillin-resistant *Staphylococcus aureus*, *Pseudomonas* spp., or any antibiotic-resistant bacteria, appropriate antibiotics must be administered for 5 days before open-airway surgery.

Temporary contraindications to open airway surgery are outlined below:

- Contraindication of open airway surgery
  - Local factors
    Severe reflux laryngitis
    Immature stenosis
    Facial skeletal anomalies causing significant airway obstruction
    Infected airway
    Aspiration
  - Systemic factors
    Cardiopulmonary disease that requires ventilatory support
    Severe neurological impairment

Expert Opinion
Anti-reflux medication for at least 1–2 weeks are strongly suggested if GERD or LPRD are suspected before and after open airway surgery. (Wei-Chung Hsu).

10.3.2 Airway Mobilization: Distal Tracheal Dissection and Infrahyoid Release

To reduce the risk of recurrent laryngeal nerve (RNL) injury, dissection against the trachea must be performed precisely, without revealing the nerves, which are frequently encased in scar tissue. Dissection can be safely performed all the way to the lower margins of the cricoid cartilage. High lateral or posterior cricoid ring dissections should be avoided, as they are prone to damaging the RNLs that run posterior to the cricothyroid joints. To avoid injury to the RLNs at the cricoid cartilage level, the cricothyroid muscles should be dissected from the cricoid cartilage and reflected laterally to protect the RLN (Fig. 10.5).

Expert Opinion

During airway stenosis surgery, damage to the recurrent laryngeal nerve (RLN) commonly occurs during the separation of surrounding soft tissue from the scar tissue around the airway. This risk is particularly high in pediatric patients, as they often have a history of multiple airway surgeries. Therefore, when separating scarred soft tissue from the airway, a powered instrument should not be used; instead, a sharp cold steel instrument should be employed. Additionally, when drilling scar tissue within the cricoid ring, the cartilage near the cricothyroid joint should not be shaved too thin, to prevent heat transfer from the drill. Adequate irrigation should be provided during the procedure to prevent heat-related nerve damage. (Tack-Kyun Kwon).

After an isthmusectomy and lateralization of the thyroid gland, Berry's ligament is meticulously dissected laterally using bipolar cauterization and a cold dissector. This procedure ensures the safe separation of the RLN from the upper trachea and cricotracheal junction. (Yoon Se Lee).

The lateral vascular supply from the tracheoesophageal grooves needs to be carefully protected to prevent tracheal ischemia, particularly if the intrathoracic trachea is extensively mobilized. The membranous trachea is dissected and separated from the anterior wall of the esophagus over a distance corresponding to the height of the cricoid plate, and dissection is performed caudally to the level of the tracheostoma. Vascular supply to the trachea should be carefully maintained beyond this lower limit. Excessive separation of the trachea from the esophagus must be avoided to maintain optimal vascular supply to the tracheal stump (Fig. 10.6).

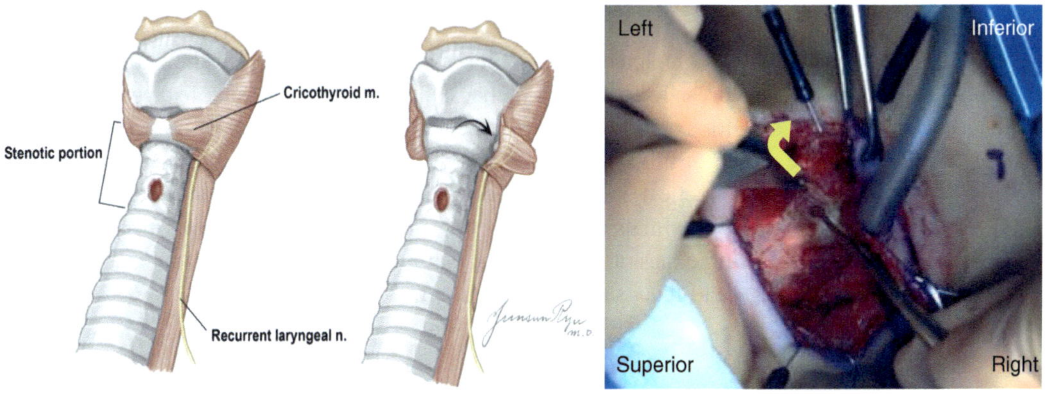

Fig. 10.5 The cricothyroid muscles are reflected laterally to protect the recurrent laryngeal nerves (black and yellow arrows). *m* muscle, *n* nerve

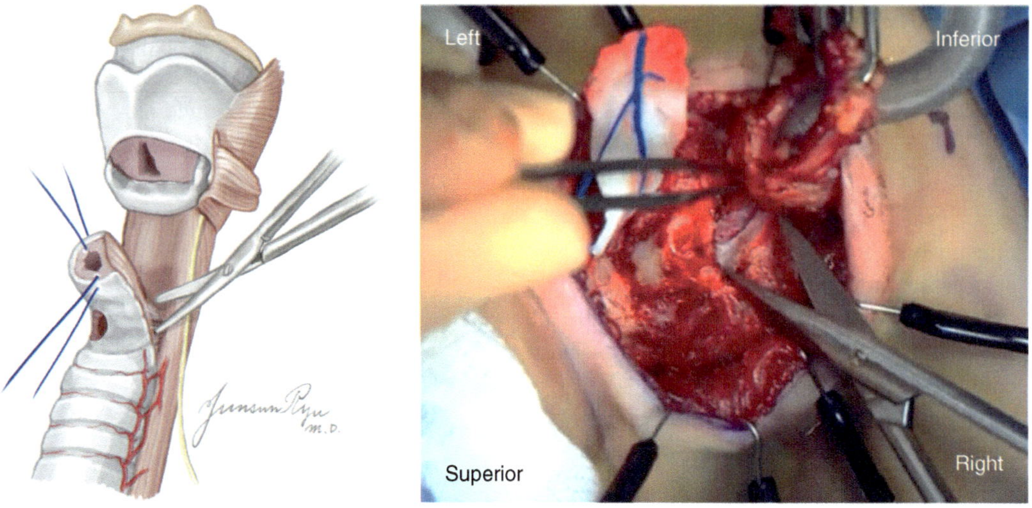

Fig. 10.6 Tracheoesophageal separation. The dissection is extended caudally to the tracheostoma level while ensuring the preservation of vascular supply to the distal tracheal stump

10.3.3 Anastomosis

Two posterolateral stitches using 3.0 Vicryl Plus must be placed to alleviate tension on the posterior suture line before conducting the posterior anastomosis, which is delicate and prone to mucosal tears. The first stitch must emerge from the submucosal plane of the inner surface of the trachea after passing through the posterolateral aspect of the second normal tracheal ring. The same stitch is then placed on the posterolateral subglottic mucosa on the laryngeal side and laterally threaded through the cricoid plate. It should arise from the outer surface of the cricoid plate in the subperichondrial plane to prevent RLN damage (Fig. 10.7).

The posterior anastomosis is completed using interrupted 5.0 Vicryl Plus sutures. To match the thickness of the thinner subglottic mucosa precisely, the stitch must be placed at full thickness through the mucosa on the tracheal side. To achieve excellent mucosal approximation, the stitch must be placed at half-thickness through the posterior cricoid cartilage and mucosa at the subglottic level (Fig. 10.8).

The anterior anastomosis is completed by placing 8–10 sutures using 4.0 Vicryl Plus through the first tracheal rings and thyroid cartilage. They must be positioned at equal intervals. All the sutures are placed before being tied outside. The anterior subcommissural defect is filled with a triangular wedge of pedicle cartilage cut to the correct size. The thyroid cartilage is subsequently sutured using two or three 5.0 Vicryl Plus sutures (Fig. 10.9).

10.3.4 Measures to Prevent Anastomotic Dehiscence and Leakage

Sterile saline is poured into the surgical field to check for anastomosis site leakage while the patient is ventilated with positive pressure. If air leakage is observed, an additional suture is placed near the leakage site. If the tension at the anastomotic site is minimal and the mucosal edge is well approximated, no additional measures are required.

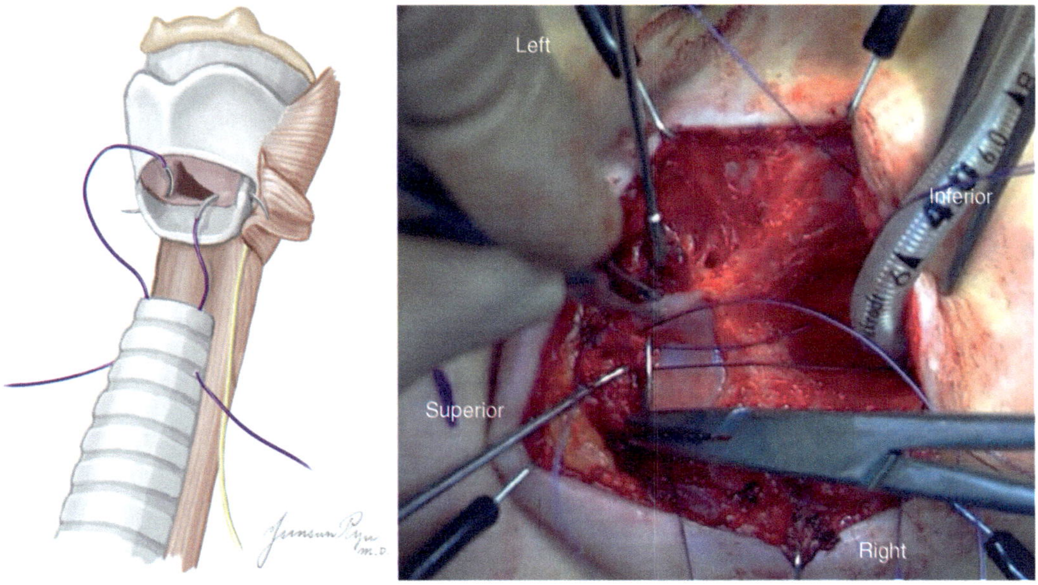

Fig. 10.7 Posterolateral stitches are the most important stitches to prevent recurrent stenosis. To protect the recurrent laryngeal nerves, they must emerge from the cricoid plate along a subperichondrial plane, having initially traversed the posterolateral subglottic mucosa

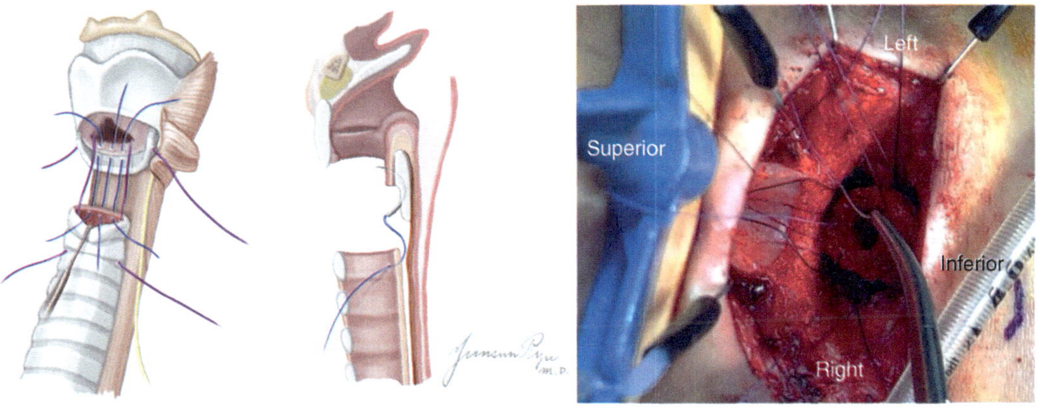

Fig. 10.8 Posterior stitches. To ensure excellent mucosal approximation, the three posterior stitches are placed full-thick through the mucosa on the tracheal side and half-thick through the posterior cricoid plate and mucosa on the laryngeal side

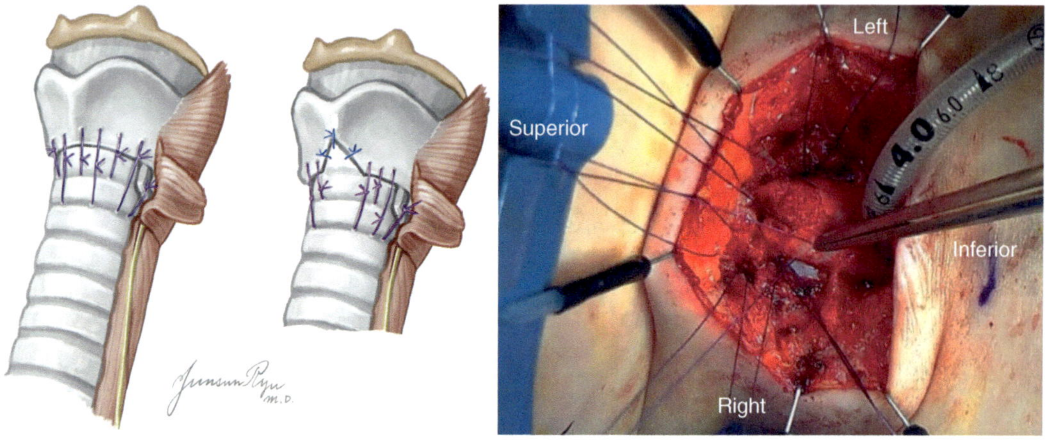

Fig. 10.9 Thyrotracheal anastomosis. Eight to 10 sutures using 4.0 Vicryl Plus are placed at an even distance. After being trimmed to the size of the subcommissural defect, the triangular wedge of the pedicled trachea is subsequently sutured in place using two or three 5.0 Vicryl Plus sutures

If some tension is present at the anastomotic site, a tension-releasing suture is placed laterally between the inferior border of the cricoid plate and the third or fourth tracheal ring.

Both lobes of the thyroid gland are mobilized and sutured over the anastomosis to prevent anastomotic leakage and to provide an enhanced vascular supply.

Expert Opinion

After checking up as described above, you may apply tissue fibrin glue (fibrin sealant) over the anastomosis site to achieve a better wound healing process. (Wei-Chung Hsu).

A sufficient release maneuver is essential to reduce tension and ischemic changes at the anastomosis site, preventing restenosis or dehiscence. Additionally, for vascularization, the remaining thyroid gland or strap muscle is used to cover the anastomosis site. (Yoon Se Lee).

10.4 KQ 10.4. How to Design and Insert the Costal Cartilage Graft to Prevent Airway Collapse, Air Leakage, and Restenosis

Seong Keun Kwon

10.4.1 Exposure of the Airway Skeleton and Anterior Incision of the Stenotic Area

Elevate the flap, including the platysma muscle, and subsequently incise the midline of the strap muscle. Carefully expose the midline of the thyroid–cricoid cartilage. Perform a central vertical incision from the lower half of the thyroid and cricoid cartilages to the first or second ring of the trachea (Fig. 10.10). If necessary, tracheal endoscopy is performed simultaneously during surgery to ensure that all stenotic areas are excised. If two or fewer normal tracheal cartilage rings from the

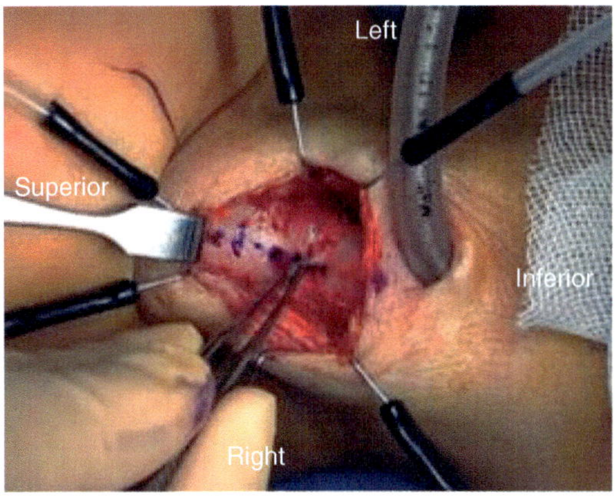

Fig. 10.10 The vertical midline incision of the airway extends through the lower half of the thyroid cartilage, cricothyroid membrane, anterior cricoid arch, and upper two or three tracheal rings

end of the stenosis to the tracheostomy are present, suprastomal collapse may occur after cartilage transplantation.

> **Expert Opinion**
> Under endoscopy-guided laryngofissure, you may precisely divide the anterior commissure of the vocal fold when the stenosis is involved up to higher larynx levels in glottic or infra-glottic levels. (Wei-Chung Hsu).
>
> Ensuring the alignment between the mucosa and the perichondrium of the graft and avoiding mucosal deficits at the anastomosis site aids in wound healing and reduces the likelihood of restenosis. (Yoon Se Lee).
>
> A reinforcement flap using the strap muscle or sternocleidomastoid muscle enhances the vascular supply to the graft. (Yoon Se Lee).

To prevent suprastomal collapse, a vertical incision can be extended to the tracheostomy site. A new tracheostomy must be performed three rings lower than the existing tracheostomy. If single-stage laryngotracheal reconstruction (Fig. 10.11a) is attempted, the tracheocutaneous tract is removed and the anterior cartilage graft is designed to cover the stoma. When two-stage laryngotracheal reconstruction (Fig. 10.11b) is planned, the size of the new tracheostomy must be minimized to prevent an A-frame deformity.

10.4.2 Cricoid Lamina Incision

The posterior wall of the airway is exposed through a gap created by an incision in the anterior part of the cricoid cartilage. A 1:100,000 epinephrine solution is injected into the anterior part of the posterior cricoid lamina using a dental syringe, and the cricoid cartilage is punctured with a needle. Epinephrine solution is also injected into the posterior part of the cricoid plate to prevent accidental incision of the mucosa posterior to the cricoid (Fig. 10.12). This measure can help prevent the posterior migration of the posterior cartilage graft.

If stenosis occurs in the interarytenoid muscle, it may also require an incision. If an incision of the interarytenoid muscle is necessary, extreme care must be taken to avoid incising the mucous membrane of the upper part of the interarytenoid muscle. This procedure prevents the transplanted cartilage from migrating to the top or back.

10.4.3 Graft Harvest and Design

The harvested costal cartilage is divided into two and designed to fit the anterior and posterior cricoid incision windows. The anterior grafted cartilage fragment is designed to be fusiform, and the posterior grafted cartilage fragment is designed to be rectangular (Fig. 10.13). The area where the perichondrium is attached is directed toward the airway to minimize the formation of granulation tissue within the airway. A flange is created at the graft edge to prevent the costal cartilage from slipping through the tracheal incision. In the case of posterior grafts, firmly suturing the cartilage graft to the posterior cricoid proves extremely difficult; therefore, it is ideal to create a wedge-shaped step to ensure that it is fixed in place with a clicking sensation (Fig. 10.14). If the fixation of

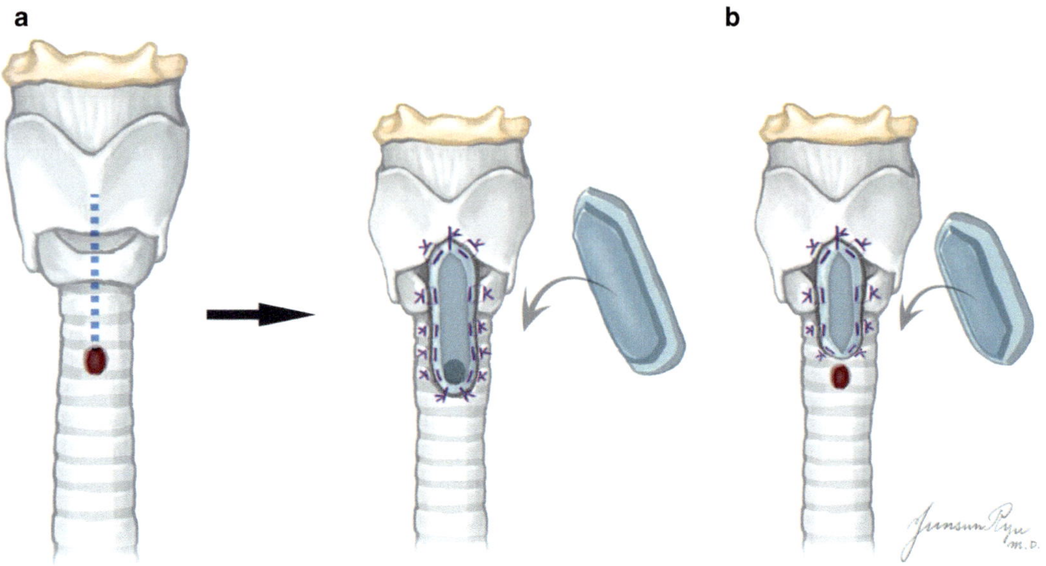

Fig. 10.11 (**a**) Single and (**b**) double-stage laryngotracheal reconstruction

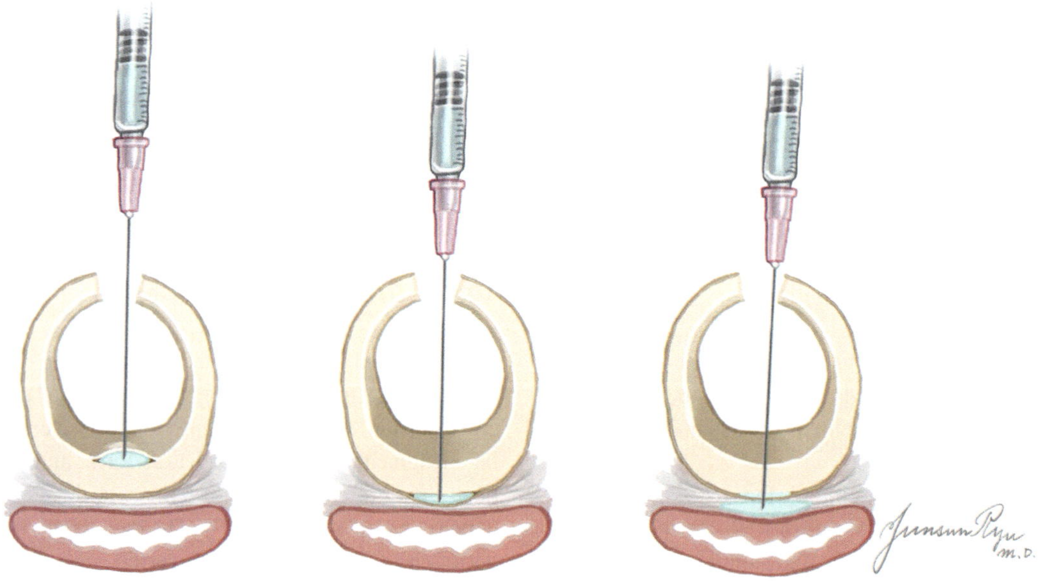

Fig. 10.12 Epinephrine injection on posterior airway before incision. A 1:100,000 epinephrine is injected with a dental syringe anterior to the cricoid plate, and the needle is punctured through the cricoid plate. Subsequently, epinephrine is injected posterior to the cricoid plate to increase the distance from the cricoid cartilage by hydrodissection. This measure can help reduce the risk of tearing the posterior mucosa during a cricoid incision

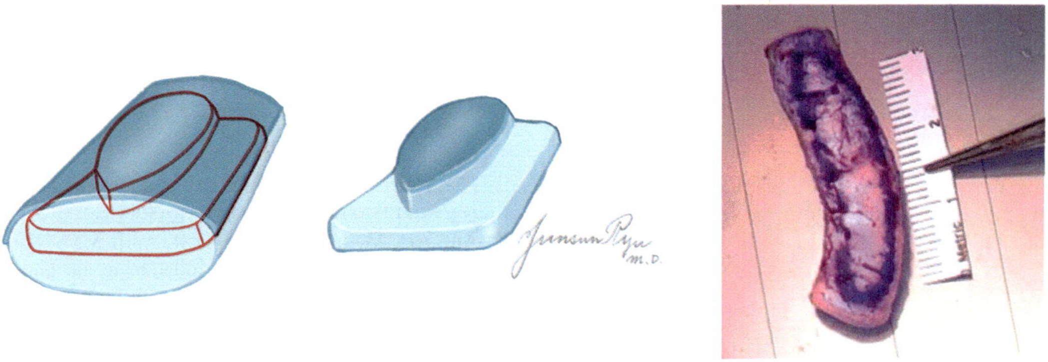

Fig. 10.13 Anterior costal cartilage graft. The area where the perichondrium is attached is directed toward the airway to minimize the formation of granulation tissue within the airway. A flange is created at the edge of the fusiform-shaped graft to prevent costal cartilage from slipping through the tracheal incision

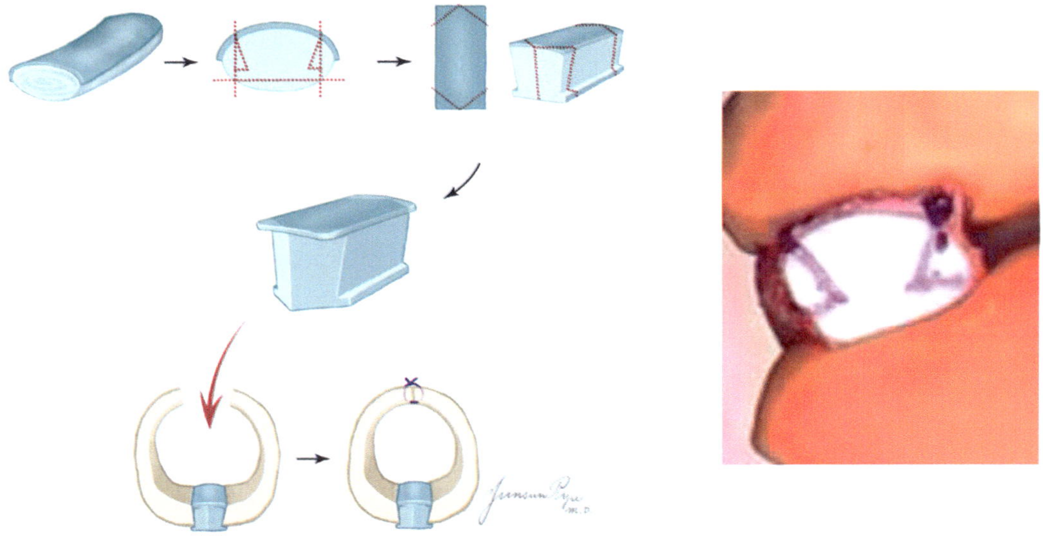

Fig. 10.14 Posterior costal cartilage graft. A wedge-shaped step is created to ensure that it is fixed in place with a clicking sensation without suture

the posterior graft cartilage is unstable, a suture is performed using 4-0 Vicryl Plus.

10.4.4 Suture of Graft

After the stent is placed and secured, the cartilage is incised anteriorly into the cricoid cartilage incision by knotting it with 4-0 Vicryl plus. The knot is placed over the thyroid, cricoid, and tracheal cartilages, rather than over the graft, when suturing the anterior grafts using the horizontal mattress technique (Fig. 10.15). The cricoid cartilage area is crucial for anchoring the anterior cartilage graft; hence, it is first stitched with sutures and then the other areas are knitted. The airway mucosa should be threaded such that it is in good contact with the perichondrium. After disinfecting the surgical site with Betadine and administering saline solution, hyperventilation

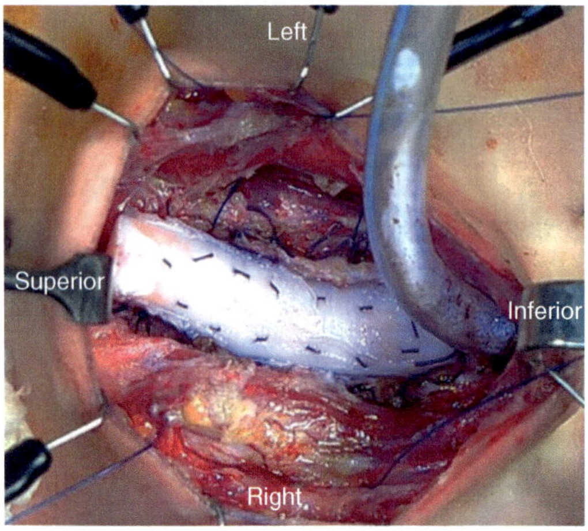

Fig. 10.15 Anterior costal cartilage graft after horizontal mattress suture. The knot is placed over the thyroid, cricoid, and tracheal cartilages rather than over the graft

should be requested from the anesthesiologist, and checks should be performed for air leaks around the cartilage graft.

> **Expert Opinion**
> Thereafter, tissue fibrin glue (a tissue sealant) may be applied over the anastomosis edges. (Wei-Chung Hsu).

References

1. Simpson GT, Strong MS, Healy GB, Shapshay SM, Vaughan CW. Predictive factors of success or failure in the endoscopic management of laryngeal and tracheal stenosis. Ann Otol Rhinol Laryngol. 1982;91(4 Pt 1):384–8. https://doi.org/10.1177/000348948209100412.
2. Ang AH, Modi VK, Raithatha R, April MM, Ward RF. A pilot study of balloon dilation in an animal model resulting in cricoid cartilage fracture: implications for the stenotic pediatric airway. Laryngoscope. 2010;120(10):2094–7. https://doi.org/10.1002/lary.21066.
3. Lee JC, Kim MS, Kim DJ, Park DH, Lee IW, Roh HJ, et al. Subglottic stenosis in children: our experience at a pediatric tertiary center for 8 years in South Korea. Int J Pediatr Otorhinolaryngol. 2019;121:64–7. https://doi.org/10.1016/j.ijporl.2019.02.044.
4. Lang M, Brietzke SE. A systematic review and meta-analysis of endoscopic balloon dilation of pediatric subglottic stenosis. Otolaryngol Head Neck Surg. 2014;150(2):174–9. https://doi.org/10.1177/0194599813510867.

Part V

Neck Dissection

Neck Dissection: Neurologic Complications

11

Dong Kun Lee and Yoon Se Lee

11.1 KQ 11.1. How to Prevent and Manage Nerve Injuries, Including Lingual, Hypoglossal, and Facial Nerves, in Level I Dissection

Dong Kun Lee

11.1.1 Facial Nerves

During elevation of the subplatysmal skin flap around the mandible, it is crucial to prevent damage to the marginal mandibular branch of the facial nerve. Hooks or army retractors assist in retracting and visualizing the skin flaps.

Maintaining a dissection plane superficial to the fascia covering the submandibular gland is essential. The facial vessels serve as a landmark for locating the facial nerve. The facial nerve is positioned deep to the fascia but superficial to the facial vessels where these vessels cross the inferior border of the mandible [1]. Accurate identification of the marginal branch of the facial nerve is vital to avoid injury.

Expert Opinion

Following neck dissection (ND), temporary apraxia occurs in 29% of cases, and persistent paralysis in 16% of cases. Temporary dysfunction typically resolves within 3–6 months. (Jun-Ook Park).

In the correct subplatysmal plane, the nerve is located within a few centimeters of the mandibular border (Fig. 11.1).

D. K. Lee (✉)
Department of Otolaryngology-Head and Neck Surgery, Dong-A University Hospital, College of Medicine, The Dong-A University, Busan, Republic of Korea

Y. S. Lee (✉)
Department of Otolaryngology—Head and Neck Surgery, Asan Medical Center, University of Ulsan, College of Medicine, Seoul, Republic of Korea
e-mail: yselee@amc.seoul.kr

K.-J. Cho, J.-O. Park (eds.), *Management of Head and Neck Surgery Complications*,
https://doi.org/10.1007/978-981-96-1860-6_11

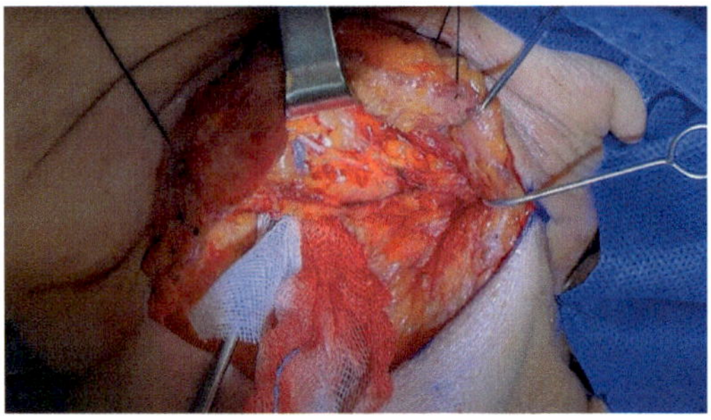

Fig. 11.1 Left level IB dissection. The marginal branch of the facial nerve is identified within 1 cm of the mandible's border

> **Expert Opinion**
> During surgery for squamous cell carcinoma in the oral tongue and floor of the mouth, thorough dissection of the lymph nodes around the marginal mandibular branch is essential; specifically, the six subgroups of level Ib (preglandular, prevascular, retroglandular, retrovascular, deep, and intraglandular). After identifying and preserving the marginal mandibular branch, meticulous removal of the lymph nodes around the facial artery and vein is required. (Jun-Ook Park).

Identifying the marginal mandibular branch can be challenging, particularly near the superior aspect of the mandibular body. The facial artery and vein run posteriorly from the submandibular gland and ascend toward its superior aspect. Generally, ligating and retracting the facial vein superiorly helps prevent injury. However, this approach is not recommended for oncological surgery, which requires complete excision of the prevascular and retrovascular lymph nodes.

Another useful landmark for identifying the marginal branch of the facial nerve is the mandibular angle. The marginal branch typically runs within a 1 cm radius of this angle. Approximately

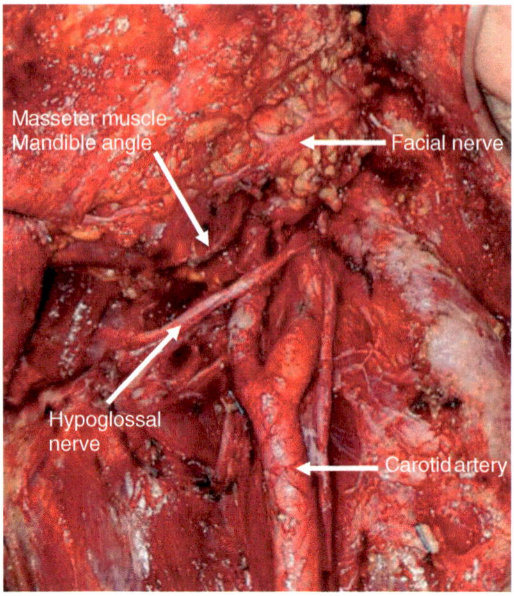

Fig. 11.2 Left level IB dissection. After removal of level IB lymph nodes, the hypoglossal nerve, masseter muscle, marginal branch of the facial nerve, carotid artery, and submandibular ganglion are identified

92% of the nerves course below the mandibular angle, whereas approximately 8% run above it. Therefore, careful dissection within a 1 cm radius around the mandibular angle is essential to prevent nerve injury [2] (Fig. 11.2). Additionally, intraoperative facial nerve monitoring can aid in locating and preserving the facial nerves during surgery.

> **Expert Opinion**
> In elderly patients with ptosis of the neck structure, the facial nerve may be 3 to 4 cm lower than its usual location, necessitating extra caution. (Jun-Ook Park).

The specimen was separated from the inferior border of the mandible to the mylohyoid muscle. The submandibular prevascular and retrovascular lymph nodes, typically located immediately below or medial to the nerve, were also exposed.

11.1.2 Lingual Nerve

After the mobilization of the submandibular gland, the contents of the submandibular triangle were dissected posteriorly. The mylohyoid muscle was retracted anteriorly to reveal the lingual nerve, Wharton's duct, and the hypoglossal nerve. The submandibular ganglion, situated just above the submandibular gland, is suspended from the lingual nerve, which is a branch of the mandibular nerve (V3), and the trigeminal nerve (cranial nerve V). When the submandibular gland is retracted posteriorly and inferiorly, the junction between the lingual nerve and the submandibular ganglion is pulled downward, causing the lingual nerve to descend in a V-shape beneath the mandible, facilitating its identification. In cases of massive lymph node metastases or severe inflammatory lesions around the lingual nerve, distinguishing the nerve from surrounding structures can be challenging. Dissecting along the proximal portion of the lingual nerve, which runs posteriorly and superiorly toward the medial pterygoid muscle, and the distal portion, which runs medially and superiorly toward the mylohyoid muscle, helps clearly identify the lingual nerve and prevent inadvertent injury. The submandibular ganglion and duct were carefully divided to ensure that the lingual nerve remained unaffected (Fig. 11.3).

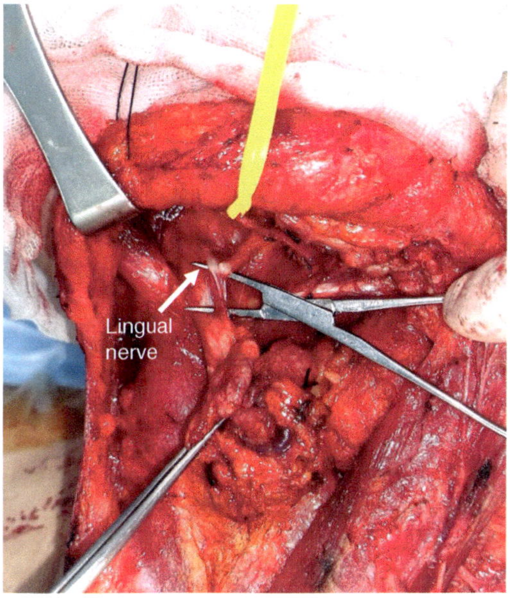

Fig. 11.3 Left level IB dissection. After retracting the mylohyoid muscle, the lingual nerve is identified before the submandibular ganglion is divided

11.1.3 Hypoglossal Nerve

The hypoglossal nerve is typically located deeper than the dissection plane. However, identifying and visualizing it helps prevent injury. At level IB, the hypoglossal nerve runs along the lateral surface of the external carotid artery at the inferior margin of the posterior belly of the digastric muscle (Fig. 11.4). Posterior progression from the digastric tendon is an effective method of identifying the hypoglossal nerve. The first prominent vein is located deep in the inferior aspect of the posterior belly, with the nerve positioned just anterior and deep to this vein. Small arterial branches retracting beneath the hypoglossal nerve may cause troublesome hemorrhage if not promptly cauterized or clipped.

> If bleeding occurs during this maneuver, avoid inadvertently clamping or cauterizing the nerve while achieving hemostasis.

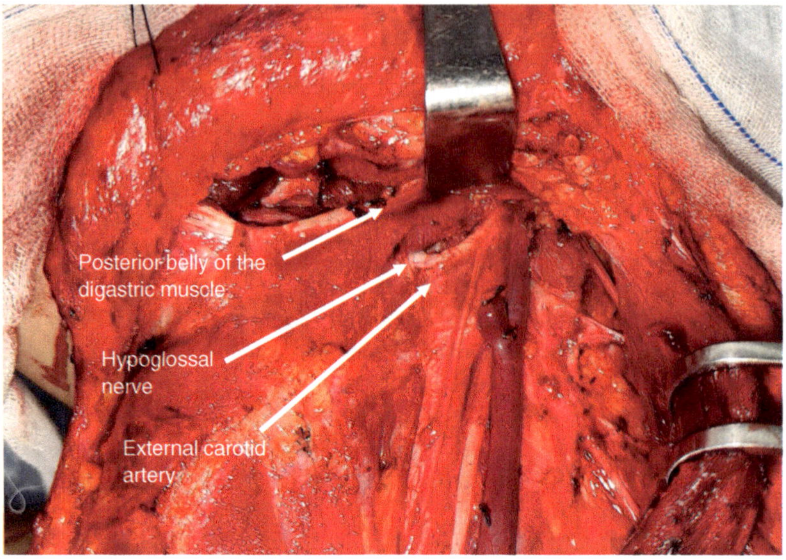

Fig. 11.4 Left level IB dissection. After retracting the posterior belly of the digastric muscle, the hypoglossal nerve is identified, crossing laterally over the external carotid artery

11.2 KQ 11.2. How Can Nerve Injuries, Including Those to the Spinal Accessory Nerve, Be Prevented and Managed During Levels II–III Dissection?

Yoon Se Lee

11.2.1 Hypoglossal Nerve

The key structures used to identify the hypoglossal nerve are the submandibular gland, the posterior belly of the digastric muscle, and the stylohyoid muscle (Fig. 11.5). The hypoglossal nerve is located beneath the posterior belly of the digastric muscle and is exposed upon elevation of the posterior belly during level IIa dissection. Neck dissection was performed either posteriorly or anteriorly around the posterior belly of the digastric muscle, subsequently exposing the internal jugular vein (IJV) [3]. Upon iatrogenic hypoglossal nerve injury, direct anastomosis and interposition grafting using the cervical plexus or greater auricular nerve should be considered. However, evidence supporting the benefits of the hypoglossal nerve reconstruction is limited [4].

> During level II dissection, the hypoglossal nerve overlying the carotid artery is identified after elevating the posterior belly of the digastric muscle using a retractor. Gentle elevation of the digastric muscle is necessary to avoid traction injury to the hypoglossal nerve.

While removing the soft tissue around the nerve, a vessel loop was used to retract the nerve, thus minimizing tension and injury (Fig. 11.6).

> When thorough dissection around the hypoglossal nerve is necessary, using vessel loops helps secure the nerve.

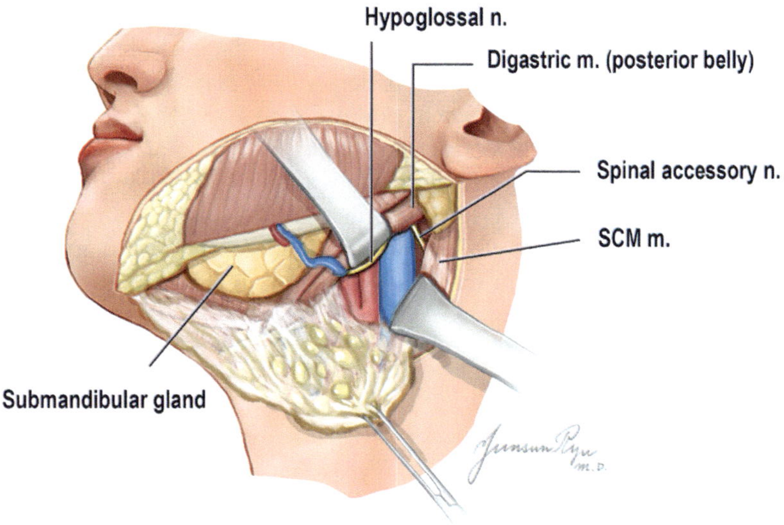

Fig. 11.5 Level II dissection. Fibro-fatty soft tissue overlying the pulling down with dissection, leaving essential structures, including the hypoglossal nerve, spinal accessory nerve, internal jugular vein, digastric muscle, and sternocleidomastoid (SCM) muscle. *n* nerve, *m* muscle

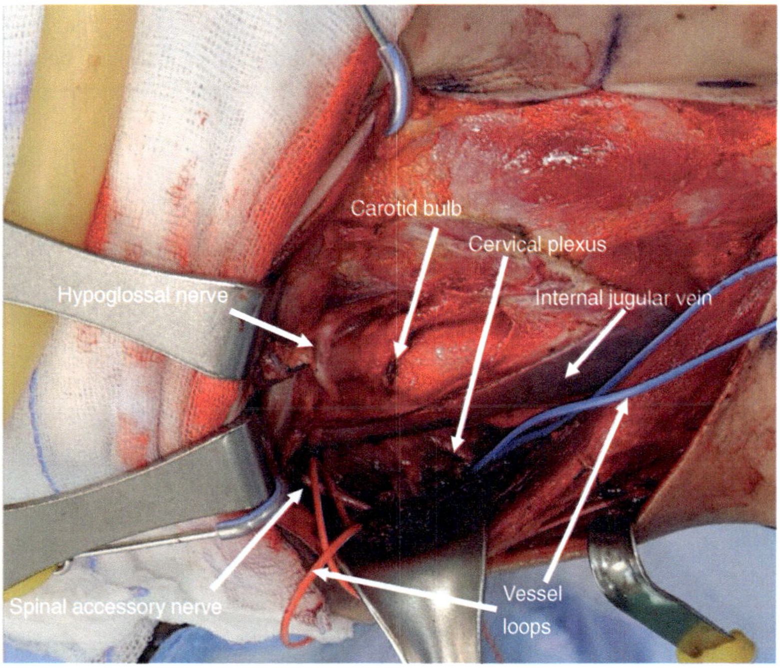

Fig. 11.6 Right level II and III dissection. The hypoglossal nerve overlying the external and internal carotid artery is identified after elevating the posterior belly of the digastric muscle. Vessel loops help in preserving the spinal accessory nerve and cervical plexus during neck dissection

Expert Opinion
The hypoglossal nerve is located deeply and is less likely to be damaged. However, when performing a modified radical neck dissection (MRND) Type I that involves resection of the IJV due to a large metastatic lymph node in level II, it is crucial to visually identify and protect the hypoglossal nerve during the neck dissection. (Sang Joon Lee).

Keep in mind the key structures for identifying SAN during level II dissection. The SAN not only runs independently but also communicates with the cervical plexus. Preserving both the SAN and its connection within the cervical plexus is necessary to prevent postoperative shoulder discomfort.

11.2.2 Spinal Accessory Nerve

The spinal accessory nerve (SAN) is usually preserved during selective neck dissection involving levels II and III or modified radical neck dissection (MRND) [5]. Assuming that the sternocleidomastoid (SCM) muscle is preserved, the key structures in identifying the SAN are the posterior belly of the digastric muscles, the IJV, and the SCM muscle (Fig. 11.7).

The SAN emerges between the posterior belly of the digastric muscle and the IJV and enters the SCM muscle. The posterior belly of the digastric muscle was easily detected by elevating the submandibular glands (SMGs). If a level Ib dissection was performed, the posterior belly of the digastric muscle was identified by pulling down the SMGs. The IJV was immediately identified deep in the posterior belly of the digastric muscle (Fig. 11.8). The SAN is typically positioned either just over, between, or posterior to the IJV (Fig. 11.7) at the posterior insertion site of the

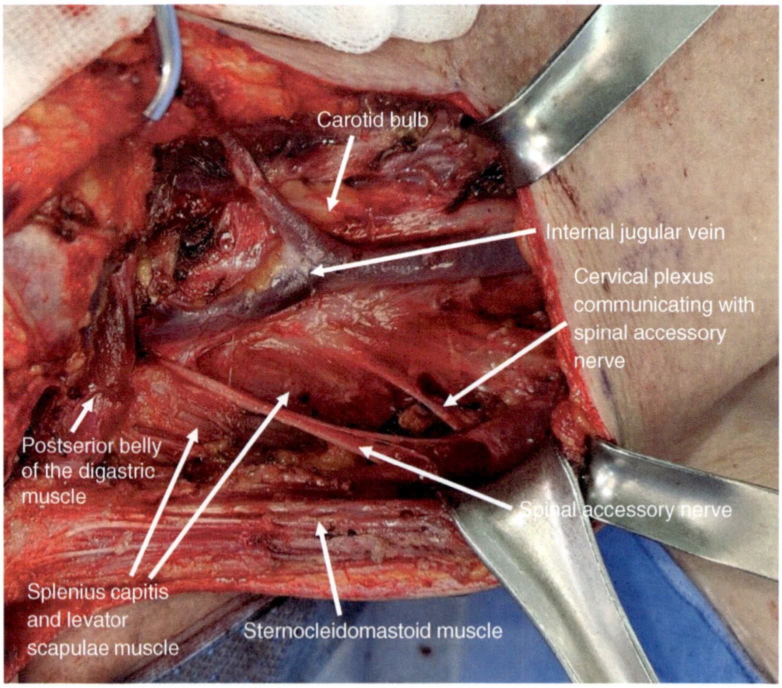

Fig. 11.7 Key structures for identifying spinal accessory nerve (SAN) during right level II and III dissection: posterior belly of the digastric muscle, sternocleidomastoid muscle, and internal jugular vein. The branch of the cervical plexus communicates with the SAN

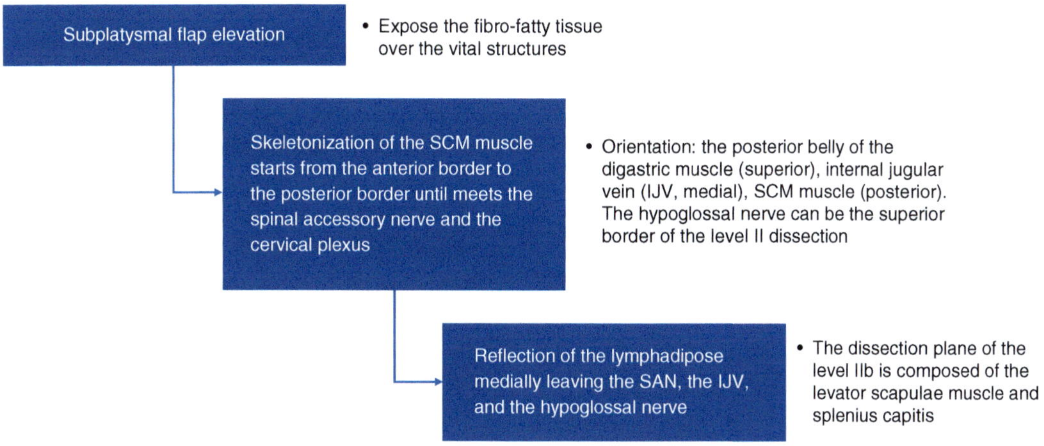

Fig. 11.8 Level IIb dissection process preserving the spinal accessory nerve. *SCM* sternocleidomastoid, *IJV* internal jugular vein, *SAN* spinal accessory nerve

digastric muscle near the mastoid tip and runs postero-downward [6]. Level II dissection usually begins by separating the SCM muscle from fibro-fatty soft tissue. To skeletonize the SCM muscle, dissection begins at its medial border and reaches the cervical plexus lying over the scalene, levator scapulae, and splenius capitis muscles, where the SAN is identified in the upper one/third region of the SCM muscle. During this procedure, the SAN can be identified without the IJV. Shoulder twitching upon electrical cautery hints at the proximity of the SAN, and cold dissection or bipolar cautery, rather than monopolar cautery, is advised to avoid incidental SAN injury to the medial portion of the SCM muscle. Additionally, bleeding obscures small structures at level II. Thus, meticulous bleeding control around the small branches of the IJV is mandatory to secure a clear operative field. The use of a vein retractor to retract the IJV medially and secure the space between the IJV and the posterior border of the SCM muscle is preferred (Fig. 11.6). The maneuver helps trace the SAN at level II [6].

Expert Opinion

To preserve the function of the SAN, it is essential to avoid unnecessary dissection around the nerve. This is particularly important when performing elective neck dissection in patients without lymph node metastasis, as avoiding unnecessary sublevel dissection is crucial for maintaining SAN function. Additionally, it is important to preserve the cervical branch of the SAN as much as possible. (Seung-Kuk Baek).

During level IIb dissection, gentle retraction of the SCM muscle (laterally), IJV (medially) and posterior belly of the digastric muscle (superiorly) help expose and preserve the SAN.

Expert Opinion
When performing MRND, one approach is to first identify the SAN 1 cm above Erb's point and then use a technique to dissect the nerve as it follows a tortuous path over the levator scapulae muscle. (Sang Joon Lee).

Postoperative shoulder dysfunction or pain is thought to occur due to traction injury to the SAN rather than a direct defect in the nerve. Although vascular insufficiency is another cause of SAN dysfunction, preventing it during neck dissection is inevitable. Considering the communication between the motor branches arising from the cervical plexus and the SAN, the cervical plexus connected to the SAN should be traced and preserved during level II neck dissection (Fig. 11.7) [7]. After identifying the oblique pathway of the SAN, the surrounding cervical plexus should be preserved. A nerve stimulator can aid in distinguishing which branches of the cervical plexus are affected by resection of fibro-fatty soft tissue. Traction damage to the nerve can be ameliorated by retracting the nerve using a vessel loop or a nerve retractor [6]. Even after preserving the SAN during neck dissection, the prevalence of shoulder pain ranges from 0%–100% and 9%–25% after modified radical and selective neck dissection, respectively, which vary according to the follow-up period and degree of discomfort [8]. Exercise intervention can relieve pain and shoulder dysfunction [9].

- The nerve stimulator can stimulate motor branches of the cervical plexus.
- Postoperative shoulder discomfort cannot be overlooked.

Expert Opinion
In contemporary head and neck surgery, classical radical neck dissections are rarely performed. Understanding the patterns of neck metastases has led to the adoption of modified or selective neck dissections. Metastases to level V are rare in most mucosal cancers. Currently, all neck dissections are performed through a single transverse incision along a natural skin crease.

During neck dissection, surgeons encounter both motor nerves (such as the marginal branch of the facial nerve, vagus, spinal accessory, hypoglossal, and phrenic nerves, as well as motor branches from the cervical roots to the scalene and levator scapulae muscles) and sensory nerves (cutaneous branches of the cervical plexus). Therefore, knowledge of anatomy and meticulous dissection techniques are crucial to prevent injury to any of these nerves.

Furthermore, when elevating the upper skin flap, meticulous attention should be paid to identify and preserve the marginal branch of the facial nerve, overlying the submandibular salivary gland.

After identifying the hypoglossal and spinal accessory nerves as discussed above, the use of nerve hooks, retractors, or vessel loops should be avoided to prevent traction injury and neuropraxia of these nerves. (Jatin Shah).

11.3 KQ 11.3. How Can We Locate and Preserve the Vagus and Phrenic Nerves During Level IV Dissection?

Yoon Se Lee

11.3.1 Vagus Nerve

At levels II–IV, the vagus nerve descends within the carotid sheath posterolateral to the internal and common carotid arteries and medial to the internal jugular vein (IJV). It is typically identified by reflecting on the specimen medially or laterally. During neck dissection at level IV, the procedure often progresses laterally to medially or vice versa (Fig. 11.9a). Most surgeons begin by dissecting the inferior portion of the IJV at level IV (Fig. 11.9b). In this study, the posterior portion of the IJV was exposed and mobilized by retraction with a vein retractor, where the thoracic duct, especially the left side of level IV, ascends. The vagus nerve, which lies over the common carotid artery (CCA), is usually exposed during this procedure (Fig. 11.9a).

Identification and retraction of the IJV facilitate the easy identification of the vagus nerve overlying the CCA.

Expert Opinion

In level IV dissection, the crucial structures to be mindful of are the vagus nerve, the phrenic nerve, and the thoracic duct on the left side and lymphatic ducts on the right side. This is particularly important when operating for metastatic carcinoma from the thyroid gland, where metastatic nodes posterior to the carotid sheath are commonly found at level IV. Meticulous dissection of these nodes requires precise identification of the thoracic duct and all other lymphatic channels, followed by their ligation to prevent chyle leakage. Injury to the branches from the thyrocervical trunk can occur, and careful identification of the arterial branches is crucial to prevent accidental bleeding. Finally, the confluence of the IJV and the subclavian vein can vary and may include additional tributaries. Undue traction on the IJV should be avoided to prevent inadvertently tenting the subclavian vein and including a portion of it in the specimen when dividing the lower end of the internal jugular vein, during resection. Such inadvertent inclusion can lead to uncontrollable bleeding from the cut end of the subclavian vein, which is challenging to ligate. (Jatin Shah).

From the hypoglossal nerve, the ansa cervicalis runs, vertically superficial to the CCA, and can be easily detected without retracting the IJV or stripping the carotid sheath. This pathway is distinct from the vagus nerve pathway (Fig. 11.10a). The IJV should be reflected laterally to secure the path of the underlying vagus nerve that courses over the CCA (Fig. 11.10b). This process is necessary in radical neck dissection to avoid ligation of the IJV to the vagus nerve. While multiple cervical sensory roots are divided into levels III and IV, some motor branches of the cervical plexus contribute to the phrenic nerve and join the spinal accessory nerve at level II, as described in the KQ 11.2.

- The vagus nerve runs between the IJV (anterolateral border) and the CCA (posteromedial border). During level III–IV dissection, retraction of the IJV exposes the vagus nerve.
- The vagus nerve should be identified and preserved before ligating the IJV upon radical neck dissection.

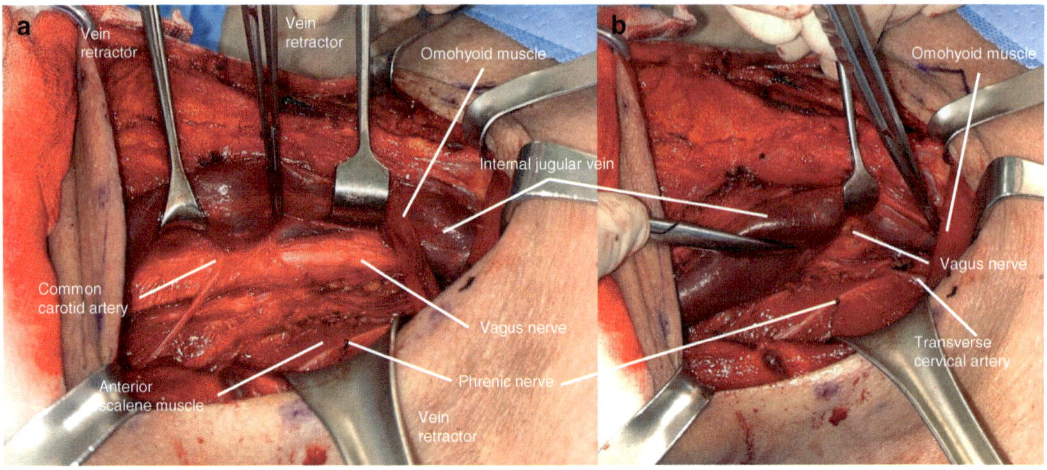

Fig. 11.9 Right levels III–IV neck dissection. (**a**) Soft tissue was removed to expose the vagus nerve on the common carotid artery and phrenic nerve on the anterior scalene muscle. (**b**) The phrenic nerve meets the transcervical artery at level IV, which is the floor of the dissection plane

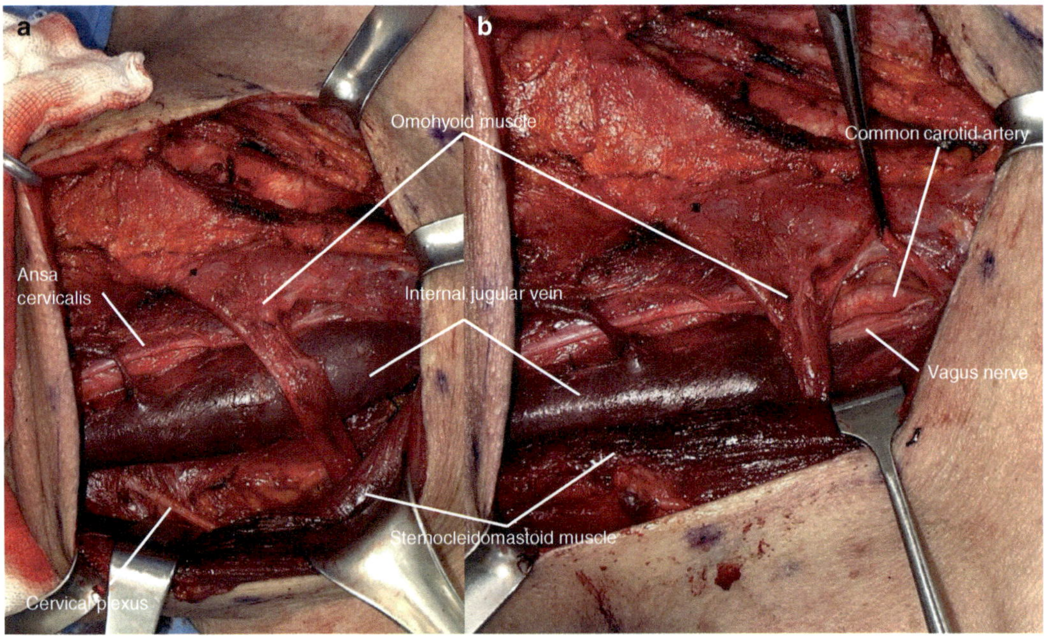

Fig. 11.10 Right levels III–IV dissection. (**a**) Ansa cervicalis superficial to the common carotid artery (CCA) and the internal jugular vein (IJV). Fibro-fatty tissue is removed superficial to the anterior scalene muscle, leaving the IJV, CCA, some cervical plexus branches, omohyoid muscle, and vagus nerve. (**b**) The vagus nerve on the lateral side of the CCA is identified upon retracting the IJV laterally

Unilateral vagus nerve injury causes unilateral vocal fold paralysis, which causes hoarseness, aspiration, dyspnea, and vocal fatigue. Upon suspicion of involvement of the vagus nerve, it is necessary to inquire about relevant symptoms in the patient and perform a laryngoscopic examination to evaluate vocal fold movement. Recovery from vagus nerve injury may be delayed, taking up to 1 year, considering that spontaneous recovery of unilateral vocal fold paralysis caused by traction injury occurs within 1–4 months [10, 11]. Hoarseness resulting from vagus nerve injury can be observed or managed through voice therapy or a surgical intervention, such as injection laryngoplasty using temporary materials. To prevent potentially lethal aspiration pneumonia, swallowing rehabilitation and medialization laryngeal surgery should be considered. Bedside swallowing, training methods include head rotation, tilting, and chin-tuck maneuvers [12]. Medialization laryngeal surgeries include injection laryngoplasty and laryngeal framework procedures such as thyroplasty type I and arytenoid adduction [13]. Additionally, tracheostomy should be considered initially in cases of bilateral vocal fold paralysis.

- Treatment of unilateral vagus nerve injuries aims to relieve dysphonia and manage aspiration, with or without dysphagia. Rehabilitation and medialization procedures encompass the available treatment options.
- Even in the absence of evident injury to the vagus nerve, vocal fold paralysis may occur. Therefore, a laryngoscopic examination is necessary to evaluate vocal fold function when patients report voice changes or dyspnea following surgery.

11.3.2 Phrenic Nerve

Identification of the floor during level IV dissection is important to avoid phrenic nerve injury. At levels II–IV, the phrenic nerve descends vertically and caudally posterolaterally to the IJV. It is situated over the anterior scalene muscle, deep to the prevertebral layer of deep cervical fascia (Figs. 11.9a and 11.11). It is unnecessary to detect and preserve the phrenic nerve unless a widely infiltrating lymph node metastasizes to the scalene muscles. Instead, level IV dissection without deterioration of the dissection plane while preserving the dissection floor or fascia carpet is essential for preserving the phrenic nerve (Fig. 11.11). The transverse cervical artery is exposed following medial retraction of the inferior portion of the IJV (Fig. 11.9b). At this stage, careful management of bleeding or chyle leakage is required to avoid inadvertent division and thermal injury to electrical or energy devices. After identifying the phrenic nerve, intraoperative monitoring using a nerve stimulator also helps to detect phrenic nerve injury [14].

Expert Opinion

Understanding the overall relationship between the cervical muscles and nerves is useful in locating the nerves accurately. The muscles forming the floor of the neck, from posterior-lateral to anterior-medial, are the splenius capitis, levator scapulae, and the scalene muscles (posterior, middle, anterior). The spinal accessory nerve (SAN) is located above the levator scapulae, the brachial plexus emerges between the anterior and middle scalene muscles, and the phrenic nerve is situated above the anterior scalene muscle. (Sang Joon Lee).

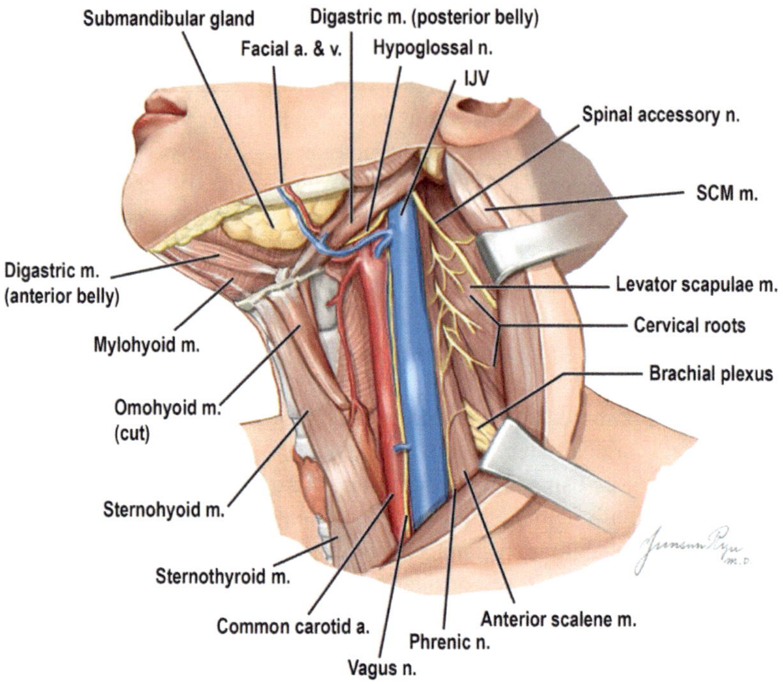

Fig. 11.11 Left levels II–IV. The phrenic nerve originates from the cervical roots. *a* artery, *v* vein, *m* muscle, *n* nerve, *IJV* internal jugular vein, *SCM* sternocleidomastoid

The incidence of phrenic nerve paralysis ranges from 0.613% to 1.035%, which is potentially underestimated because of ambiguous symptoms, including mild dyspnea or chest discomfort post-surgery [15]. Thus, unilateral phrenic nerve palsy is diagnosed through chest radiography or ultrasonography, which reveals unilateral diaphragmatic palsy (elevation) and an increase in basal lobe atelectasis and pulmonary infiltration (Fig. 11.12). Although unilateral phrenic nerve palsy is usually asymptomatic, bilateral phrenic nerve paralysis is a rare but serious complication of neck dissection, potentially leading to postoperative respiratory failure and prolonged ventilator dependence. Thus, the early detection of bilateral phrenic nerve paralysis using chest radiography or ultrasonography is critical. For uncompensated diaphragmatic palsy, interventions such as diaphragmatic plication and phrenic nerve reconstruction by a thoracic surgeon improve functional restoration [16, 17].

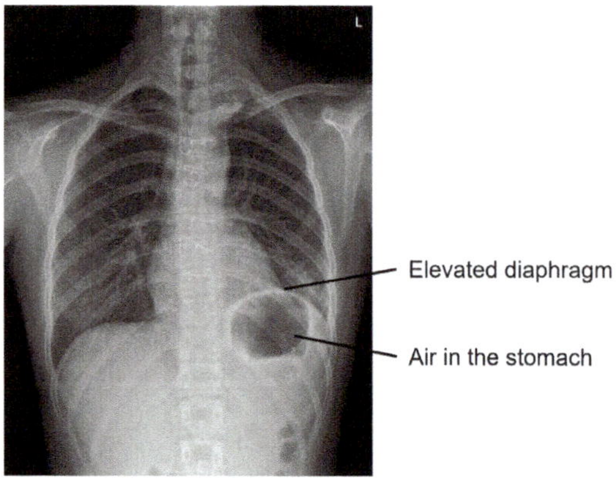

Fig. 11.12 Left diaphragmatic palsy caused by left phrenic nerve injury

Unilateral diaphragmatic palsy induced by unilateral phrenic nerve injury is usually asymptomatic. Chest X-ray and sonography are available methods to evaluate phrenic nerve injury. However, bilateral diaphragmatic palsy should be managed by a thoracic surgeon.

11.3.3 Spinal Accessory Nerve at Level V

Several methods are available for detecting the spinal accessory nerve (SAN) at level V. The subplatysmal and skin flaps were elevated at level V. The plastysmal muscle layer disappears at this level, and the thin skin flap needs to be elevated to expose level V until the trapezius muscle is identified without injuring the SAN. Twitching of the trapezius muscle during dissection with a monopolar body can indicate the location of the SAN. Locating the SAN 1–1.5 cm above the greater auricular nerve, which encircles the posterior border of the SCM muscle (Erb's point), is preferred (Fig. 11.13). As the SAN usually runs parallel to the external jugular vein (EJV), an imaginary line parallel to the EJV, above Erb's point, helps identify the SAN, with the depth of dissection being the primary concern. The trapezius branch of the SAN entering the trapezius muscle can originate from either a branch in the SCM or the SAN [18]. While dissecting the anterior border of the trapezius muscle, the SAN innervating the trapezius muscle can be located at the junction of the upper two-thirds and lower one-third.

The multiple large nerves observed at level V upon dissection and detection of the SAN can be confusing. The course and depth of the nerve are clues for sacrifice. The nerves located superficial to the trapezius muscle, or those that course horizontally, are sensory nerves that can be divided during neck dissection. Additionally, a nerve stimulator can be useful in discriminating the SAN from other sensory branches of the cervical plexus (Fig. 11.14). After identifying the SAN, it should be carefully dissected at level V. Nerve hooks and vessel loops are used to dissect the soft tissue around the SAN, avoiding either traction injury or devascularization.

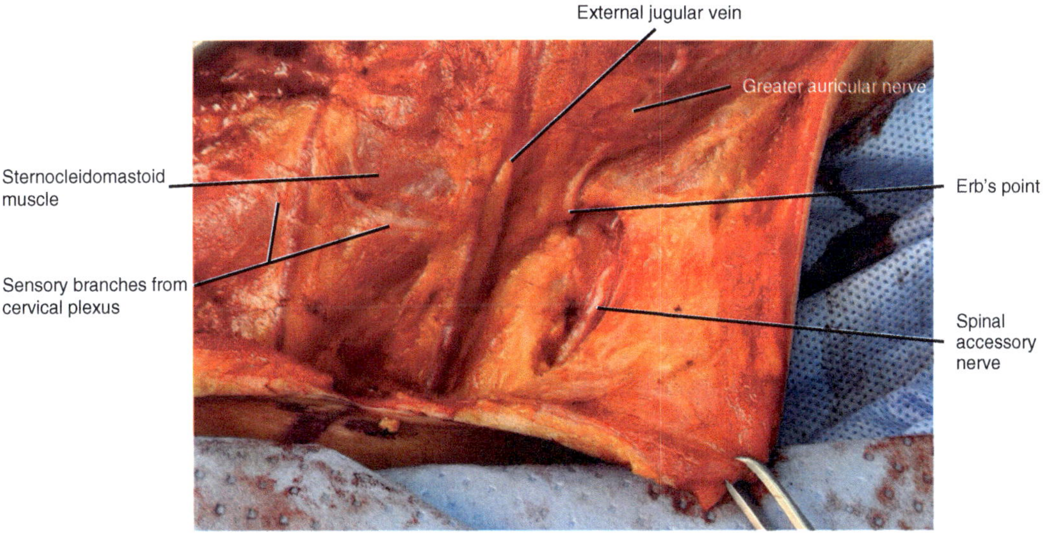

Fig. 11.13 Left level V dissection. After elevating the skin and subplatysmal flap to expose the external jugular vein and the greater auricular nerve, dissection starts by identifying the spinal accessory nerve (SAN). SAN runs from 1 to 2 cm above the Erb's point at the posterior border of the sternocleidomastoid muscle to the upper margin of the inferior one-third of the trapezius muscle

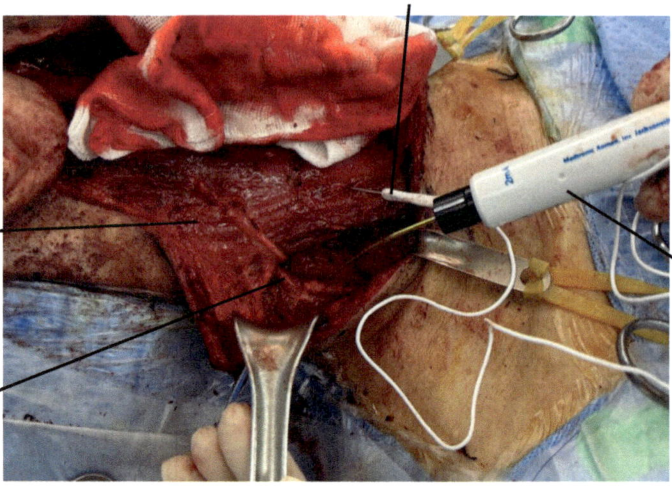

Fig. 11.14 Nerve stimulator (locator). Portable nerve stimulator (Medtronic 8,562,010 VARI-STIM II® nerve locator) helps to trace motor nerve at level V

Expert Opinion
In level V dissection, avoid circumferential dissection around the SAN to prevent ischemic injury to the nerve. It is best to leave the nerve in its position and avoid dissecting posterior and lateral to the nerve. (Jatin Shah).

Reconstruction of the SAN at level V involves an end-to-end anastomosis and the use of an interposition graft. Interpositional grafting using a branch of the cervical plexus reduced postoperative shoulder discomfort. Additionally, various shoulder exercises after level V-neck dissection can help alleviate shoulder discomfort [18].

- In level V, Erb's point and the IJV are good indicators of the SAN. The nerve stimulator helps to confirm nerve integrity.
- Branches from the SAN to the trapezius and SCM muscles may differ. Preserving the SAN at level IIb does not always guarantee the preservation of the SAN to the trapezius muscle.
- Upon injury to the SAN, neurotization through interposition grafts and direct anastomosis are viable options to reconstruct nerve continuity.

Expert Opinion
To prevent neurologic complications during neck dissection, it is crucial to have a thorough anatomical knowledge of the nerves that can be encountered at each level. When removing any structures, it is essential to identify and verify the nerves that may be present in the surrounding area before proceeding, in order to avoid nerve damage. (Seung-Kuk Baek).

References

1. Andersen PE. Modified radical neck dissection. In: Cohen JI, Clayman GL, editors. Atlas of head & neck surgery. 1st ed. Amsterdam: Elsevier; 2011. p. 183–4.
2. Marolt C, Freed B, Coker C, Steele R, Johnson K, Arellanes R, Gordon V, Wright B, Stephens R, Surek CC. Key anatomical clarifications for the marginal mandibular branch of the facial nerve: clinical significance for the plastic surgeon. Aesthet Surg J. 2021;41:1223–8. https://doi.org/10.1093/asj/sjaa368.
3. Khafif A. Lateral neck dissection. Oper Tech Otolaryngol. 2004;15(3):160–7.
4. Avitia S, Osborne RF. Surgical management of iatrogenic hypoglossal nerve injury. Ear Nose Throat J. 2008;87:672–6.
5. Holmes JD. Neck dissection: nomenclature, classification, and technique. Oral Maxillofac Surg Clin North Am. 2008;20(3):459–75.
6. Cohen JI, Clayman GL. Atlas of head and neck surgery E-book: expert consult-online and print. Amsterdam: Elsevier; 2011.
7. Lanisnik B, Zargi M, Rodi Z. Identification of three anatomical patterns of the spinal accessory nerve in the neck by neurophysiological mapping. Radiol Oncol. 2014;48(4):387–92.
8. Gane EM, Michaleff ZA, Cottrell MA, et al. Prevalence, incidence, and risk factors for shoulder and neck dysfunction after neck dissection: a systematic review. European Journal of Surgical Oncology. 2017;43:1199–218.
9. Carvalho AP, Vital FM, Soares BG. Exercise interventions for shoulder dysfunction in patients treated for head and neck cancer. Cochrane Database Syst Rev. 2012;18:CD008693.
10. Lee YS, Kim YH, Kwon M, Ryu IS, Jung GE, Kim ST, et al. Short-term treatment results for unilateral vocal fold palsy induced by mediastinal lesions. J Voice. 2014;28(6):809–15.
11. Liu MY, Chang CP, Hung CL, Hung CJ, Huang SM. Traction injury of recurrent laryngeal nerve during thyroidectomy. World J Surg. 2020;44(2):402–7.
12. Park JS, Hwang NK. Chin tuck against resistance exercise for dysphagia rehabilitation: a systematic review. J Oral Rehabil. 2021;48(8):968–77.
13. Dhar SI, Ryan MA, Davis AC, Jedlanek E, Pietsch K, Price C, et al. Does medialization improve swallowing function in patients with unilateral vocal fold paralysis? A systematic review. Dysphagia. 2022;37(6):1769–76.
14. Duque CS, Dueñas JP, Marulanda M, Pérez D, Londoño A, Roy S, Khadem MA. Phrenic nerve stimulation during neck dissection for advanced thyroid cancer involving level IV: is it worth doing it? Updat Surg. 2017;69:83–7.
15. Lee MFH, Gan JY, Zhang M, Stokan MJ, Palme CE. The phrenic nerve; the forgotten nerve in head and neck surgery. ANZ J Surg. 2023;93(3):500–5.
16. Gazala S, Hunt I, Bédard EL. Diaphragmatic plication offers functional improvement in dyspnoea and better pulmonary function with low morbidity. Interact Cardiovasc Thorac Surg. 2012;15(3):505–8.
17. Kaufman MR, Elkwood AI, Colicchio AR, CeCe J, Jarrahy R, Willekes LJ, et al. Functional restoration of diaphragmatic paralysis: an evaluation of phrenic nerve reconstruction. Ann Thorac Surg. 2014;97(1):260–6.
18. Sakamoto K, Ozawa H, Shimanuki M, Kida A, Kitama T, Iwabu K, et al. Trapezius muscle branch of the spinal accessory nerve without penetrating the sternocleidomastoid muscle as a pitfall in neck dissection: prevalence in a Japanese institution and a protocol for the prevention of iatrogenic injury. Acta Otolaryngol. 2021;141(8):825–9.

Neck Dissection: Others

12

Jeon Yeob Jang, Jeongkye Hwang,
Sang-Yeon Kim, and Dong Jin Lee

12.1 KQ 12.1. How Should Chyle Leakage Be Managed Post-Surgery?

Jeon Yeob Jang

Chyle leakage can be recognized either during surgery or the early postoperative period.

In a surgical setting, the presence of a chyle leak may be suspected if clear or milky fluid is observed in the operative field, particularly in the supraclavicular area. If a chyle leak is discovered during the procedure, the surgeon should temporarily halt neck dissection and attempt to manage the leak by ligating the thoracic duct. Employing surgical loupes can improve visualization. Even if no chyle leak is found during the operation, a meticulous inspection of the level IV area is recommended before concluding the surgery. Placing the patient in the Trendelenburg position and applying an intraoperative Valsalva maneuver (achieved by requesting the anesthesiologist to apply positive airway pressure, thereby

> ◆ **Intraoperative identification and management of a chyle leakage**
> ◆ During lower neck dissections, any signs of a chyle leak should be promptly investigated (Fig. 12.1). The Trendelenburg position and intraoperative Valsalva maneuver can aid in finding the locations of the chylous fistula. In case a chyle leakage is found, ligating the thoracic duct or its branches surrounding the leakage area with ties, sutures, or surgical clips is recommended (Video 12.1).

Supplementary Information The online version contains supplementary material available at https://doi.org/10.1007/978-981-96-1860-6_12.

J. Y. Jang (✉)
Department of Otolaryngology, Ajou University School of Medicine, Ajou University Hospital, Suwon, Republic of Korea

J. Hwang (✉)
Department of Vascular & Transplant Surgery, Eunpyeong St. Mary's Hospital, College of Medicine, The Catholic University of Korea, Seoul, Republic of Korea
e-mail: jjungyong@catholic.ac.kr

S.-Y. Kim
Department of Otolaryngology—Head and Neck Surgery, Seoul St. Mary's Hospital, College of Medicine, The Catholic University of Korea, Seoul, Republic of Korea

D. J. Lee (✉)
Department of Otolaryngology-Head and Neck Surgery Kangnam Sacred Heart Hospital, College of Medicine, Hallym University of Korea, Seoul, Republic of Korea
e-mail: djlee@hallym.or.kr

K.-J. Cho, J.-O. Park (eds.), *Management of Head and Neck Surgery Complications*,
https://doi.org/10.1007/978-981-96-1860-6_12

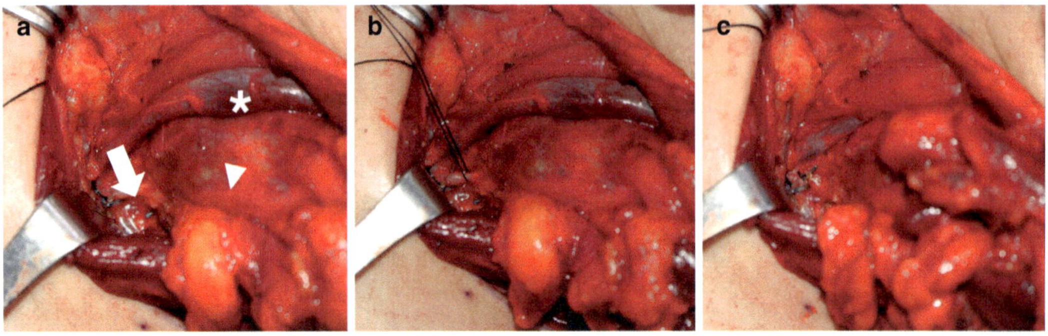

Fig. 12.1 Intraoperative identification and ligation of the thoracic duct during left radical neck dissection. (**a**) The panel shows the identified thoracic duct (arrow) during the neck dissection. The asterisk indicates the internal jugular vein. The arrowhead indicates the surgical specimen during neck dissection. (**b**) The panel shows the ligation of the identified thoracic duct using a tie. (**c**) The panel shows the thoracic duct after ligation, separated from the specimen

increasing the intrathoracic pressure) may assist the surgeon in locating the origin of the leak.

Expert Opinion
When residual tissue remains in the operative bed, a figure-of-eight suture is more effective than a simple knot. If no residual tissue is present and the vessel wall is torn, coaptation can be facilitated using a commercially available surgical pledget. (Yun-Sung Lim)

Expert Opinion
The best management strategy for a chyle leak is "prevention." Although the thoracic duct is situated on the left side of the neck, nearly similar sized lymphatic ducts are present in a similar location on the right side of the neck. Therefore, it is important to remember that accessory lymphatic ducts may be present alongside the thoracic duct and can contribute to postoperative chyle leaks. Therefore, meticulous attention should be given to identifying and carefully ligating all the lymphatic ducts. Finally, it should be a routine practice to check the area posterior to the carotid sheath with a Valsalva maneuver prior to closure of the wound. (Jatin Shah)

In the postoperative period, chyle leaks were typically identified when feeding was resumed. Most of these leaks can be clinically diagnosed in the presence of an unexpected accumulation of white fluid in the drainage or if the drainage output suddenly increases following feeding. Signs of a chyle leak may include wound erythema and, occasionally, palpable fluid accumulation in the supraclavicular area. Furthermore, triglyceride (TG) levels >100 mg/dL in the drainage fluid or levels that exceed those in the serum are indicative of a chyle leak in cases where the diagnosis is uncertain.

◆ **Clinical signs and tests for diagnosing a chyle leakage postoperatively**
◆ Clinical sign: Increase in drain output with color change from serosanguinous to milky (Fig. 12.2).
◆ Biochemical study: TG levels in the drainage output >100 mg/dL or exceeding the serum TG level.
◆ Chest radiography: Rule out concurrent chylothorax.

The treatment of postoperative chyle leaks can be classified into two main categories: conservative management and surgical intervention. The initial

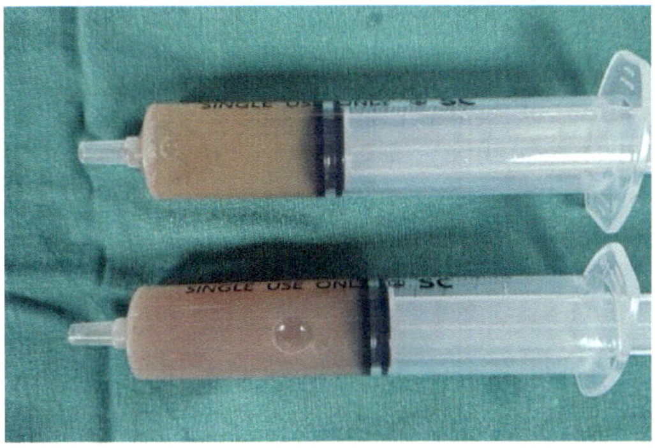

Fig. 12.2 The color of the drain has turned milky in chyle leakage

treatment approach usually comprises conservative methods that are frequently successful in decreasing chyle leakage. Closed drainage to facilitate the adherence of skin flaps and pressure dressings can effectively induce spontaneous closure of most fistulas. Dietary adjustments, such as switching to a low-fat diet or incorporating medium-chain TGs (MCTs), are also part of the treatment. MCTs, which are largely water-soluble, enter the circulatory system primarily through the liver, thereby bypassing the gastrointestinal lymphatic system. However, dietary changes alone may not completely inhibit the chyle flow. Total parenteral nutrition (TPN), which circumvents the gastrointestinal-lymphatic system and delivers all the necessary nutrients, is an alternative, especially in high-output leaks or when dietary modification is ineffective. Some clinicians prefer TPN as the primary treatment. It is important to constantly replenish electrolytes, vitamins, and trace elements during the treatment.

◆ **Conservative treatments are warranted for most chyle leakages.**
◆ **Nutritional management is one of the essential aspects of conservative treatments.**
◆ Low-fat or a medium-chain TG diet.
◆ TPN if indicated.
◆ Daily correction of electrolytes, vitamins, and trace elements.

Expert Opinion

In addition to these conservative treatments, sclerotherapy, which involves aspiration of chyle and injection of picibanil, can be useful. By inducing a surrounding inflammatory response, delayed closure of the thoracic duct can be achieved without surgical treatment. (Yun-Sung Lim)

There are various criteria for deciding on the surgical treatment for chyle leakage, but in ambiguous cases, I generally prefer to resolve the issue quickly with surgical intervention rather than opting for conservative treatments. (Chul-Ho Kim)

Adjunctive pharmacological treatments can effectively reduce chyle leakage. These included the use of octreotide, a long-lasting somatostatin hormone analog, and orlistat, a pancreatic lipase inhibitor. The administration of octreotide at a dose of 100 μg subcutaneously three times daily has proven beneficial, as evidenced by notably reducing hospital stays [1, 2]. Although the exact mechanism of action of octreotide in treating a chyle leak is not fully understood, it is thought to function primarily by reducing secretions in the gastrointestinal tract and pancreas, lowering hepatic venous pressure, and decreasing splanchnic blood flow. In contrast, orlistat blocks pancreatic enzymes, thereby preventing the absorption and intestinal circulation of lipids. Orlistat was effective at a dose of 120 mg three times daily, as reported in a previous case series [3].

◆ **Adjunctive pharmacological methods are beneficial in reducing leakage.**
◆ The long-acting analog of the hormone somatostatin (octreotide) proved to be effective in prospective clinical trials and a systematic review.
◆ Pancreatic lipase inhibitor (orlistat) is reported to be effective based on case series studies.

Surgical intervention is recommended for chyle leaks unresponsive to conservative medical management, particularly high-output leaks. These are often characterized by a daily output of 500–1000 mL lasting over 5 days, although the specific criteria may vary among clinicians. [4]. In addition, patients with chylomas who do not respond to needle aspiration or pressure dressings may require surgery. The objective of surgical intervention is to securely close the thoracic duct using ties, clips, or sutures while carefully avoiding damage to adjacent structures such as the phrenic nerve or internal jugular vein. Identifying the thoracic duct can be challenging during re-exploration, owing to factors such as local inflammation from the leaked chyle or adhesions from prior surgeries. Techniques such as Trendelenburg positioning and the Valsalva maneuver, used in the initial surgery, can help locate the leak site. Additionally, employing local flaps, such as sternocleidomastoid muscle flaps, is often effective. Lymphangiography with thoracic duct embolization has recently gained popularity as either a salvage or primary treatment, with reported success rates ranging from 40% to 75% [5, 6]. Due to its low morbidity and fair success rate, it is a feasible alternative to surgical exploration, contingent on the availability of appropriate equipment and personnel in the interventional radiology department.

◆ **After conservative management, high-output leaks that lack improvements require surgical intervention.**
◆ **Surgical intervention**: Securely close the leakage site using a tie, clipping, or suture; a locoregional flap could be helpful.
◆ **Alternative:** Lymphangiography with thoracic duct embolization.

In cases where exploratory surgical repair fails, video-assisted thoracoscopic ligation is an effective rescue procedure that targets the proximal end of the thoracic duct. This method is typically considered the final option when other treatments fail to manage chyle leaks, although some clinicians recommend it as the primary option for high-output leaks [7].

The summary of Chyle leakage management is as follows. (Fig. 12.3.)

(1) During lower neck dissections, it is important to examine any indications of a chyle leak immediately.
 ① Upon detecting a chyle leak during the procedure, the surgeon should pause the neck dissection and attempt to control the leak by ligating the thoracic duct.
 ② If no chyle leak is found during surgery, it is recommended to closely inspect the level IV area before finishing. The Trendelenburg position and an intraoperative Valsalva maneuver may assist in identifying any hidden leak sources.
(2) In the postoperative period, chyle leaks can manifest as unexpected white fluid accumulation in the drainage or a sudden increase in drainage output after feeding.
 ① When uncertain, a chyle leak can be indicated by TG levels exceeding 100 mg/dL in the drainage fluid or by levels that surpass those in the serum.
(3) The initial treatment typically involves conservative methods
 ① Low-fat diet or a medium-chain TG diet
 ② Consider TPN in high-output leakage
 ③ Maintain closed drainage with/without pressure dressing
 ④ Consider octreotide administration
 ⑤ Chest radiography to rule out concurrent chylothorax
(4) An interventional approach is recommended for chyle leaks that do not improve with conservative medical treatment, particularly high-output

(continued)

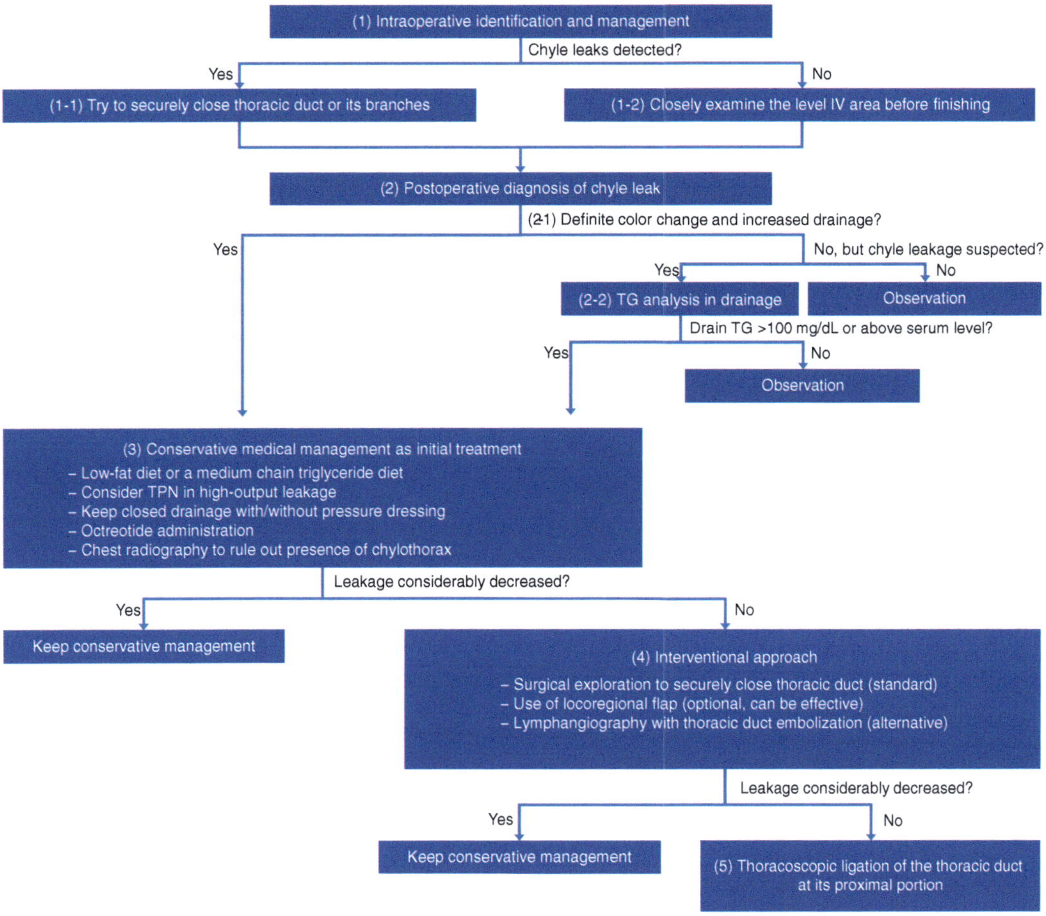

Fig. 12.3 Algorithm for managing chyle leakage

leaks with a daily discharge of 500–1000 mL for more than 5 days.

① Surgical exploration securely aims to close the thoracic duct using ties, clips, or sutures, with careful attention to avoid damaging nearby structures.

② Lymphangiography with thoracic duct embolization could be considered alternatively depending on the institutional setting.

(5) In cases where an interventional approach has failed, video-assisted thoracoscopic ligation is an effective rescue procedure, targeting the thoracic duct at its proximal end.

12.2 KQ 12.2. How to Manage Patients After Bilateral Internal Jugular Vein Ligation?

Jeon Yeob Jang

Radical neck dissection (RND), which involves *en bloc* cervical lymphadenectomy along with the associated essential structures, including the internal jugular vein (IJV), sternocleidomastoid, and spinal accessory nerve, has been used to treat metastatic head and neck cancers since it was first reported by Crile [8]. Although modified RND or selective neck dissections, which lower surgical morbidity, have largely substituted RND recently, extensive neck disease still requires RND, which involves the removal of the IJV.

The IJVs are the largest channels for venous outflow from the cranial cavity; thus, bilateral ligation of the IJV inevitably increases intracranial pressure [9]. Bilateral RND decompensates the extracranial venous circulation, causing facial congestion and cyanosis. These changes are largely resolved by collateral drainage systems such as vertebral vessels. However, in some patients with poorly developed collateral vessels, serious and potentially fatal complications may occur, including blindness owing to prolonged papilledema, life-threatening laryngeal edema, stroke, and death.

◆ **Ligation of bilateral IJV results in varying degrees of sequelae, which can be fatal.**
◆ Prolonged intracranial hypertension and subsequent neurological sequelae.
◆ The severity of such changes depends on individual anatomical variations, including the number and size of the existing anastomoses and collateral vessels.

12.2.1 Preoperative Consideration

During bilateral neck dissection, preservation of at least one IJV is recommended to prevent severe complications. If ligation of both IJVs is anticipated, the decision between simultaneous and staged RNDs remains debatable. Although some studies have claimed that simultaneous bilateral RND carries a low risk of life-threatening complications, the consensus favors staged dissections, preferably with a 1-month gap between neck dissections, to promote the development of collateral venous drainage [10, 11]. However, staged neck dissections may also lead to marked increases in intracranial pressure. Importantly, staged neck dissection carries a risk of spreading viable cancer cells. Furthermore, this approach may delay the initiation of adjuvant treatment, particularly in patients with a locally advanced disease.

Careful preoperative evaluation is required when simultaneous bilateral RND is performed. This includes an assessment of the burden of lymph node metastasis on each side of the neck and its relationship with the surrounding essential structures, particularly the IJV. Reconstruction of the resected IJV may be affected by the extent of the remaining vessels, and the site with the least metastasis is generally selected for reconstruction. Consultations with a neurologist and ophthalmologist may help assess baseline findings for comparison with potential postoperative deficits.

◆ **The decision between staged and simultaneous bilateral RND is a matter of debate.**
◆ Staged bilateral RND could enable the development of collateral venous drainage, reducing the risk of life-threatening complications.
◆ Staged bilateral RND may increase the risk of viable tumor spread during the interval between neck dissections and could delay the timing of adjuvant treatment.

Expert Opinion

If there is a possibility of ligating both internal jugular veins, I prefer to first operate on the area with less extensive invasion, and if it is possible to remove only the part of the internal jugular vein invaded by the cancer, I perform a partial resection and use primary closure for the resected area. This approach can achieve a narrowing of the internal jugular vein but still provides an effect similar to reconstruction with an external jugular vein (EJV). If complete resection of both veins is necessary, I do not favor a staged operation. Instead, I prefer to remove both sides and use an autologous bypass graft, such as an EJV or the contralateral internal jugular vein (IJV), for reconstruction (Chul-Ho Kim).

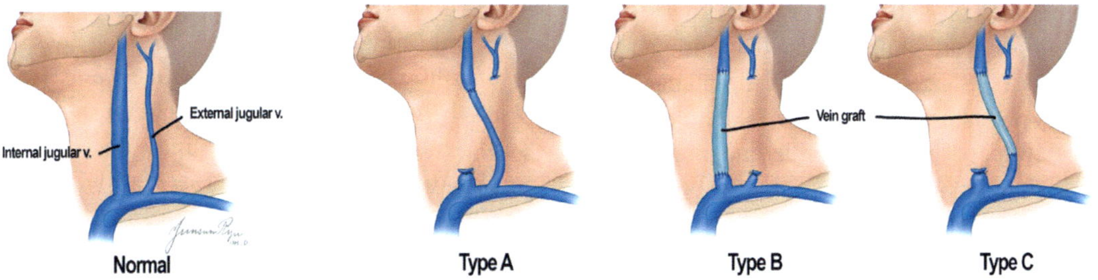

Fig. 12.4 Three categories of internal jugular vein reconstruction techniques proposed by Katsuno et al. v, vein. This illustration is modified from the original image published by Katsuno et al. [12]

12.2.2 Intraoperative Management

To address the risk of increased intracranial pressure, a range of reconstruction techniques for venous drainage systems have been proposed. Reconstruction of the IJVs using the external jugular vein (EJV) or a graft from the greater saphenous vein has also been described. In 2000, Katsuno et al. classified IJV reconstruction into three categories [12]. In type A reconstruction, the upper segment of the EJV is connected to the upper stump of the IJV. By contrast, types B and C involve the use of interposed vein grafts to bridge either the IJVs or the IJV and EJV, respectively. (Fig. 12.4)

Various other modified methods of IJV reconstruction have been reported, including anastomosis with the upper stump of the anterior jugular vein, the use of a portion of the contralateral IJV as a bypass graft, and the use of synthetic materials [13]. Identifying sufficient working space for vascular clamping of the upper or lower IJV stump is essential for proper surgical planning. Determining whether the EJV should be preserved is crucial. Furthermore, the availability of a skilled microvascular surgeon, capable of performing either end-to-end anastomosis or end-to-side venotomy procedures, is critical.

- **If feasible, reconstruction of the venous drainage system is recommended after bilateral internal jugular vein (IJV) ligation.**
- **Various techniques have been reported.**
- IJV–external jugular vein (EJV) anastomosis (superior IJV stump–EJV as a recipient vein).
- Bypass graft using autologous vein (EJV or greater saphenous vein or contralateral IJV).
- Bypass graft using synthetic material.
- IJV-anterior jugular vein (AJV) anastomosis (superior IJV stump–AJV as a recipient vein).

12.2.3 Postoperative Management

Following bilateral IJV ligation, patients should be closely monitored for signs and symptoms of increased intracranial pressure, such as headache, nausea, vomiting, altered mental status, and visual disturbances. Monitoring may include regular neurological assessments and intracranial pressure monitoring in high-risk patients, including those of advanced age, those with a history of cerebrovascular disease, or those with poorly developed vertebral vessels. Consulting a neurologist is strongly recommended, and if required, an ophthalmologist should be consulted. Therefore, postoperative brain imaging should be considered.

This situation is uncommon, and there is no high-quality evidence regarding its postoperative management. The consensus advocates elevating the patient's head to aid brain venous outflow. Careful management of the fluid balance is crucial. Overhydration can exacerbate cerebral edema, whereas dehydration can lead to venous thrombosis. Given the risk of thrombosis after vein ligation, appropriate venous thromboembolism prophylaxis should be considered [14]. In cases of marked cerebral edema, corticosteroids may be used to reduce inflammation and edema. Careful monitoring of oxygen saturation and the identification of dyspnea symptoms are required for potentially severe laryngeal edema and subsequent airway stenosis. Elective tracheostomy can be considered when simultaneous bilateral RND is performed.

◆ **Postoperative management should be multidisciplinary.**
◆ Close monitoring of the signs and symptoms of increased intracranial pressure.
◆ Consultation with a neurologist for an objective assessment and management.
◆ Head elevation, appropriate fluid management, and consideration of diuretics.
◆ Prophylaxis for venous thrombosis and consideration of anticoagulation.

Bilateral ligation of the IJVs can have devastating consequences. Appropriate preoperative surgical planning and postoperative management are important for mitigating unexpected results. A multidisciplinary team approach is crucial, involving surgical oncologists, microvascular surgeons, neurologists, critical care specialists, and ophthalmologists, if necessary.

Expert Opinion

Sacrifice of both internal jugular veins is rarely necessary, but if such a circumstance presents itself, appropriate intra operative planning and ancillary measures should be considered as discussed above. The only venous drainage after such an event is from the prevertebral plexus of veins, and those along the central compartment laryngo pharyngeal complex. In that setting, conservative management may be enough to manage the patient, until satisfactory new venous channels develop along the prevertebral plexus. However, if bilateral IJV sacrifice with radical neck dissections and total pharyngo laryngectomy are performed, the intracranial venous drainage will be compromised, and consideration should be given to restoring intracranial venous drainage with a vein graft (Jatin Shah).

12.3 KQ 12.3. What Is the Appropriate Management for Unintentional Carotid Artery Injury?

Jeongkye Hwang and Sang-Yeon Kim

Rare unintentional injuries to the carotid artery during head and neck surgery may have disastrous consequences. Intraoperative injury to the carotid artery can rapidly lead to exsanguinating hemorrhage. Vascular control may be straightforward or extremely challenging, depending on the location of the injury. Management of a life-threatening situation initially focuses on maintaining the airway, breathing, and circulation. Management of circulatory compromise due to hemorrhage involves simultaneous fluid resuscitation and procedures to achieve hemostasis. These are essential for preventing cerebral damage due to massive bleeding [15]. Appropriate management of unintentional carotid artery injuries requires a comprehensive understanding of the injury, the patient's condition, and the available interventions. Both non-surgical and surgical options have merits, and the choice should be tailored to individual cases to optimize outcomes and minimize complications. The central question in the management of unintentional carotid artery injury concerns whether to ligate the vessel or to restore blood flow [16]. The pathophysiology, clinical presentation, and various management options for unintentional carotid artery injuries are discussed below.

Expert Opinion

In the event of unexpected and sudden damage to the carotid artery during surgery, it is crucial to collaborate with a vascular surgeon who is experienced in this field. If the damage is not severe, primary repair could be a good approach. Depending on the type and the extent of the vascular injury, various methods should be considered in order to determine the most suitable surgical technique for the patient. (Chul-Ho Kim)

Injury to the carotid artery can lead to a catastrophic situation and may even lead to fatal hemorrhage. Therefore, the potential risk to the artery should be preoperatively anticipated and appropriately studied with cerebral angiography in order to assess cross circulation. These situations include massive metastatic disease surrounding or contiguous to the carotid system in the upper neck, previously radiated neck with large volume disease in the upper neck. Proper planning includes well monitored anesthesia, with controlled blood pressure, availability of vascular instruments, and the availability of a vascular surgeon on standby. Intraoperatively, blunt dissection in the vicinity of the artery, particularly in a radiated neck, should be avoided, as well as traction and the use of retractors on the vessel. (Jatin Shah)

Generally, factors associated with carotid artery injuries include the presence of tumors around the carotid artery, previous radiation therapy, presence of infection, history of prior surgeries, and the surgeon's expertise level [15]. Carotid artery injuries during surgery can occur for various reasons, including accidental incision, improper retraction, inadequate exposure, anatomical variations, and unexpected bleeding. The type and severity of carotid artery injuries that can occur during head and neck surgery are summarized as follows. (1) Intimal injury (intimal flap) due to inadvertent contact with surgical instruments or retraction tools. (2) Pseudoaneurysm, a localized pulsating swelling that develops at the arterial injury site. Blood leaks out of the damaged artery and collects in the surrounding tissues, forming a sac-like structure. Pseudoaneurysms are prone to rupture and can cause rapid and severe bleeding. (3) Partial laceration. This may cause significant bleeding. However, the artery may still be partially functional, allowing some blood to flow to the brain. Prompt surgical intervention to repair the lacerated artery is crucial for preventing complications. (4) Complete transection of the carotid artery. This results in profuse medial bleeding, leading to a rapid decrease in blood pressure. A lack of blood supply to the brain can quickly cause neurological deficits, and in some cases, unconsciousness. Emergency surgical repair is essential to restore the blood flow promptly to prevent catastrophic consequences [17, 18].

◆ **The type and severity of carotid artery injuries**

- Intimal injury (intimal flap)
- Pseudoaneurysm
- Partial laceration
- Complete transection

When a carotid artery injury is suspected or identified during surgery, immediate action to control bleeding, repair the artery, and restore normal blood flow is necessary. Surgeons may perform vascular repair using various techniques, such as suturing the damaged artery and providing synthetic grafts to bypass the injured segment. Coordination between the vascular surgeons and interventional radiologists may be required in complex cases. Timely management is crucial to prevent further complications. Initial interventions include stabilizing the patient's hemodynamics, ensuring airway patency, and controlling bleeding, if present [19]. Hemostasis can often be achieved using direct pressure or endovascular techniques, such as embolization. Endovascular interventions are increasingly used to manage carotid artery injuries. Angioplasty and stent placement can restore blood flow and prevent further damage. These minimally invasive approaches offer reduced morbidity compared to surgical options.

◆ **Rapid Response to Injury**: Immediate actions are required when carotid artery injury occurs during surgery. To prevent catastrophic outcomes, aim to control bleeding, repair the artery, and restore blood flow.

◆ **Surgical and Non-Surgical Options:** The choice between ligation and restoring blood flow through repair or grafts should be based on the injury type, the condition of the patient, and surgical expertise.

Bleeding may be external and/or internal (hypopharynx or mouth). If possible, direct pressure with a finger at the hemorrhagic site is the best temporizing maneuver. Digital control of the bleeding site is maintained while dissection is performed to obtain both proximal and distal control of the carotid artery and its branches [20]. Passing a Fogarty catheter (Fig. 12.5a) into or through the site of rupture and inflating a balloon may help temporize the injury, allowing the surgeon to obtain vascular control [15].

◆ **Techniques for Hemostasis**: Direct pressure and endovascular techniques, such as embolization, angioplasty, and stent placement, are pivotal for managing bleeding and restoring blood flow.

Rapid but meticulous dissection of the carotid sheath is of utmost importance to preserve its structure. It is easier to locate the common carotid artery at the base of the neck, facilitated by an omohyoid transection. This maneuver, performed using a 45-degree angled DeBakey vascular clamp (Fig. 12.5b), provides rapid proximal vascular control. These clamps

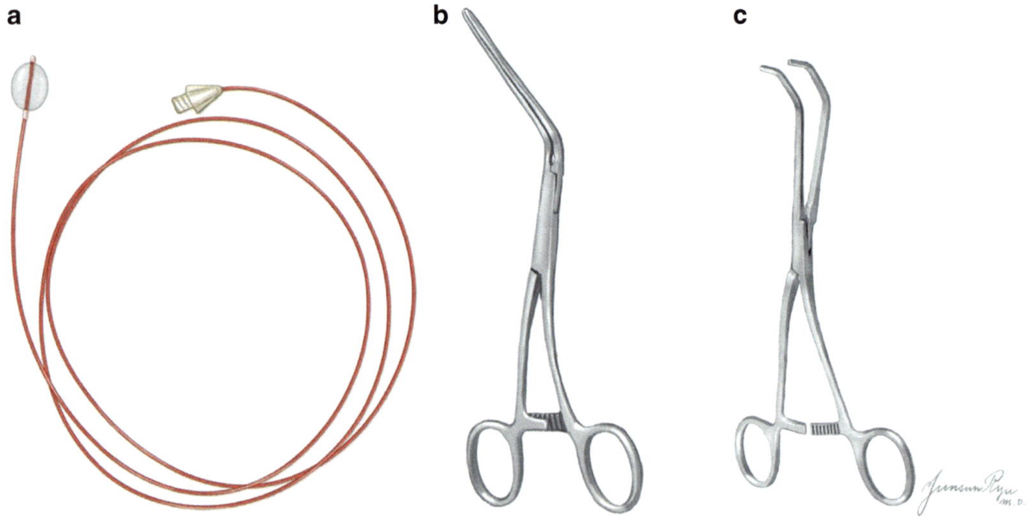

Fig. 12.5 (**a**) Fogarty catheters. (**b**) DeBakey peripheral vascular clamp. (**c**) Kitzmiller clamps

can be used to achieve proximal control of the internal and external carotid arteries. The total control of these three vessels is very important. In particular, the right and left Kitzmiller clamps were optimal for obtaining high proximal control of the internal carotid artery (Fig. 12.5c).

Surgical repair aims to restore blood flow, thereby preventing complications and preserving neurological functions. The choice of surgical technique depends on the extent of the injury, the patient's overall health, and the surgeon's expertise. To find the carotid artery injury when the vessel is no longer pulsating (e.g., a hematoma injury or proximal interruption), the external carotid branches may be followed in a retrograde manner from the superior thyroid artery at the superior cornu of the thyroid cartilage [21]. After obtaining vascular control, the decision to repair is based on the extent of injury, patient stability, and the availability of an appropriately sized conduit [22]. For small partial lacerations, primary repair should be undertaken with or without patch angioplasty (Fig. 12.6) [23]. For patch angioplasty with an autogenous vein, bovine pericardium or a prosthetic alternative may be necessary.

Simple closure can be accomplished with interrupted (Fig. 12.7a) or continuous monofilament sutures (Fig. 12.7b) if the lumen of the carotid vessel is not compromised [24].

The repair of more extensive injuries requires an interposition or bypass graft. Vein grafts are the conduit of choice, given their decreased rate of infection compared to prosthetic grafts. Polytetrafluoroethylene and Dacron grafts are often appropriate for common carotid artery injuries. In contrast, the autogenous vein is a better choice for the internal carotid artery because of its vessel size and better patency rate (Fig. 12.8) [25].

In situations where primary repair or grafting is not feasible, bypass procedures can be performed using a segment of a different blood vessel (such as the saphenous vein) to reroute blood flow around the injured segment (Fig. 12.9) [26].

An external carotid artery flap provides an alternative method for repairing common carotid artery injuries in young patients when primary repair is not possible (Fig. 12.10) [27].

For injuries near the carotid bulb, another option is to perform an external carotid artery transposition to the distal internal carotid artery (Fig. 12.11) [22, 28]. Patients presenting with injuries at the base of the skull often require carotid artery ligation, which is associated with a 45% risk of mortality [29]. Ligation of the common or internal carotid is generally reserved for irreparable injuries.

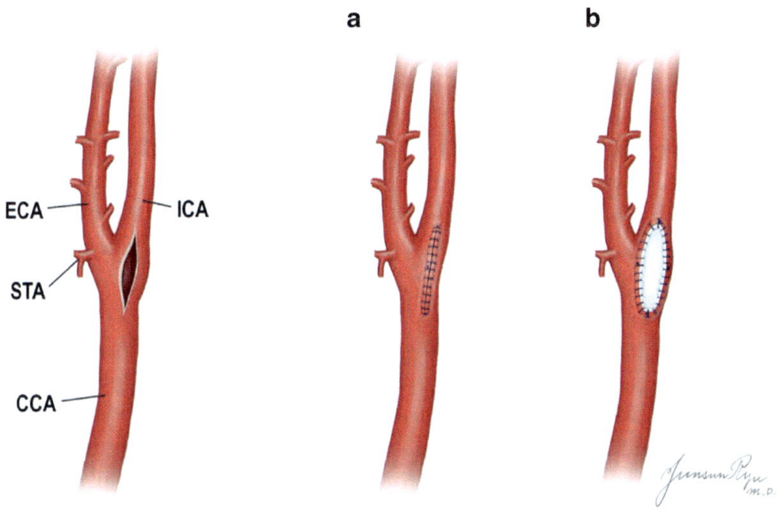

Fig. 12.6 (**a**) Primary repair. (**b**) A patch angioplasty. ECA, external carotid artery; ICA, internal carotid artery; STA, superior thyroid artery; CCA, common carotid artery

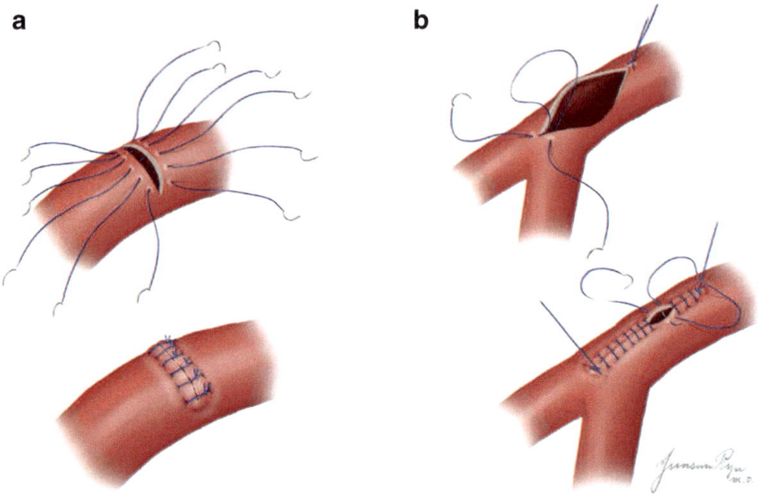

Fig. 12.7 (**a**) An interrupted suture technique. (**b**) A continuous running suture technique

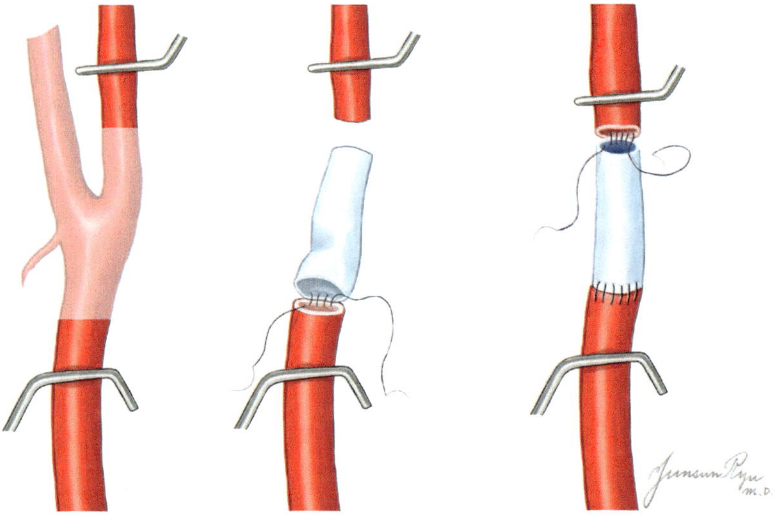

Fig. 12.8 Carotid graft replacement

◆ **Surgical Techniques for Repair:** Depending on the extent and type of the injury, options include primary repair, patch angioplasty with autogenous vein or synthetic materials, and bypass grafting using a vein or a synthetic conduit.

◆ **Emergency Preparedness:** Surgeons must be ready for quick, decisive actions, including ways to obtain proximal and distal vascular control and selecting the appropriate surgical technique to repair the artery.

Carotid artery surgery requires specialized skills owing to the delicate nature of the procedure and the risk of neurological complications. Surgical intervention should be performed promptly to minimize the risk of stroke, infection, and other complications. To select the most appropriate surgical approach, a comprehensive assessment of the patient's medical history, coexisting conditions, and imaging findings is essential. Neurological monitoring during surgery can also be useful for detecting changes in cerebral perfusion and facilitating prompt intervention if needed.

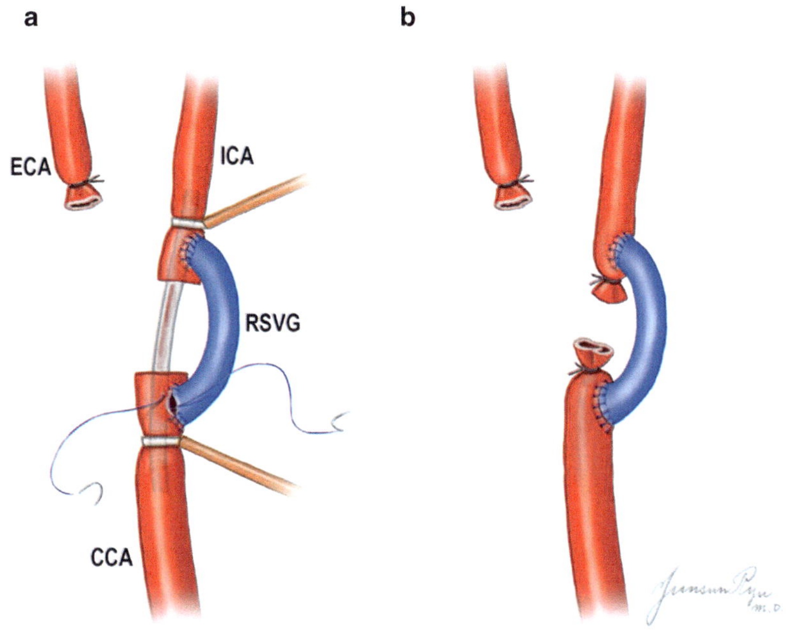

Fig. 12.9 (**a**) Injured carotid artery containing the shunt is bypassed with a reversed saphenous vein graft (RSVG). (**b**) After anastomoses are completed, the shunt is removed, and carotid stumps are ligated. ECA, external carotid artery; ICA, internal carotid artery; CCA, common carotid artery

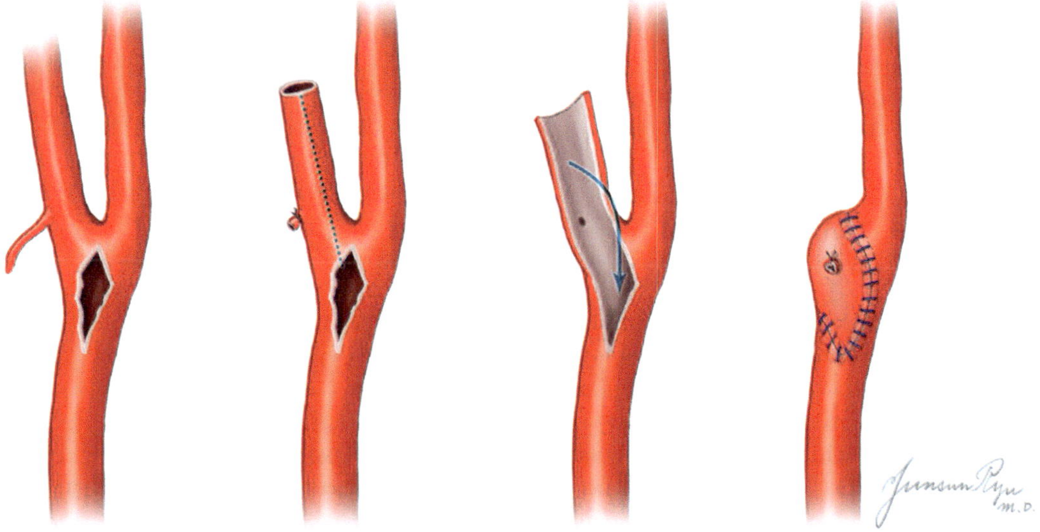

Fig. 12.10 The external carotid artery flap is rotated down over the defect in the common carotid artery

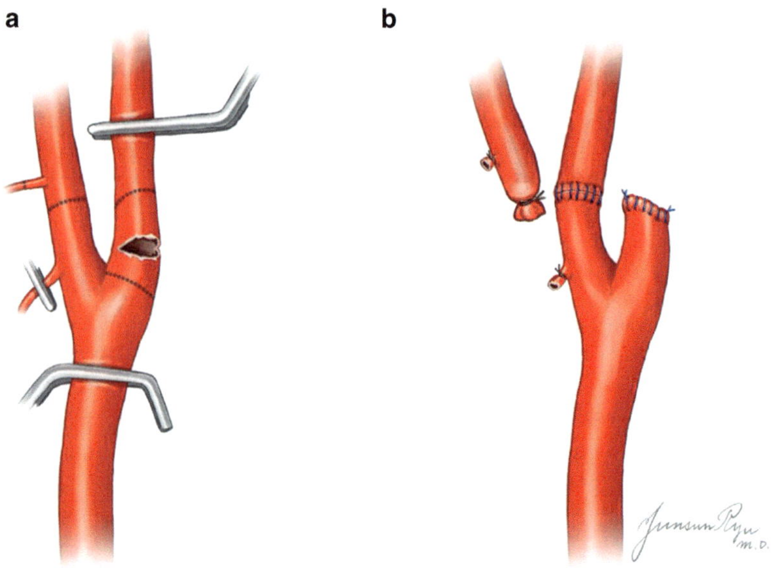

Fig. 12.11 (**a**) Internal carotid injury near the carotid bulb. (**b**) External carotid artery transposition to the internal carotid artery

◆ **Postoperative Monitoring:** Vigilance for cerebrovascular complications is essential, given the critical role of the carotid artery in cerebral perfusion. Neurological monitoring during and after surgery can help ensure the detection of adverse changes and timely intervention.

In managing carotid artery injuries during surgery, maintaining the circulating volume and minimizing the risk of cerebrovascular complications are both important. The carotid artery is the major blood vessel that supplies oxygenated blood to the brain. It comprises internal and external branches, each of which plays a crucial role in cerebral perfusion. The underlying mechanisms of cerebrovascular complications due to carotid artery injuries are as follows. (1) Direct mechanical disruption to the carotid artery leads to structural damage, compromising blood flow, and potentially causing thrombotic or embolic events. (2) Carotid artery injury may result in bleeding, leading to reduced cerebral perfusion and potentially causing ischemic events. (3) Swelling, hematoma, or anatomical distortion can lead to compression of adjacent blood vessels, impeding blood flow and causing an ischemic episode. (4) Carotid artery injury can trigger an inflammatory cascade, promoting thrombus formation and vessel wall damage and contributing to cerebrovascular complications. These various considerations should be addressed during surgery, and postoperative monitoring of their occurrence is necessary.

12.4 KQ 12.4. What Is the Appropriate Management for Skin Flap Necrosis After Neck Dissection?

Dong Jin Lee

Skin flap necrosis is a rare side effect of surgical procedures, including neck dissection. Skin necrosis occurs when the blood supply to the skin is interrupted or damaged. This limits the

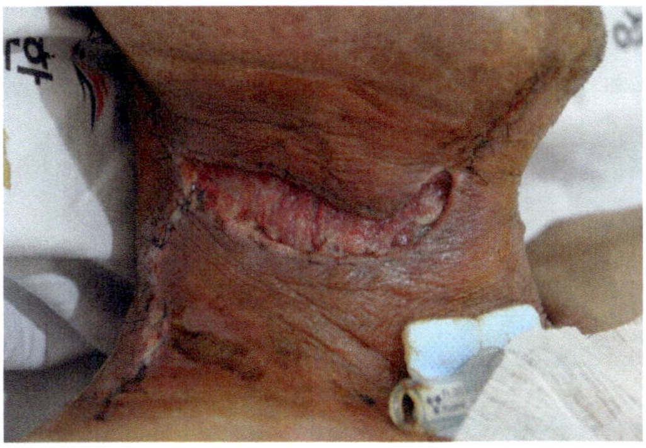

Fig. 12.12 Wound dehiscence after skin flap necrosis

delivery of oxygen and nutrients, resulting in the death of skin tissue. Skin necrosis after neck dissection usually causes wound dehiscence and requires additional surgical treatment (Fig. 12.12).

The skin of the neck is supplied by the facial artery and its branches through the platysma from the superior to the inferior direction. The lower neck is supplied by the transverse cervical artery and its branches, while the midportion and posterior neck skin are supplied by the superior thyroid and occipital arteries, respectively. Transverse and anterior incisions placed well within the platysma provide the best cosmetic outcomes and prevent skin necrosis [30].

Signs and symptoms of skin necrosis can appear as early as 2–4 days post-surgery and may progress hourly. Therefore, it is important to closely monitor patient healing because early identification offers the best chance for recovery (Table. 12.1).

◆ Signs and symptoms of skin flap necrosis include dark, blue, or black discoloration at the incision site; increased pain, swelling, or redness; fever or warmth in the incision area; and an open wound that does not appear to be healing.

Algorithm for the management of skin flap necrosis (Fig. 12.13)

Table. 12.1 Signs and symptoms of skin flap necrosis

Signs and symptoms of skin flap necrosis
Dark, blue, or black discoloration at the incision site
Increase in pain, swelling, or redness
Fever or warmth in the incision area
Open wound that does not appear to be healing

12.4.1 Prevention

Patients with head and neck cancer who require neck dissection surgery invariably have multiple barriers to wound healing. A comprehensive approach is necessary to optimize outcomes and avoid complications. Predispositions for poor wound healing and skin necrosis are innate; however, certain factors such as nutrition, blood sugar control, smoking, and alcohol abuse can be optimized before surgery [31]. Tobacco and alcohol cessation counseling should be provided. Although non-smokers have shown improved healing outcomes post-surgery compared with smokers, even short-term perioperative tobacco cessation is associated with lower postoperative infection rates [32]. Significantly more wound-related complications occurred in patients with excessive alcohol consumption. Nutritional referrals or encouragement to maximize nutrition should be routine. In some patients, preoperative gastrostomy tube placement is prudent. Finally, consultation or communication with other medical providers is essential to optimize a patient's medical condition. Controlling blood sugar levels, managing immunosuppressant medications, optimizing thyroid glucose levels, and improving pulmonary function are all factors that can be optimized preoperatively to promote skin healing and prevent skin necrosis postoperatively [31].

In addition, conforming to the vascular supply and planning the incision along watershed lines ensures optimal access to all structures without compromising skin approximation and healing. A single incision without a trifurcation point is preferable for preventing skin necrosis. Macfee incisions and the hockey stick 'J' incisions are preferred to avoid flap breakdown at trifurcation points. Proper approximation of the platysma during wound closure ensures complete closure of the neck and prevents skin necrosis [30].

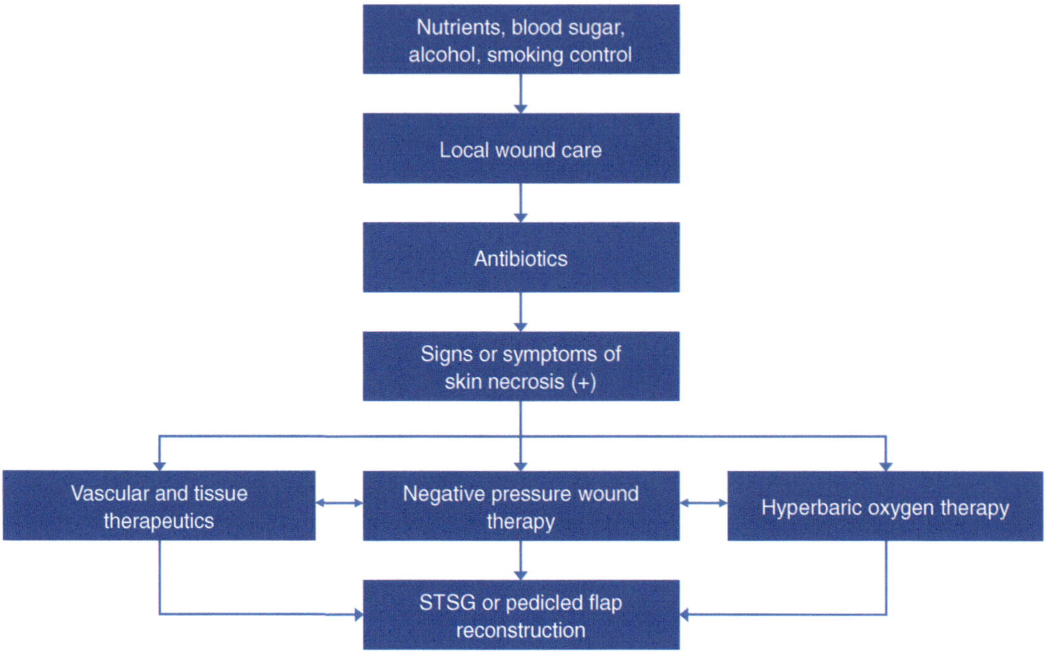

Fig. 12.13 Algorithm for the management of a skin flap necrosis. STSG, split-thickness skin graft

Particular attention should be paid during skip flap closure to mitigate complications, especially in patients with a history of radiation, previous surgeries, excessive skin tension, or large dead spaces underneath the skin flap. These factors increase the risk of skin flap necrosis and necessitate careful management.

◆ Some predispositions to poor wound healing and skin necrosis are innate, but certain factors such as nutrition, blood sugar levels, smoking, and alcohol abuse can be optimized prior to the surgery. Additionally, aligning the incision with the vascular supply and planning it along the watershed lines will provide optimal access to all structures without compromising skin approximation and healing.

Expert Opinion

Necrosis of a skin flap is very rare; therefore, it is crucial to thoroughly identify and clarify the underlying cause of this complication. It is important to address and correct any fundamental or underlying conditions or diseases. If the wound area is necrotic, major structures such as the carotid artery are exposed, and no specific contraindications exist for continuing the surgery, surgical intervention for wound care and management is necessary. (Chul-Ho Kim)

Compressive dressings can potentially cause skin necrosis by restricting blood flow to the skin underneath if applied too tightly or if there is inadequate monitoring of the patient's condition. (Yun-Sung Lim)

12.4.2 Local Wound Care

The general principles of local wound healing involve decontamination, prevention of further trauma, and optimization of the wound bed environment. In severe cases, the affected tissue must be removed through surgery or other means. Chronic wounds often exhibit bacterial colonization, and increased bacterial counts are associated with delayed wound healing and skin necrosis [33]. Wounds are thoroughly washed to reduce the bacterial load. Various topical treatments and dressings, including sodium hypochlorite, topical antibiotics, and silver-based dressings, reported a decrease in colonization [34]. Furthermore, several topical treatments have been used to optimize the local tissue environment. Topical therapies, including hydrocolloids, alginates, and other foams and gels, have demonstrated efficacy in promoting a moist environment conducive to healing and preventing skin necrosis [35]. Traditionally, wet-to-dry dressing changes have been used for the debridement of nonviable tissue and are frequently used by surgeons to promote granulation tissue.

12.4.3 Antibiotics

Perioperative antibiotics should be administered, especially when considering head and neck surgery, which typically involves a clean, contaminated field. Methicillin-resistant *Staphylococcus aureus* (MRSA) infections have been linked to postoperative wound infections and skin necrosis during head and neck surgery [36]. Studies have shown that a short perioperative antibiotic course is as effective as a prolonged course in primary head and neck surgery for preventing surgical site infections and skin necrosis. Prolonged courses are associated with an additional risk of antibiotic-resistant infections [37].

12.4.4 Vascular and Tissue Therapeutics

Treatments and modalities involve mediators of inflammation, vasodilation, cytokines, and other growth factors to aid in preserving the skin flap and wound healing. Examples include the study of platelet-rich plasma and fibrin glue applied in rat pharyngotomies, which showed higher inflammatory and fibroblastic activities than controls [38]. Prostaglandin E1 is a mediator for vasodilation that has primarily been used in vascular surgery as well as in the head and neck free flap literature. Its application in salvage laryngectomy to avoid pharyngocutaneous fistulas and other wound-healing complications has been successful in a small case series [39].

12.4.5 Hyperbaric Oxygen Treatment

Hypoxia and hypoperfusion are underlying etiologies of poor wound healing and skin necrosis, particularly in previously treated tissues. Hyperbaric oxygen (HBO) increases tissue oxygen tension and promotes angiogenesis, collagen formation, and antimicrobial properties [40]. HBO can be used preoperatively to improve tissue oxygenation to prevent skin necrosis or aid wound healing. HBO is primarily indicated as an adjunct to conservative wound care strategies and can work synergistically with local wound therapy for skin necrosis.

12.4.6 Negative Pressure Wound Therapy

Recent review highlights that the use of negative pressure wound therapy (NPWT) after open ventral hernia repair can reduce the incidence of hernia recurrence, infection, and wound dehiscence simultaneously [41]. However, NPWT has no visible effect on other complications such as seroma, hematoma, or skin necrosis. Nonetheless, a limitation of this review is the significant heterogeneity among the studies, possibly attributable to differences in article quality and NPWT techniques.

12.4.7 Split-Thickness Skin Graft or Pedicled Reconstruction

Split-thickness skin graft (STSG) has traditionally been the treatment of choice for skin necrosis after neck dissection, owing to its technical simplicity. Other regional flaps, such as the submental island and supraclavicular flaps, have also been used. Muscle coverage has been shown to promote wound healing owing to its high vascularity, ability to close dead spaces, and expression of growth factors [42].

◆ The general principles of local wound healing involve decontamination, preventing further trauma, and optimizing the environment of the wound bed. Perioperative antibiotics should be administered, especially considering head and neck surgery typically involves a clean-contaminated field. Vascular therapeutics such as prostaglandin E1, hyperbaric oxygen treatment, NPWT, STSG, or pedicled reconstruction can be applied if skin necrosis occurs.

12.5 KQ 12.5. What Is an Effective Strategy to Manage Severe Peripheral Lymphedema?

Dong Jin Lee

Lymphedema is a prevalent side effect of direct tumor invasion, radiation therapy (RT), or surgical resection, all of which disrupt lymphatic drainage (Fig. 12.14) [43]. It generally begins and progresses gradually 8–12 weeks after the initiation of RT and can persist indefinitely [44]. It can be external (skin and soft tissue) or internal (pharyngeal and laryngeal mucosa) and can induce sensations of heaviness and achiness, potentially resulting in skin alterations. Furthermore, it can cause difficulties in breathing, congestion, visual impairment, motor function disruption (e.g., reduced neck motion, jaw tightness or trismus, and chest tightness), ear pain, sensory limitations, problems related to speech, voice, or swallowing (e.g., inability to use an electrolarynx, difficulty in articulation, drooling, and loss of food from the mouth), and emotional issues (e.g., depression, frustration, and embarrassment).

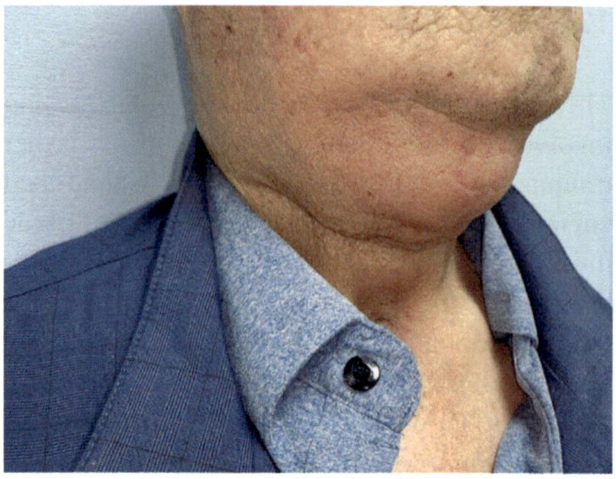

Fig. 12.14 Lymphedema after postoperative radiation therapy

Lymphedema comprises several stages [45]:

- Stage 0: No visible swelling but a sensation of heaviness in the neck.
- Stage 1a: Mild visible swelling without pitting. Reversible.
- Stage 1b: Mild visible swelling with pitting. Reversible.
- Stage 2: Irreversible firm-pitting swelling, with no visible changes in the tissue.
- Stage 3: Irreversible changes in the tissue, with scarring and fibrosis.

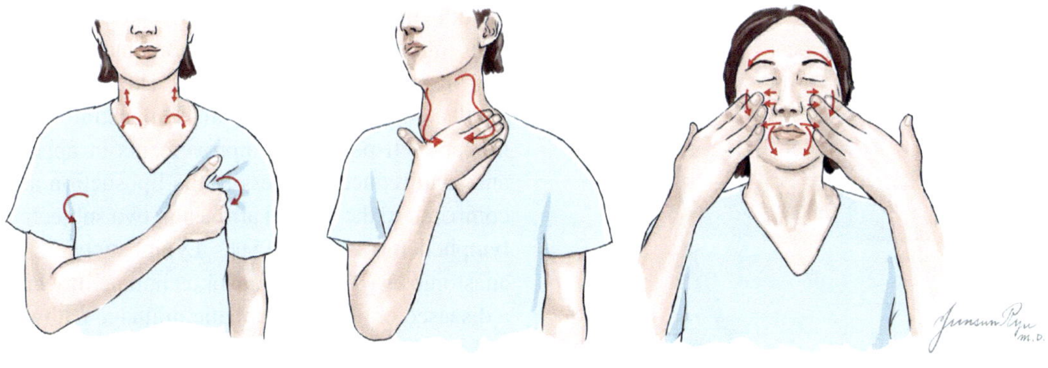

Fig. 12.15 Manual lymphatic drainage

Expert Opinion
Lymphedema is an extremely common complication that arises when local blood and lymphatic circulation are compromised following surgery or chemoradiation therapy. I generally advise patients to engage in massages and exercises and appropriately use head-compression garments. Additionally, some studies suggest that devices such as vibrators or ultrasound machines can be beneficial. (Chul-Ho Kim)

Cosmetic sequelae remain the most common complications of head and neck lymphedema (HNL), with 84% of patients reporting complaints regarding their appearance (Fig. 12.15). Moreover, 33% of the patients reported functional deficits such as pain, dysphagia, and dysphonia [44].

The diagnosis and measurement of HNL are challenging; achieving reproducible measurements is problematic owing to inconsistent and often obscure reference points in affected patients [46]. Management of HNL includes manual lymphatic drainage (MLD), complete decongestion therapy (CDT), the use of selenium compounds and liposuction, and microvascular surgery.

◆ Cosmetic sequelae remain the most prevalent complication of HNL, with 84% of patients reporting complaints regarding their appearance. However, 33% of patients also report functional deficits such as pain, dysphagia, and dysphonia. The management of HNL includes MLD, CDT, the use of selenium compounds and liposuction, and microvascular surgery.

1. Manual Lymphatic Drainage

   MLD is recommended as a first-line therapy for HNL according to American Cancer Society guidelines [47]. Originally developed by Dr. Vodder, it involves tissue massage, joint manipulation, and stretching exercises performed by a trained therapist [48].

2. Complete decongestion therapy

   CDT, a relatively recent treatment, has become the predominant approach for the management of HNL because of its effectiveness. CDT is integrated with MLD using custom compression garments, physical exercise, and skincare routines [49]. However, despite being commonly recommended by healthcare providers, compliance with the use of compression garments for HNL is a barrier for many patients who seek alternative therapies (Fig. 12.16).

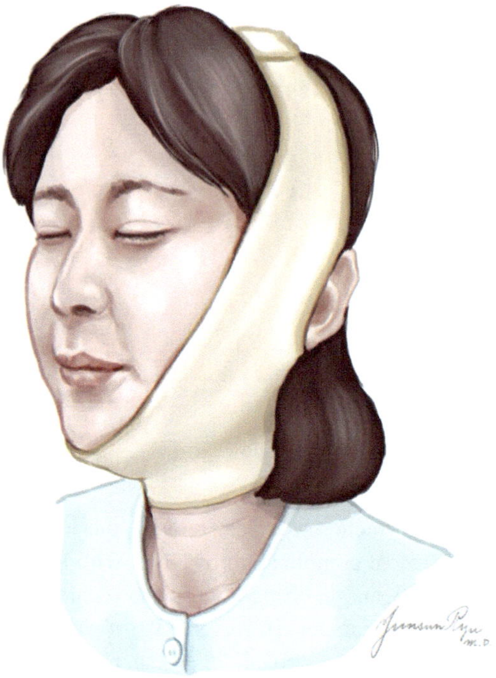

Fig. 12.16 Head-compression garments for complete decongestion therapy

3. Selenium compounds

Selenium compounds, which are thought to reduce lymphedema by increasing the activity of enzymes responsible for clearing reactive oxygen species, have been studied as alternatives and adjuncts to compressive therapy. However, their adoption remains limited [50]. The use of orally administered sodium selenite was investigated in a few studies on HNL. In a randomized controlled trial (RCT) conducted by Zimmermann et al., the efficacy of 1000 μg of sodium selenite in reducing postoperative HNL was evaluated, showing a significant reduction in lymphoma 1 week post-treatment; however, no significant difference was observed compared to placebo at 2 weeks post-treatment [50].

4. Liposuction and microvascular surgery

Surgical management is increasingly employed in refractory cases. These procedures include liposuction and microvascular surgery. Only one RCT investigated submental liposuction in patients with HNL [51]. The 2018 RCT conducted by Alamoudi et al. demonstrated significant self-perceived improvements in appearance and reduced distress in the liposuction arm compared to the control arm using two subjective lymphedema scales [51]. Lymphaticovenular anastomosis (LVA) is a novel technique in which a diseased or absent lymphatic drainage pathway is bypassed by identifying locally functioning lymphatic vessels and surgically anastomosing them to a suitable venule to create a functional drainage pathway [52].

◆ 1. MLD and CDT are recommended as first-line therapies for HNL. Selenium compounds, thought to reduce lymphedema by increasing the activity of reactive oxygen species-clearing enzymes, have been studied as alternatives and adjuncts to compressive therapy. Recently, surgical management, including liposuction and microvascular surgery, has been increasingly employed to treat refractory cases.

Expert Opinion

Unlike lymphedema in the extremities following axillary or groin dissection, HNL is a relatively less morbid phenomenon. It is particularly seen in patients who underwent bilateral neck dissections and pre- or postoperative radiotherapy. With the increasing use of modified and selective neck dissection strategies, it is now a rare complication. Most patients with a moderate degree of lymphedema are effectively managed with manual massage therapy. Only in rare instances surgical intervention with venous lymphatic microsurgery is required. The potential role of lymph node transplantation is currently under investigation, and may show some promise. (Jatin Shah)

References

1. Jain A, Singh SN, Singhal P, Sharma MP, Grover M. A prospective study on the role of octreotide in management of chyle fistula neck. Laryngoscope. 2015;125(7):1624–7.
2. Magoo S, Bhate K, Santhosh Kumar SN, Kakodkar P, Gajul M, Mastud S. Effect of octreotide in stopping post surgical chyle leak in neck dissection-a systematic review. J Oral Biol Craniofac Res. 2022;12(5):737–41.
3. Belloso A, Saravanan K, de Carpentier J. The community management of chylous fistula using a pancreatic lipase inhibitor (orlistat). Laryngoscope. 2006;116(10):1934–5.
4. Delaney SW, Shi H, Shokrani A, Sinha UK. Management of chyle leak after head and neck surgery: review of current treatment strategies. Int J Otolaryngol. 2017;2017:8362874.
5. Kim PH, Tsauo J, Shin JH. Lymphatic interventions for chylothorax: a systematic review and meta-analysis. J Vasc Interv Radiol. 2018;29(2):194–202 e4.
6. Kim J, Bang DH, Choi TW, Won JH, Kwon Y. Lymphangiography and lymphatic embolisation for the treatment of chyle leaks after neck surgery: assessment of lymphangiography findings and embolisation techniques. Br J Radiol. 2023;96(1149):20220831.
7. Wilkerson PM, Haque A, Pitkin L, Soon Y. Thoracoscopic ligation of the thoracic duct complex in the treatment for high-volume chyle leak following modified radical neck dissection: safe, feasible, but underutilised. Clin Otolaryngol. 2014;39(1):73–4.
8. Crile G. Excision of cancer of the head and neck. JAMA. 1906;47:1780–6.
9. Jones RK. Increased intracranial pressure following radical neck surgery. AMA Arch Surg. 1951;63(5):599–603.
10. Moore OS, Frazell EL. Simultaneous bilateral neck dissection: experience with 151 patients. Am J Surg. 1964;107:565–8.
11. Razack MS, Baffi R, Sako K. Bilateral radical neck dissection. Cancer. 1981;47(1):197–9.
12. Katsuno S, Ishiyama T, Nezu K, Usami S. Three types of internal jugular vein reconstruction in bilateral radical neck dissection. Laryngoscope. 2000;110(9):1578–80.
13. Farlow JL, McCrary HC, Li M, Old MO. Internal jugular vein reconstruction: an algorithm for reconstructive surgeons. Oral Oncol. 2023;145:106523.
14. Zhou D, Ding JY, Ya JY, Pan LQ, Yan F, Yang Q, et al. Understanding jugular venous outflow disturbance. CNS Neurosci Ther. 2018;24(6):473–82.
15. Tisherman SA. Management of major vascular injury: open. Otolaryngol Clin North Am. 2016;49(3):809–17. https://doi.org/10.1016/j.otc.2016.02.004.
16. Sobol SM, Freeman R, Thawley S, Little J, Beven E. Management of inadvertent injury to the carotid artery during head and neck surgery. Head Neck Surg. 1982;4(6):475–82. https://doi.org/10.1002/hed.2890040606.
17. DuBose JJ, Savage SA, Fabian TC, et al. The American Association for the Surgery of Trauma PROspective Observational Vascular Injury Treatment (PROOVIT) registry: multicenter data on modern vascular injury diagnosis, management, and outcomes. J Trauma Acute Care Surg. 2015;78(2):215–22.; discussion 222-3. https://doi.org/10.1097/TA.0000000000000520.
18. Creager MA, Beckman JA, Loscalzo J. Vascular medicine: a companion to Braunwald's heart disease. 3rd ed. Elsevier; 2019. p. 960.
19. Verdonck P, de Schoutheete JC, Monsieurs KG, Van Laer C, Vander Poorten V, Vanderveken O. Penetrating and blunt trauma to the neck: clinical presentation, assessment and emergency management. B-ENT. 2016;26(2):69–85.
20. Asensio JA, Vu T, Mazzini FN, et al. Penetrating carotid artery: uncommon complex and lethal injuries. Eur J Trauma Emerg Surg. 2011;37(5):429. https://doi.org/10.1007/s00068-011-0132-3.
21. Flint PW, Haughey BH, Lund VJ, Robbins KT, Thomas JR, Lesperance MM, Francis HW. Cummings otolaryngology: head and neck surgery, vol. 3. 7th ed. Elsevier; 2020.
22. Stafforini NA, Singh N. Management of vascular injuries in penetrating trauma. Surg Clin North Am. 2023;103(4):801–25. https://doi.org/10.1016/j.suc.2023.04.018.
23. Marsman MS, Wetterslev J, Jahrome AK, et al. Carotid endarterectomy with patch angioplasty versus primary closure in patients with symptomatic and significant stenosis: a systematic review with meta-analyses and trial sequential analysis of randomized clinical trials. Syst Rev. 2021;10(1):139. https://doi.org/10.1186/s13643-021-01692-8.
24. Sidawy AN, Perler BA. Rutherford's vascular surgery and endovascular therapy. 10th ed. Elsevier; 2022. p. 28–36.
25. Igor Koncar NI, Dragas M, Banzic I, Markovic M, Kostic D, Davidovic L. Vascular surgery—principles and practice. IntechOpen; 2012.
26. Sunar H, Canbaz S, Edis M, Duran E. A different repair technique for carotid artery injury. EJVES Extra. 2002;4:35–6.
27. Asfar S, Al-Ali J, Ben-Nakhi M. Repair of common carotid artery injury with an external carotid artery flap. Med Princ Pract. 2004;13(5):292–4. https://doi.org/10.1159/000079531.
28. Moore EE, Feliciano DV, Mattox KL. Trauma. 7th ed. McGraw Hill; 2013. p. 471–2.
29. Weaver FA, Yellin AE, Wagner WH, Brooks SH, Weaver AA, Milford MA. The role of arterial reconstruction in penetrating carotid injuries. Arch Surg. 1988;123(9):1106–11. https://doi.org/10.1001/archsurg.1988.01400330082013.
30. Kerawala CJ. Complications of head and neck cancer surgery—prevention and management. Oral Oncol. 2010;46(6):433–5.

31. Kwon D, Genden EM, de Bree R, Rodrigo JP, Rinaldo A, Sanabria A, et al. Overcoming wound complications in head and neck salvage surgery. Auris Nasus Larynx. 2018;45(6):1135–42.
32. Sorensen LT. Wound healing and infection in surgery. The clinical impact of smoking and smoking cessation: a systematic review and meta-analysis. Arch Surg. 2012;147(4):373–83.
33. Edwards R, Harding KG. Bacteria and wound healing. Curr Opin Infect Dis. 2004;17(2):91–6.
34. Lin YH, Hsu WS, Chung WY, Ko TH, Lin JH. Silver-based wound dressings reduce bacterial burden and promote wound healing. Int Wound J. 2016;13(4):505–11.
35. Singer AJ, Dagum AB. Current management of acute cutaneous wounds. N Engl J Med. 2008;359(10):1037–46.
36. Jeannon JP, Orabi A, Manganaris A, Simo R. Methicillin resistant Staphylococcus aureus infection as a causative agent of fistula formation following total laryngectomy for advanced head & neck cancer. Head Neck Oncol. 2010;2:14.
37. Simo R, French G. The use of prophylactic antibiotics in head and neck oncological surgery. Curr Opin Otolaryngol Head Neck Surg. 2006;14(2):55–61.
38. Eryilmaz A, Demirci B, Gunel C, Kacar Doger F, Yukselen O, Kurt Omurlu I, et al. Can tissue adhesives and platelet-rich plasma prevent pharyngocutaneous fistula formation? Auris Nasus Larynx. 2016;43(1):62–7.
39. Shiga K, Tateda M, Saijo S. Complication-free laryngeal surgery after irradiation failure with prostaglandin E1 administration. Ann Otol Rhinol Laryngol. 2002;111(9):783–8.
40. Thom SR. Hyperbaric oxygen: its mechanisms and efficacy. Plast Reconstr Surg. 2011;127(Suppl 1):131S–41S.
41. Xu Y, Shao S, Gong Z, Ri H, Xu Z, Kang H, et al. Efficacy of prophylactic negative pressure wound therapy after open ventral hernia repair: a systematic review meta-analysis. BMC Surg. 2023;23(1):374.
42. Chan JK, Harry L, Williams G, Nanchahal J. Soft-tissue reconstruction of open fractures of the lower limb: muscle versus fasciocutaneous flaps. Plast Reconstr Surg. 2012;130(2):284e–95e.
43. Deng J, Murphy BA, Dietrich MS, Wells N, Wallston KA, Sinard RJ, et al. Impact of secondary lymphedema after head and neck cancer treatment on symptoms, functional status, and quality of life. Head Neck. 2013;35(7):1026–35.
44. Smith BG, Hutcheson KA, Little LG, Skoracki RJ, Rosenthal DI, Lai SY, et al. Lymphedema outcomes in patients with head and neck cancer. Otolaryngol Head Neck Surg. 2015;152(2):284–91.
45. Executive Committee of the International Society of Lymphology. The diagnosis and treatment of peripheral lymphedema: 2020 Consensus Document of the International Society of Lymphology. Lymphology. 2020;53(1):3–19.
46. Tacani PM, Franceschini JP, Tacani RE, Machado AF, Montezello D, Goes JC, et al. Retrospective study of the physical therapy modalities applied in head and neck lymphedema treatment. Head Neck. 2016;38(2):301–8.
47. Cohen EE, LaMonte SJ, Erb NL, Beckman KL, Sadeghi N, Hutcheson KA, et al. American cancer society head and neck cancer survivorship care guideline. CA Cancer J Clin. 2016;66(3):203–39.
48. Kasseroller RG. The Vodder school: the Vodder method. Cancer. 1998;83(12 Suppl American):2840–2.
49. Gradalski T, Ochalek K, Kurpiewska J. Complex decongestive lymphatic therapy with or without Vodder II manual lymph drainage in more severe chronic postmastectomy upper limb lymphedema: a randomized noninferiority prospective study. J Pain Symptom Manage. 2015;50(6):750–7.
50. Zimmermann T, Leonhardt H, Kersting S, Albrecht S, Range U, Eckelt U. Reduction of postoperative lymphedema after oral tumor surgery with sodium selenite. Biol Trace Elem Res. 2005;106(3):193–203.
51. Alamoudi U, Taylor B, MacKay C, Rigby MH, Hart R, Trites JRB, et al. Submental liposuction for the management of lymphedema following head and neck cancer treatment: a randomized controlled trial. J Otolaryngol Head Neck Surg. 2018;47(1):22.
52. Yamamoto T, Yoshimatsu H, Yamamoto N, Yokoyama A, Numahata T, Koshima I. Multisite lymphaticovenular anastomosis using vein graft for uterine cancer-related lymphedema after pelvic lymphadenectomy. Vasc Endovascular Surg. 2015;49(7):195–200.

Part VI

Thyroid/Parathyroid

Thyroid Surgery: Neurologic Complications

13

Yong Bae Ji and Seung-Won Lee

13.1 KQ 13.1. What to Do If a Loss of Signal Is Encountered in the Nerve Monitoring System During Thyroidectomy?

Yong Bae Ji

Loss of signal (LOS) is a condition in which electromyography (EMG) signals are not observed or appear weak despite stimulation of the recurrent laryngeal nerve (RLN). According to the International Neural Monitoring Study Group, LOS is defined as EMG changes from initial satisfactory amplitude to no or low response (i.e., 100 μV or less) with stimulation at 1–2 mA on dry field [1]. When LOS occurs, it is crucial to determine whether it results from nerve impairment or technical and/or equipment issues. To verify this, laryngeal twitching is assessed. This method provides an initial and rapid assessment approach. During nerve stimulation, the operator touches the back of the cricothyroid joint with a finger to detect muscle twitching.

◆ When a loss of signal occurs, the initial step is laryngeal twitching.

Expert Opinion

Injury to the RLN in thyroid surgery can cause vocal cord paralysis and potentially interfere with breathing. Using intraoperative neuromonitoring (IONM), the surgeon can evaluate the real-time laryngeal EMG response, representing the functional status of RLN. At times, there may be partial or total loss of EMG signal (LOS), indicating that RLN stress or injury has occurred; the surgeon can also evaluate the surgical maneuver that produced the impending or actual RLN injury. By elucidating the mechanism of RLN injury and the surgical pitfalls, IONM can help surgeons improve surgical techniques, predict recovery outcomes, and plan intra- and post-operative management. The widespread use of IONM

(continued)

Supplementary Information The online version contains supplementary material available at https://doi.org/10.1007/978-981-96-1860-6_13.

Y. B. Ji (✉)
Department of Otolaryngology-Head and Neck Surgery, College of Medicine, Hanyang University, South Korea, Seoul, Republic of Korea
e-mail: jyb20000@hanyang.ac.kr

S.-W. Lee (✉)
Department of Otolaryngology-Head and Neck Surgery, SoonChunHyang University Hospital, Bucheon, South Korea
e-mail: lsw0922@schmc.ac.kr

K.-J. Cho, J.-O. Park (eds.), *Management of Head and Neck Surgery Complications*,
https://doi.org/10.1007/978-981-96-1860-6_13

in thyroid surgery has revealed the need to develop reliable strategies for cases in which LOS occurs during planned total thyroidectomy. In addition, false LOS and LOS recovery may occur and may lead to an unnecessary staged operation. This chapter provides an overview of LOS analysis and management to assist surgeons in clinical decision-making. (Wu Chewei)

13.1.1 Presence of Laryngeal Twitch

If a laryngeal twitch is observed, the stimulation segment is functioning correctly, and there are no issues with muscle relaxation or nerve conduction. However, the problem lies in the recording segment. The most prevalent cause of these instances is incorrect tube positioning [2]. Even if the electrode designed to make contact with the larynx is initially placed accurately, the electrode attached to the surgical tube may shift over time owing to traction of the larynx or trachea caused by thyroid manipulation during surgery. Thus, the most common reason for signal loss without impairment of nerve function is the failure of neuromonitoring owing to changes in the position of the tube electrode.

In this scenario, it is necessary to check and rectify the position of the tube in collaboration with the anesthesiologist, even during surgery. Adjustments may involve inserting the tube deeper or slightly withdrawing it. This change in electrode position can arise not only from changes in tube depth but also from rotation, which is a factor contributing to false positives. Thus, it was beneficial to verify the impedance values. If tube displacement is suspected intraoperatively, confirmation can be obtained via translaryngeal stimulation. In this situation, a stimulation current of 3–5 mA is required to pass through the cartilage. The location of the electrodes in the airway is determined by electrically stimulating the thyroid cartilage, cricothyroid membrane, and cricoid cartilage. For instance, a maximum response in the cricoid area indicates excessive intubation depth.

Occasionally, issues may arise from a dislodged ground electrode or a problem in the connection between the ground electrode and interface connector box, especially when surface electrodes are utilized. Therefore, it is crucial to inspect these contacts.

Contralateral vagus nerve stimulation is required when LOS occurs in the ipsilateral RLN. If EMG signals cannot be obtained from the contralateral vagus nerve, it could signify a problem on the recording side. Conversely, a signal observed in the contralateral vagus nerve indicates potential damage to the ipsilateral nerve.

◆ If a laryngeal twitch occurs during the stimulation of the RLN, it indicates the proper functioning of the stimulation segment. The most prevalent cause of signal loss without impairment of nerve function is typically the displacement of the EMG tube. Additionally, issues might arise from the ground electrode or its connection to the interface connector box.

◆ To discern a false positive, stimulation of the contralateral vagus nerve can provide clarification.

Expert Opinion

As mentioned above, angulation can be one cause of false-positive LOS, and this requires confirmation with video laryngoscopy. (Hok Nam Li)

If adjustment is needed, moving the tube in or out might be insufficient, as rotation or angulation can be the problem, and translaryngeal stimulation through cartilage may not be accurate due to high impedance. Therefore, if adjustment is needed, the anesthesiologist should use the video laryngoscope and make adjustments according to the visual position of the tube EMG electrode. (Hok Nam Li)

(continued)

If LOS detected in the contralateral vagus nerve, this could also be an angulation problem. In my experience, anesthesiologists tend to choose a smaller tube size to reduce pressure or the risk of damage; however, the trachea is relatively large, and if there is too much space between the EMG tube and the trachea during surgery after manipulation of the enlarged thyroid, the tube can point at the contralateral vocal cord or tracheal wall, without touching the ipsilateral vocal cord, causing false-positive LOS. This requires confirmation with video laryngoscopy (Hok Nam Li)

If a laryngeal twitch occurs during the stimulation of the RLN, it indicates that the stimulation segment is functioning properly. The most common cause of this twitch is typically the displacement of the EMG tube. Additionally, issues may arise from the ground electrode or its connection to the interface connector box. (Kang Dae Lee)

To differentiate a false-positive result, stimulating the contralateral vagus nerve can help clarify the situation. (Kang Dae Lee)

13.1.2 Absence of Laryngeal Twitch

When a laryngeal twitch is not observed, problems with the stimulator should be ruled out. Specifically, scenarios in which the current from the stimulation probe might not have been adequately delivered should be considered. To confirm the integrity of the system, contractions should be provoked by stimulating nearby strap muscles or checking the current return (Video 13.1). The occurrence of muscle twitch or normal current returns can help to exclude abnormalities within the stimulation segment.

However, an appropriate current level must be applied accurately. The depolarization threshold of the RLN ranges from 0.3 to 0.4 mA, with maximum depolarization achieved at approximately 0.8 mA [3]. Therefore, the initial stimulation current is typically set to 1.0 mA. It is important to acknowledge that if the nerve is not fully exposed owing to the presence of blood or fascia, a normal EMG signal might not be obtained.

If there is no current return, this indicates an issue on the stimulation side. At this point, it is essential to examine the stimulation probe, interface connector box, and ground electrode errors. If no errors are identified, the ipsilateral vagus nerve should be stimulated again to rule out the possibility that the stimulated tissue is not neural tissue. If all potential errors are ruled out, neuromonitoring can be confirmed as effective, and this can be regarded as ipsilateral nerve damage. The information provided above is summarized and presented in a schematic format in Fig. 13.1.

Table 13.1 summarizes situations that can lead to false-positive or false-negative outcomes, ultimately leading to neuromonitoring failure.

◆ If a laryngeal twitch is not observed, the problem on the stimulator side should be ruled out first by checking the strap muscle twitch, current return, and stimulation current.

13.1.3 Alternative Techniques

Alternative methods have been developed to address the issue of frequent false positives arising from misplacement of the EMG tube or inadequate contact with the vocal cords. One method involves intraoperative neuromonitoring (IONM) using transcartilage needle electrodes [4] or skin-adhesive electrodes [5] (Fig. 13.2). These approaches offer the benefit of consistent EMG signal acquisition because they maintain continuous contact, even in the presence of thyroid gland manipulation or changes in position. Furthermore, the transcartilage needle electrode has the additional advantage of enabling sensitive monitoring because it can yield higher sig-

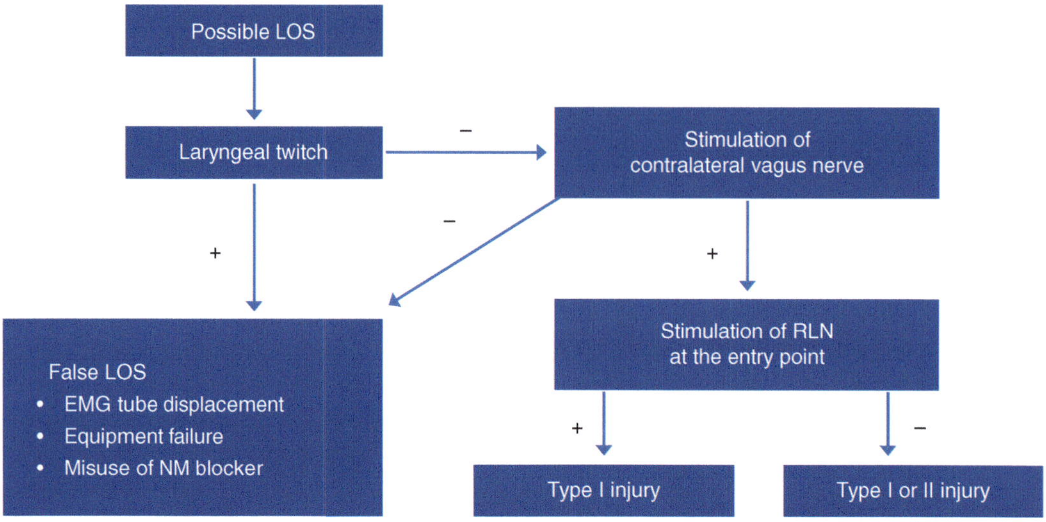

Fig. 13.1 Troubleshooting algorithm in loss of signal (LOS). EMG, electromyography; NM, neuromuscular; RLN, recurrent laryngeal nerve

Table 13.1 Causes of false-positive or false-negative results in intraoperative neuromonitoring

False positive (normal vocal cord function with EMG signal loss)
Equipment failure including tube malposition
Nerve covered by blood or connective tissues
Misuse of neuromuscular blocking agent
Insufficient stimulation current
False negative (abnormal vocal cord function with EMG signal)
Stimulation distal site to injured site
Injury after last stimulation
Delayed injury
Injury of posterior branch of recurrent laryngeal nerve
Cricoarytenoid dislocation
Significantly lower EMG amplitude than the initial

EMG, electromyography

nal amplitudes than an EMG tube. However, there is a limitation in that it is difficult to apply to endoscopic or robotic thyroid surgery. In addition, in patients with special airway conditions, such as pediatric groups or patients with difficult tracheal tumors or tracheostomies, in whom the EMG tube is unsuitable, the trans-cartilage method provides an ideal alternative. Conversely, skin-adhesive electrodes are noteworthy for their cost-effectiveness; however, they have the drawback of lower signal amplitudes owing to the contact resistance posed by the skin.

◆ Transcartilage needle electrodes or skin adhesive electrodes serve as valuable alternative techniques to circumvent tube malposition problems, which are frequently the primary cause of false positives.

Expert Opinion

The benefits of using needle or skin electrodes, which are commonly employed as alternative methods, include:

1. Electrode contact remains stable despite changes in the patient's posture or position, ensuring consistent amplitude.
2. They can be applied quickly and easily without requiring an anesthesiologist, thus reducing preparation time.
3. They are readily usable during surgery, even if not prepared beforehand.
4. They are suitable for use in tracheostomy cases or with pediatric patients.
5. They are unaffected by secretions in the trachea.
6. They are cost-effective in Korea, where insurance coverage for EMG endotracheal tubes is limited.(Byung-Joo Lee)

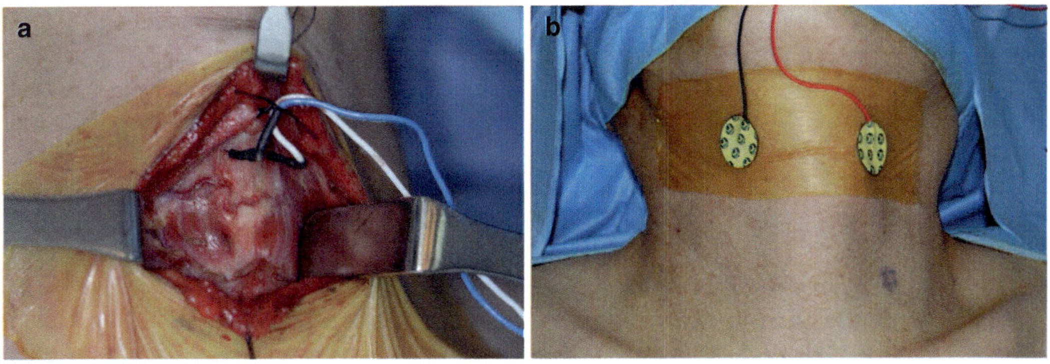

Fig. 13.2 (**a**) Transcartilage needle electrode. (**b**) Skin adhesive electrode

13.1.4 Types of Injury and Prognosis

When one side of the nerve is injured, surgeons should evaluate the location and cause of nerve injury. This evaluation facilitates feedback on the technique and guides the timing of surgery on the contralateral side.

The injury site should be identified using a probe that starts from the distal part of the ipsilateral RLN, which is the entry point. The surgeon traces the dissected nerve toward its proximal part to pinpoint the site of the injury. Through this process, the causes of nerve injury, such as traction, cauterization, or ligation, can be inferred. In addition, this procedure aids in determining the type of nerve injury involved. If a distinct injured area is clearly identified, it is categorized as a type 1 or segmental injury. Conversely, if the damaged area is not discernible and the nerve injury diffuses over the entire length, it is classified as type 2 or global injury [1].

Traction injuries are commonly reported to be the primary cause of both type 1 and type 2 injuries, whereas injuries resulting from cauterization or ligation are predominantly type 1 injuries. Recovery of nerve function tends to occur earlier in type 2 injuries than in type 1 injuries, with permanent damage more frequently reported in type 1 injuries [6, 7].

Further investigations into nerve injury and recovery have yielded findings indicating that even if the criteria for LOS are not met, a high likelihood of vocal cord paralysis exists if the EMG amplitude reduction is >60% between the proximal and distal parts of the RLN [8].

> ◆ If nerve injury occurs, the surgeon should evaluate the location and cause of the injury and determine the timing of surgery on the contralateral side.

13.1.5 Staged Thyroidectomy

To date, evidence has shown that staged thyroid surgery reduces bilateral vocal fold paralysis or tracheotomy when LOS is detected on one side using IONM. In a study involving over 2600 nerves, Goretzki et al. found that the incidence of bilateral vocal cord paralysis was 17% when LOS was disregarded, whereas it was 0% when the surgery was stopped or staged surgery was performed on the contralateral side [9]. Similarly, Melin et al. reported that bilateral vocal cord paralysis was observed in 16% of cases when the second operation proceeded after the initial LOS, whereas staged surgery resulted in a 0% occurrence [10]. In a subsequent study encompassing 3426 nerves, they reported a 28.6% contralateral nerve damage rate after LOS on one side [11]. In another study by Sadowski et al. involving a cohort of 220 patients and employing a staged approach upon signal loss on the first side, the incidence of bilateral vocal cord paralysis was significantly reduced [12].

13.2 KQ 13.2. How to Prevent Superior Laryngeal Nerve Injury During Thyroidectomy and What to Do If It Occurs?

Yong Bae Ji

13.2.1 Anatomy of the External Branch of the Superior Laryngeal Nerve

The superior laryngeal nerve, a branch of the vagus nerve, typically branches off at the nodose ganglion and is divided into internal and external segments. The external branch of the superior laryngeal nerve (EBSLN) descends dorsolaterally to the carotid sheath and crosses medially. Subsequently, it traverses the superior thyroid artery and vein situated above the superior thyroid pole and extends toward the larynx, carrying motor fibers to the cricothyroid (CT) muscle. The CT muscle contributes to voice modulation by elevating pitch, which is achieved by elongating and tensioning the vocal cords. Consequently, damage to the EBSLN leads to alterations in the voice quality, particularly at higher pitch ranges. Although the symptoms of EBSLN injury may be subtle, they pose significant problems to professional voice users [13–15].

The EBSLN is vulnerable to damage owing to anatomical variations in its proximity to the superior pole of the thyroid gland. Patients with large goiters and thyroid tumors located in the superior pole, short neck, or lower-lying nerves, such as Cernea types 2a and 2b, are at an elevated risk of nerve damage [16] (Fig. 13.3).

Expert Opinion
In the Cernea classification of EBSLN, type I is more common among Western populations, whereas types 2a and 2b are more frequently observed in Asians. Therefore, greater caution is necessary during thyroid surgery in Asian patients. (Byung-Joo Lee)

13.2.2 Avoiding Injury to the External Branch of the Superior Laryngeal Nerve

Owing to the lack of effective treatments for EBSLN injuries, the prevention of such injuries is important. Various techniques have been used to preserve the EBSLN during superior pole dissection in thyroidectomy: (1) visual identification

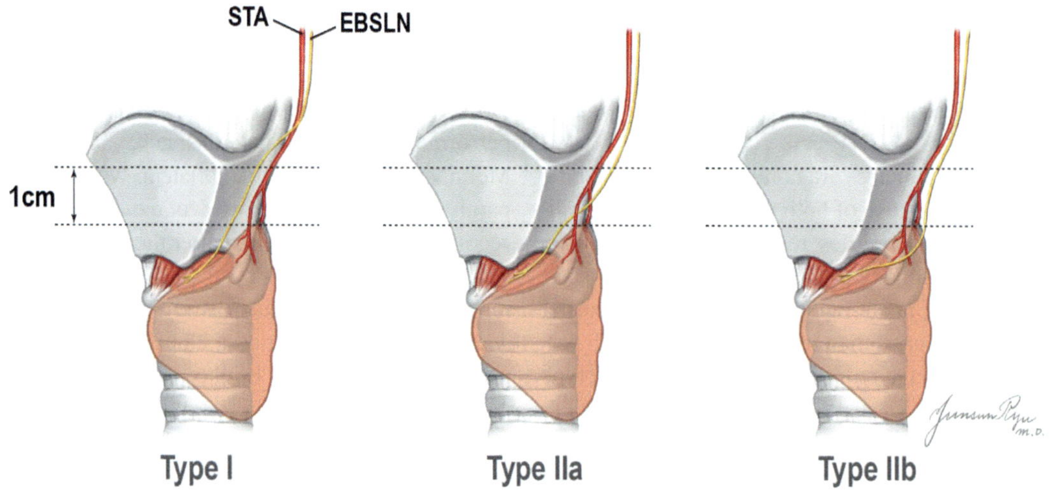

Fig. 13.3 Anatomy of the external branch of the superior laryngeal nerve. STA, superior thyroidal artery; EBSLN, external branch of the superior laryngeal nerve

of the EBSLN before ligation of the superior thyroid vessels; (2) individual dissection and ligation of the superior thyroid vessels in close proximity to the thyroid gland without identification of the nerve; and (3) electrical mapping of the sternothyroid-laryngeal triangle to assess the cricothyroid muscle (CTM) twitch or evoked EMG response using IONM.

Although visual identification of the nerve is a safe way to preserve it during thyroid surgery, it cannot be visually identified in some patients due to anatomical variations [13, 15]. The reported visual identification rate of the EBSLN without nerve monitoring varies from 10% to 88.4% [17–20] (Video 13.2).

Some authors have reported that individual ligation of the superior thyroid vessels adjacent to the thyroid gland capsule without visual identification of the nerve is a safe technique to prevent EBSLN injury and that the prevalence of nerve injury with this technique is similar to that with routine nerve identification [14]. However, other authors reported that the risk of EBSLN injury is higher when it is not visually identified during surgery [15, 16, 21]. Cernea et al. reported that EBSLN injury occurred in 12% of cases handled by experts and in 28% of cases handled by residents when the superior thyroid pole was dissected without visual identification of the EBSLN, whereas no injury occurred when the superior pole was dissected by an expert and the EBSLN was identified visually [16]. A prospective laryngeal EMG study comparing 50 patients without visual identification and 50 patients with visual identification of the EBSLN showed that EBSLN injury was significantly higher in the group without nerve identification (50% vs. 26%) [21].

Fortunately, recent reports have shown that IONM improves the identification and preservation of the EBSLN during conventional thyroidectomy. Barczynski et al. conducted a randomized controlled trial to compare visual identification alone and visual identification with IONM. The identification rate of the nerve was significantly higher (34.3% vs. 83.8%, $p < 0.001$), and the voice parameters were better in the IONM group [17]. Another study reported that the EBSLN was identified in only 36.9% of cases with visual identification alone and in 95.2% with the addition of IONM [22]. A prospective comparative study conducted on 240 nerves at risk (NARs) showed that the EBSLN was identified in 234 NARs (97.5%) using IONM, whereas 190 EBSLNs (79.1%) were identified visually (odds ratio = 10.35, 95% confidence interval 4.37–24.65) [23].

Moreover, it is not always imperative to directly confirm the presence of EBSLN using IONM. Even in cases in which the nerve was not identified using the IONM probe, the absence of the nerve in the stimulated region was indicated. IONM is useful not only for identifying and preserving the nerve but also for surgical procedures because it indicates that blood vessels can be safely ligated even when the nerve is not identified. Therefore, efforts to visually confirm the EBSLN or meticulous individual ligation of the superior thyroid vessels close to the superior pole of the thyroid gland, to identify the nerve, or to confirm its absence before ligation of the vessels are the best ways to prevent nerve injury.

◆ IONM of the EBSLN is helpful to map, identify, and preserve the nerve and dissect the superior pole. Even in cases where the EBSLN is not identified using IONM, the surgeon can divide the superior thyroid vessels safely after confirming the absence of the nerve.

Expert Opinion

EBSLN can be confirmed using IONM through two methods:

1. By observing twitching of the cricothyroid muscle, which is detectable in all patients.
2. By recording an EMG glottic response, which is identifiable in approximately 70%–80% of cases.

(continued)

When using IONM to preserve the EBSLN, a detectable magnetic nerve probe can be attached to the surgical instrument. This method is advantageous over traditional nerve stimulators owing to its convenience and speed, as it does not require any changes to the instrument. During surgery, when dissecting the upper pole of the thyroid, the superior thyroid artery or vein is ligated in areas where cricothyroid muscle twitching is not observed. Thus, the surgery proceeds only after confirming the absence of EBSLN, rather than verifying its presence. (Byung-Joo Lee)

Nevertheless, voice changes are the main symptoms when an EBSLN injury occurs. However, this effect is variable and subtle. Moreover, voice changes, including arytenoid injury and cricothyroid or strap muscle dysfunction, are common and multifactorial after thyroid surgery. Therefore, it is difficult to confirm EBSLN injury based on clinical and endoscopic findings. Several findings of EBSLN injury have been reported, including bowing of the vocal cords, inferior displacement of the vocal cords, and posterior glottic rotation toward the affected side. However, these findings were neither specific nor uniform [14].

In the case of unilateral EBSLN injury, the symptoms of most patients improve to varying degrees within 3 months owing to compensation by the healthy side. However, when the bilateral EBSLN is injured, the patient may experience cricothyroid and inferior pharyngeal constrictor muscle dysfunction, dysphonia, dysphagia, and choking.

Various treatment options have been suggested, including steroids, voice therapy, and surgery. Voice therapy, such as the glissando maneuver (continuous sliding or gliding between two or more pitches to strengthen the adductor muscles), is the most common and preferred treatment option for persistent voice abnormalities. Treatment ultimately aims to strengthen the cricothyroid muscles, although treatment results vary [24].

Although surgical treatment for SLN injuries is not commonly performed, several studies have reported procedures such as cricothyroid approximation and reinnervation using the nerve-muscle pedicle technique [25, 26].

◆ Voice therapy is preferred, although no optimal treatment is available when EBSLN injury occurs.
◆ In cases of considerable voice changes, especially in professional voice users, surgical treatment might be considered.

Expert Opinion

Damage to the EBSLN can produce variable voice changes, which can negatively affect a patient's quality of life, as well as cause a premature ending of a professional career. Recently, IONM techniques have been shown to increase the rates of EBSLN identification and have allowed the surgeon to verify the integrity of the nerve. This chapter gives surgeons an overview of the EBSLN anatomy, injury prevention strategy, and management. (Wu Chewei)

13.3 KQ 13.3. What Is the Appropriate Management for Inadvertent Recurrent Laryngeal Nerve Transection During Surgery?

Seung-Won Lee

◆ Conventionally, medialization thyroplasty with or without arytenoid adduction is the gold standard for treating permanent unilateral vocal fold paralysis after thyroid surgery. Primary intraoperative recurrent

(continued)

laryngeal nerve (RLN) reinnervation during thyroid surgery has been confirmed to be an ideal approach. It possesses the potential to restore a normal or near-normal voice while preserving laryngeal anatomy, ultimately providing stable voice outcomes for a lifetime.

Thyroplasty can pose a burden to both patients and doctors due to the need for additional neck incisions and surgery. In recent years, similar to thyroplasty, injection laryngoplasty (IL) has gained popularity among patients and doctors, as it is a simple and safe procedure performed under local anesthesia without the need for neck incisions [28]. However, long-term follow-up data indicate that it is generally less effective in patients with large posterior glottal gaps, and its effectiveness diminishes over time due to the absorption of injected materials [29].

Expert Opinion

Primary reinnervation is necessary to maintain the muscle tone and better voice outcome, but it cannot replace injection laryngoplasty. Nerve reconnection requires a long period of time, and the outcome of reinnervation is variable as in all nerve reinnervation. Primary reinnervation in long term can help voice outcome and lessen the need of repeating IL. However, primary reinnervation cannot replace IL at the early post-op period, particularly in patients with voice symptoms and phonation gap. (Hok Nam Li)

RLN reinnervation is necessary if the nerve is transected to allow for a better long term outcome, but the first approach in the early post-op period is IL. If the patient experiences voice symptoms or phonation gap, the results of IL are more promising. IL can also be performed in the clinic under local anesthesia, and it is less invasive than open medialization thyroplasty or arytenoid adduction. (Hok Nam Li)

IL for large gap can be less effective, but it can be improved by injecting a larger volume until the true cord is medialized to the midline and the patient's voice is improved. (Hok Nam Li)

Primary intraoperative recurrent laryngeal nerve (RLN) reinnervation possesses several advantages over thyroplasty and IL. This technique can be safely performed during surgery without compromising the airway, thus eliminating the need for additional skin incisions or IL. The 2020 Guidelines for the Management of Unilateral Vocal Fold Paralysis by the Korean Society of Laryngology, Phoniatrics, and Logopedics recommend considering intraoperative RLN reinnervation if direct laryngeal nerve injury occurs during surgery [30].

The reinnervation technique, whether direct or ansa-RLN, depends on the length of the RLN defect and the tension of the anastomosis. Direct reinnervation was suitable for shorter defects (Fig. 13.4), whereas ansa-RLN reinnervation was used for segmental defects to prevent excess tension [31] (Fig. 13.5). Subsequent medialization procedures may be avoided by performing intraoperative reinnervation during surgery, thus eliminating the need for foreign body implantation and reducing the risk of potential airway compromise [32].

Expert Opinion

In my experience, it can be categorized into direct anastomosis, cable graft, and ansa-RLN. Additionally, a cable graft may be feasible if it meets a certain length requirement. (Byung-Joo Lee)

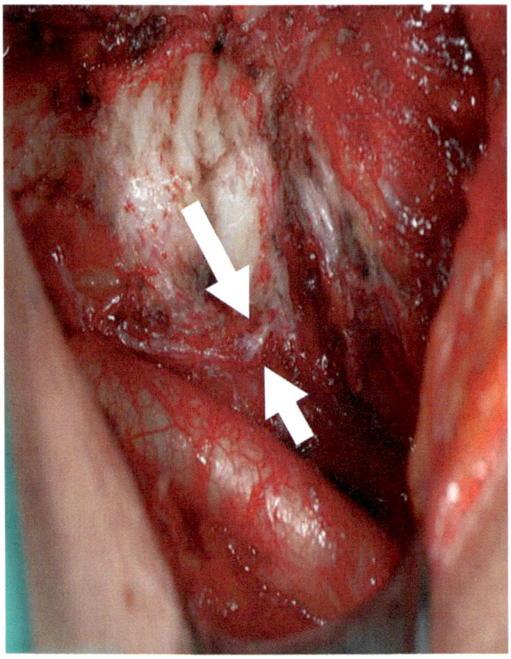

Fig. 13.4 Representative photograph demonstrating the direct reinnervation of the right recurrent laryngeal nerve (arrows)

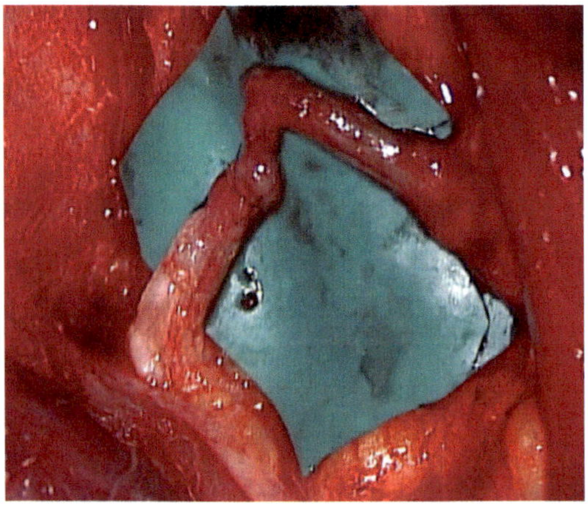

Fig. 13.5 Representative photograph demonstrating the reinnervation of the right ansa cervicalis to the right recurrent laryngeal nerve

For ansa-RLN reinnervation, the ipsilateral sternocleidomastoid muscle was retracted laterally, and the ansa cervicalis overlying the internal jugular vein was identified. After identifying the branches of the ansa cervicalis supplying the sternohyoid and sternothyroid muscles, they were transected into the lateral aspect of the strap muscle. Subsequently, the ansa cervicalis was mobilized, and four to five interrupted 9-0 nylon epineural sutures were placed for complete anastomosis with the recurrent laryngeal nerve (RLN).

While intraoperative RLN reinnervation may require 3–6 months to become effective, long-term outcomes indicate favorable results without deterioration of voice parameters [30]. A study by Lee et al. in 19 patients undergoing thyroid surgery demonstrated statistically significant improvements in voice parameters at 12 months post-surgery with stability up to 36 months and surpassing the outcomes of IL [33].

At 24 and 36 months after surgery, the RLN reinnervation group exhibited greater improvements in voice parameters than did the IL group. Long-term absorption of the injected materials in the IL may have contributed to these differences. Lee concluded that both RLN reinnervation and IL provided statistically significant voice improvements at 36 months postoperatively, with RLN reinnervation exhibiting better results after 3 years (Fig. 13.6).

Expert Opinion

For long-term absorption problems, calcium hydroxyapatite (Radiesse) is better than hyaluronic acid (Restylane), and in the long-term and even in response to small amounts of absorption, the contralateral true cord approach typically exhibits better compensation with time. Thus, not many patients require repeated injections. (Hok Nam Li)

Based on my experience, intraoperative RLN reinnervation can sometimes require longer than 3–6 months to exhibit effects, and the results can vary. (Hok Nam Li)

The authors' long-term voice results 10 years, after the primary intraoperative RLN reinnervation, demonstrated stable voice outcomes. Moreover, there is a positive trend toward improved voice parameters for up to 10 years after reinnervation [34].

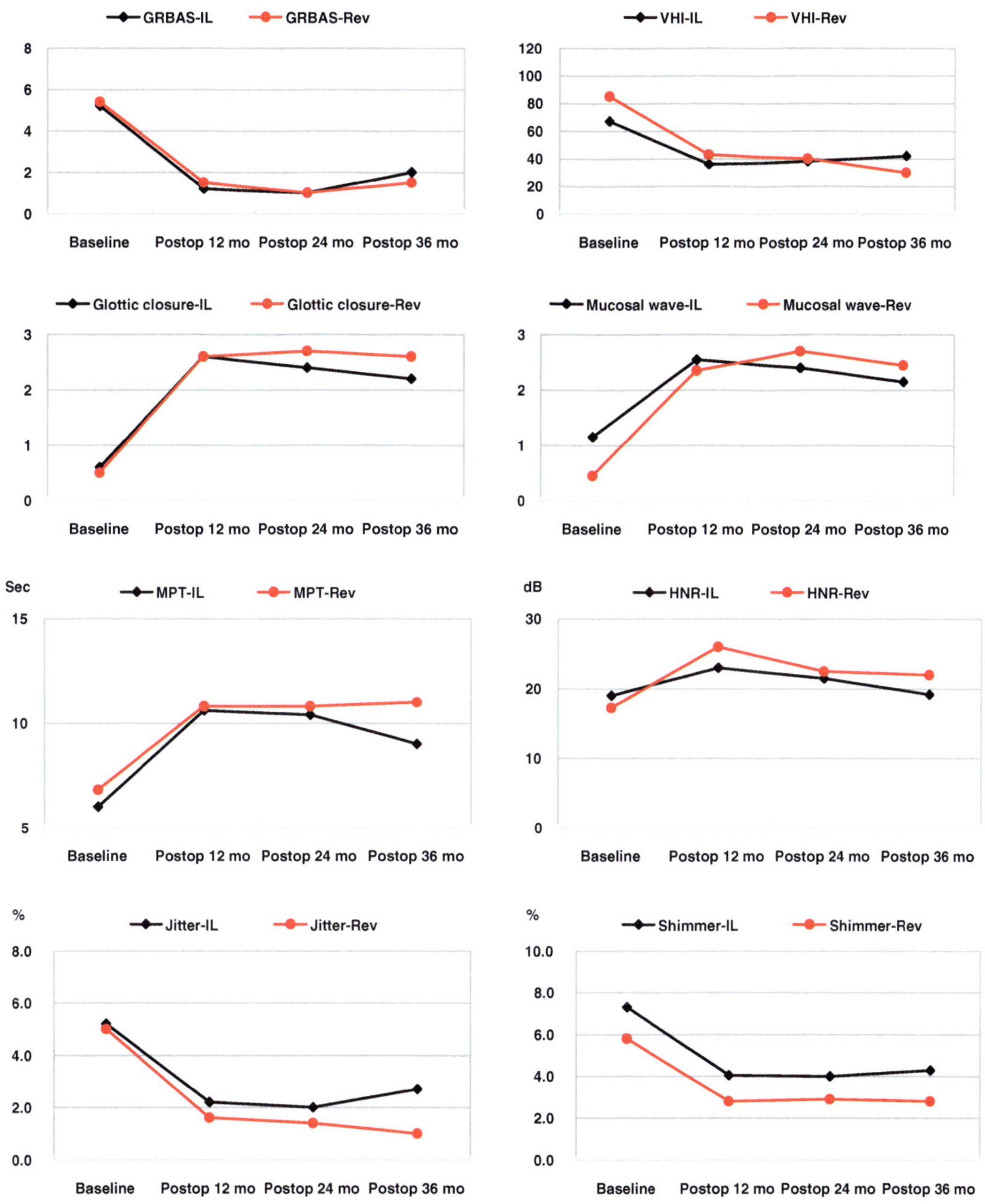

Fig. 13.6 Comparative results of voice analysis between injection laryngoplasty and recurrent laryngeal nerve reinnervation. Postop, postoperative; GRBAS, grade, rough, breathy, asthenic, strained; IL, injection laryngoplasty; Rev, recurrent laryngeal reinnervation; VHI, Voice Handicap Index; MPT, maximum phonation time; HNR, harmonic to noise ratio

When advanced thyroid cancer invades the recurrent laryngeal nerve (RLN) at the laryngeal entry point, reinnervation may be challenging, particularly if the distal portion of the RLN is difficult to locate. RLNs are frequently compromised near Berry's ligament due to thyroid cancer invasion. In cases with involvement near the laryngeal entry point, incision of the inferior constrictor muscle to facilitate RLN lateralization can offer increased exposure for effective RLN

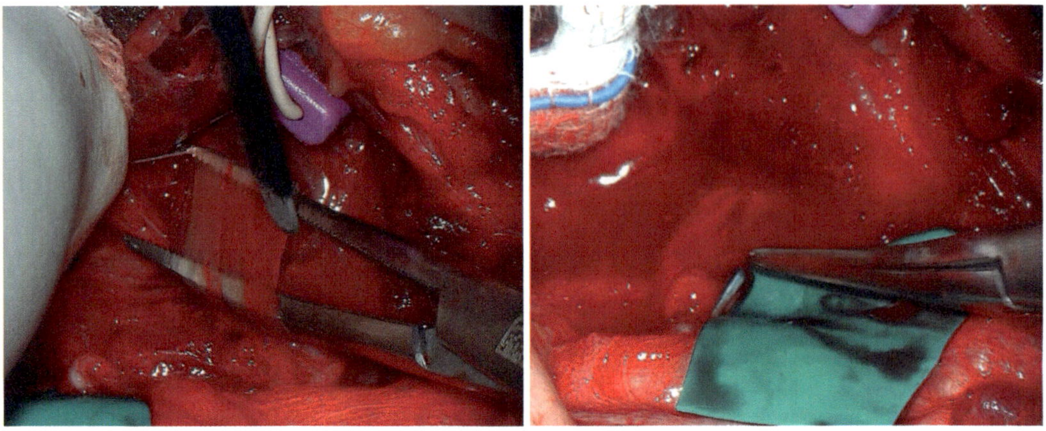

Fig. 13.7 Intralaryngeal dissection of the recurrent laryngeal nerve. In cases involving the laryngeal entry point, incising the inferior constrictor to facilitate recurrent laryngeal nerve (RLN) lateralization can offer enhanced exposure for RLN management

management. Intra-laryngeal nerve dissection may be required to identify the fine branches of the RLN [35] (Fig. 13.7).

◆ When the recurrent laryngeal nerve is resected during surgery, intraoperative reinnervation of the nerve is preferentially recommended, as it can ensure long-term stable voice outcomes without postoperative airway compromise.

Expert Opinion

For advanced thyroid cancer with RLN invasion and if pre-op VC is mobile, for a better patient outcome attempt to preserve the RLN if possible, as no method such as IL or reinnervation is 100% promising. At post op RAI or RT typically allows for good microscopic residual control. For pre-op VC palsy, the RLN must be sacrificed to allow for complete tumor resection. (Hok Nam Li)

During intra-laryngeal nerve dissection it is not easy to locate fine branches, and it is easy to cause injury during dissection. Additionally, if a surgeon reinnervates a larger nerve to fine branches, the results can be less effective. (Hok Nam Li)

The RLN is one of the most frequent sites of invasion for locally advanced thyroid cancer. In cases where RLN cannot be preserved or is inadvertently transected during surgery, emerging primary intraoperative RLN reinnervation techniques have been demonstrated to offer several advantages over conventional medialization thyroplasty and injection laryngoloplasty (IL) such as maintaining long-term tension and volume of the reinnervated thyroarytenoid muscle, and this eliminates the need for foreign body implants for voice rehabilitation. (Wu Chewei)

Considering the long-term survival of patients with thyroid cancer, intraoperative RLN reinnervation is recommended as the primary treatment when RLN resection is performed during thyroid surgery. Its stability and efficacy make it a favorable treatment for permanent post-thyroidectomy unilateral vocal fold paralysis (UVFP) without the need for revision surgery. When intraoperative reinnervation is not possible, postoperative IL or conventional medialization thyroplasty can be considered as second-line treatment [33] (Fig. 13.8).

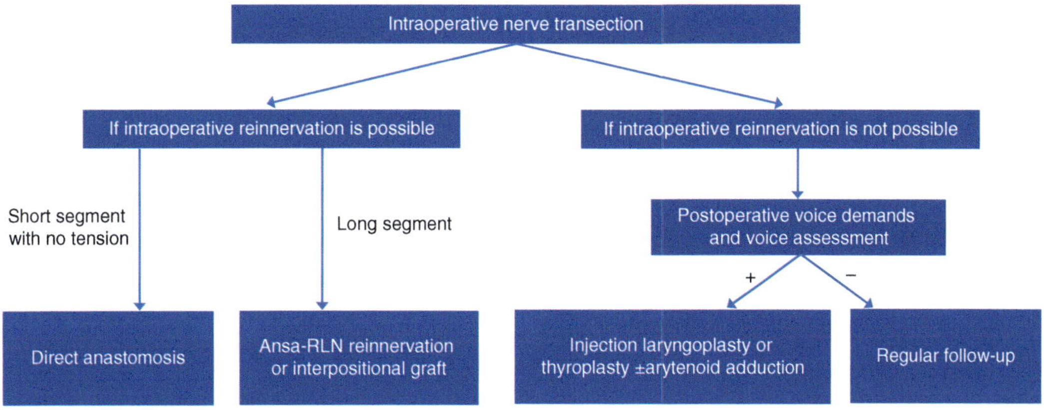

Fig. 13.8 Author's treatment algorithm for intraoperative nerve transection. RLN, recurrent laryngeal nerve; regular follow-up, regular endoscopic follow-up

◆ When thyroid cancer invades the recurrent laryngeal nerve (RLN) at the laryngeal entrance and the distal portion of the RLN cannot be located, intralaryngeal dissection of the RLN can be performed to locate the distal portion and perform reinnervation.

Expert Opinion
The most important takeaway from this chapter should be the need for prevention. In particular, transection should not happen when surgery is performed by an experienced thyroid surgeon. For tumors that require transaction or in the case of traction injury, IL is more appropriate for the patient, reinnervation is highly important but remains supplementary to IL. (Hok Nam Li)

13.4 KQ 13.4. How to Prevent and Manage Hypoparathyroidism After Total Thyroidectomy

Seung-Won Lee

Hypoparathyroidism occurs after thyroidectomy due to devascularization or unintentional resection of the parathyroid glands. Considering their varied embryology and anatomy, preservation is crucial. Blood supply to both parathyroid glands commonly originates from the inferior thyroid artery, thus emphasizing the need to separate these vessels from the thyroid capsule during surgery to maintain proper blood flow and function.

The arterial blood supply to the parathyroid glands is provided by a single terminal artery in 80% of cases. In 20% of the cases, two to four separate arteries are present. The inferior thyroid artery frequently supplies the superior and inferior glands. In 15% of patients, the superior parathyroid gland receives blood from the superior thyroid artery, and in 10%, ananastomotic communication of both systems can be observed [36].

Extracapsular dissection of the thyroid gland is recommended to preserve parathyroid glands *in situ*. To preserve the blood supply to the parathyroid glands during thyroidectomy, individual ligation of the peripheral branches of the inferior thyroid artery is performed rather than ligation of the main trunk of the vessel [37].

The upper parathyroid glands were deep, and the lower parathyroid glands were superficial to the coronal plane of the recurrent laryngeal nerve (Fig. 13.9).

The location of the parathyroid glands varies, with the superior glands typically located deeper relative to the mid-portion of the superior pole of the thyroid. The inferior glands are more variable but are often located inferior, posterior, or lateral to the lower thyroid pole.

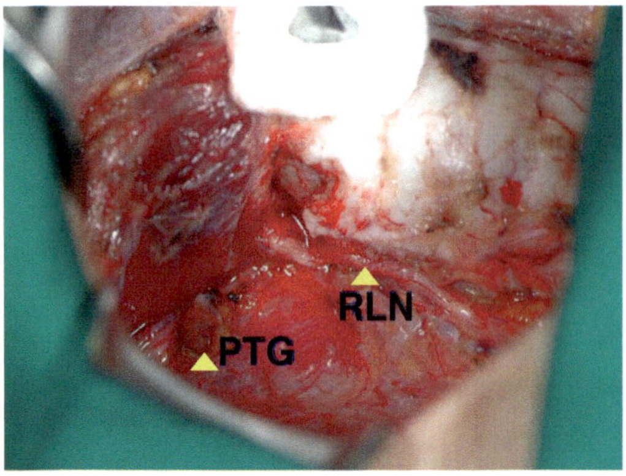

Fig. 13.9 Location of superior parathyroid gland and recurrent laryngeal nerve. The superior parathyroid gland (PTG) is located deep to the recurrent laryngeal nerve (RLN)

◆ Generally, the upper parathyroid glands are located deep, while the lower parathyroid glands are situated superficially in relation to the coronal plane of the recurrent laryngeal nerve. The parathyroid gland is vascularized by a single terminal artery, referred to as the parathyroid artery. Preservation of the parathyroid artery necessitates extracapsular dissection.

Expert Opinion

The typical location of superior parathyroid gland should be next to the RLN insertion site. (Hok Nam Li)

Identification and preservation of parathyroid glands remain challenging despite advances in thyroid surgical techniques; therefore, understanding the embryology, anatomy, and proper surgical and imaging techniques for parathyroid gland preservation is essential. (Wu Chewei)

To preserve the parathyroid gland during surgery, it is crucial to verify its presence and condition. While the color, shape, and vascular hilum of the gland are key indicators, certain hospitals also consider near-infrared parathyroid autofluorescence imaging to be important for confirmation. Additionally, to ensure proper postoperational function of the parathyroid gland, it is essential to not only locate the gland accurately but also to carefully preserve the blood vessels supplying it. Parathyroid dysfunction is common after central cervical lymph node dissection following a total thyroidectomy, so understanding the anatomical relationship between the recurrent laryngeal nerve and the inferior thyroid artery is vital for prevention. (Byung-Joo lee)

While "capsular dissection" and "extracapsular dissection" may be conceptually similar, the former typically refers to dissection along the true capsule, whereas the latter pertains to dissection along the inner surface of the false capsule or thyroid sheath. (Kang Dae lee)

Most parathyroid glands can be distinguished from the surrounding tissues based on their color, surface, and consistency. Typically, these glands exhibit a light brown to tan color, reflecting their fat content, vascularity, and proportion of oxyphil cells. The yellow hue may occasionally be mistaken for the surrounding fat. A distinct hilar vessel was also observed, provided that the surrounding fat did not obscure the hila of the glands [38].

In terms of surface characteristics, the parathyroid gland is notably discrete, encapsulated, and smooth, thus separating it from the more lobular surface of the thyroid. In contrast, lymph nodes exhibited mottled and pitted surfaces. Palpation revealed that the parathyroid gland was softer than the thyroid or nodal tissues (Fig. 13.10 and Table 13.2).

Understanding the variability in the locations of the parathyroid glands, particularly the superior and inferior glands, is vital during dissection. Devascularized or unintentionally resected parathyroid tissue should be identified, frozen, biopsied, confirmed as a normal parathyroid gland,

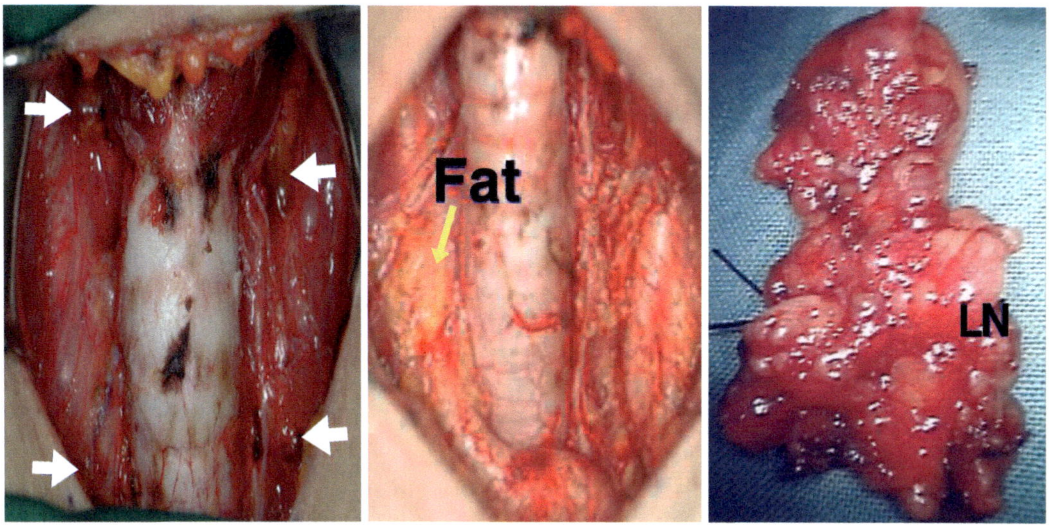

Fig. 13.10 Comparative surgical photos of gross appearances of the parathyroid gland (white arrows), fat (yellow arrow), and lymph node (LN)

Table 13.2 Characteristics of the parathyroid gland, fat, and lymph nodes

	Color	Shape	Vascular hilum
Parathyroid gland	Tan, brown color	Elliptical, flat	Yes
Fat	Bright yellow	Amorphous	No
Lymph node	White gray to red	Spherical to elliptical	No

and reimplanted, as in parathyroid autotransplantation. This involves creating a pocket in the sternocleidomastoid muscle and transplanting minced parathyroid tissue [39].

Parathyroid autotransplantation is clinically and biochemically effective, with a functional graft survival rate of 93% [40].

In conclusion, understanding the embryology, anatomy, and proper surgical techniques for parathyroid gland preservation is essential to prevent hypoparathyroidism after total thyroidectomy.

Expert Opinion

In practice, the survival rate of parathyroid autotransplantation may be lower. (Hok Nam Li)

Recent advancements in fluorescence techniques such as near-infrared autofluorescence (NIRAF) and indocyanine green (ICG) imaging have proven valuable for identifying and assessing the perfusion of the parathyroid glands during thyroid surgery. While traditional identification relies on the surgeon's experience that can be subjective, NIRAF imaging allows for earlier detection of parathyroid glands in a significant percentage of cases. However, NIRAF does not provide information regarding gland viability post-resection. Conversely, ICG fluorescence angiography enables intraoperative identification of critical blood vessels and allows for assessment of parathyroid perfusion after resection. Combining these techniques with a surgeon's expertise and thorough anatomical knowledge can help to reduce the risk of postoperative hypoparathyroidism following total thyroidectomy [27]. (Wu Chewei, Kang Dae Lee)

References

1. Schneider R, Randolph GW, Dionigi G, et al. International neural monitoring study group guideline 2018 part I: staging bilateral thyroid surgery with monitoring loss of signal. Laryngoscope. 2018;128(Suppl 3):S1–S17.
2. Lu IC, Chu KS, Tsai CJ, et al. Optimal depth of NIM EMG endotracheal tube for intraoperative neuromonitoring of the recurrent laryngeal nerve during thyroidectomy. World J Surg. 2008;32:1935–9.
3. Wu CW, Wang MH, Chen CC, et al. Loss of signal in recurrent nerve neuromonitoring: causes and management. Gland Surg. 2015;4(1):19–26.
4. Jung SM, Tae K, Song CM, Lee SH, Jeong JH, Ji YB. Efficacy of transcartilaginous electrodes for intraoperative neural monitoring during thyroid surgery. Clin Exp Otorhinolaryngol. 2020;13(4):422–8.
5. Lee HS, Oh J, Kim SW, et al. Intraoperative neuromonitoring of recurrent laryngeal nerve during thyroidectomy with adhesive skin electrodes. World J Surg. 2020;44(1):148–54.
6. Schneider R, Randolph G, Dionigi G, et al. Prospective study of vocal fold function after loss of the neuromonitoring signal in thyroid surgery: the International Neural Monitoring Study Group's POLT study. Laryngoscope. 2016;126:1260–6.
7. Schneider R, Sekulla C, Machens A, Lorenz K, Thanh PN, Dralle H. Dynamics of loss and recovery of the nerve monitoring signal during thyroidectomy predict early postoperative vocal fold function. Head Neck. 2016;38(Suppl 1):E1144–51.
8. Wu CW, Hao M, Tian M, et al. Recurrent laryngeal nerve injury with incomplete loss of electromyography signal during monitored thyroidectomy-evaluation and outcome. Langenbecks Arch Surg. 2017;402:691–9.
9. Goretzki PE, Schwarz K, Brinkmann J, Wirowski D, Lammers BJ. The impact of intraoperative neuromonitoring (IONM) on surgical strategy in bilateral thyroid diseases: is it worth the effort? World J Surg. 2010;34:1274–84.
10. Melin M, Schwarz K, Lammers BJ, Goretzki PE. IONM-guided goiter surgery leading to two-stage thyroidectomy—indication and results. Langenbecks Arch Surg. 2013;398:411–8.
11. Melin M, Schwarz K, Pearson MD, Lammers BJ, Goretzki PE. Postoperative vocal cord dysfunction despite normal intraoperative neuromonitoring: an unexpected complication with the risk of bilateral palsy. World J Surg. 2014;38:2597–602.
12. Sadowski SM, Soardo P, Leuchter I, Robert JH, Triponez F. Systematic use of recurrent laryngeal nerve neuromonitoring changes the operative strategy in planned bilateral thyroidectomy. Thyroid. 2013;23:329–33.
13. Sulica L. The superior laryngeal nerve: function and dysfunction. Otolaryngol Clin North Am. 2004;37(1):183–201.
14. Teitelbaum BJ, Wenig BL. Superior laryngeal nerve injury from thyroid surgery. Head Neck. 1995;17(1):36–40.
15. Cernea CR, Ferraz AR, Furlani J, et al. Identification of the external branch of the superior laryngeal nerve during thyroidectomy. Am J Surg. 1992;164(6):634–9.
16. Cernea CR, Ferraz AR, Nishio S, Dutra A Jr, Hojaij FC, dos Santos LR. Surgical anatomy of the external branch of the superior laryngeal nerve. Head Neck. 1992;14(5):380–3.
17. Barczyński M, Konturek A, Stopa M, Honowska A, Nowak W. Randomized controlled trial of visualization versus neuromonitoring of the external branch of the superior laryngeal nerve during thyroidectomy. World J Surg. 2012;36(6):1340–7.
18. Jonas J, Bähr R. Neuromonitoring of the external branch of the superior laryngeal nerve during thyroid surgery. Am J Surg. 2000;179(3):234–6.
19. Dionigi G, Boni L, Rovera F, Bacuzzi A, Dionigi R. Neuromonitoring and video-assisted thyroidectomy: a prospective, randomized case-control evaluation. Surg Endosc. 2009;23(5):996–1003.
20. Loré JM Jr, Kokocharov SI, Kaufman S, Richmond A, Sundquist N. Thirty-eight-year evaluation of a surgical technique to protect the external branch of the superior laryngeal nerve during thyroidectomy. Ann Otol Rhinol Laryngol. 1998;107(12):1015–22.
21. Hurtado-Lopez LM, Pacheco-Alvarez MI, Montes-Castillo MDIL, Zaldivar-Ramirez FR. Importance of the intraoperative identification of the external branch of the superior laryngeal nerve during thyroidectomy: electromyographic evaluation. Thyroid. 2005;15(5):449–54.
22. Uludag M, Aygun N, Kartal K, Besler E, Isgor A. Is intraoperative neural monitoring necessary for exploration of the superior laryngeal nerve? Surgery. 2017;161(4):1129–38.
23. Hurtado-López L-M, Díaz-Hernández PI, Basurto-Kuba E, Zaldívar-Ramírez FR, Pulido-Cejudo A. Efficacy of intraoperative neuro-monitoring to localize the external branch of the superior laryngeal nerve. Thyroid. 2016;26(1):174–8.
24. Orestes MI, Chhetri DK. Superior laryngeal nerve injury: effects, clinical findings, prognosis, and management options. Curr Opin Otolaryngol Head Neck Surg. 2014;22(6):439–43.
25. Shaw G, Searl J, Hoover L. Diagnosis and treatment of unilateral cricothyroid muscle paralysis with a modified Isshiki type 4 thyroplasty. Otolaryngol Head Neck Surg. 1995;113:679–88. [PubMed: 7501377].
26. El-Kashlan HK, Carroll WR, Hogikyan MD, et al. Selective cricothyroid muscle reinnervation by muscle-nerve-muscle neurotization. Arch Otolaryngol Head Neck Surg. 2001;127:1211–5.
27. Silver Karcioglu AL, Triponez F, Solorzano CC, Iwata AJ, Abdelhamid Ahmed AH, Almquist M, et al. Emerging imaging technologies for parathyroid gland identification and vascular assessment in thyroid surgery: a review from the American Head and Neck Society endocrine sur-

gery section. JAMA Otolaryngol Head Neck Surg. 2023;149(3):253–60.
28. Lee SW, Kim JW, Chung CH, Mok JO, Shim SS, Koh YW, et al. Utility of injection laryngoplasty in the management of post-thyroidectomy vocal cord paralysis. Thyroid. 2010;20(5):513–7.
29. Kwon TK, Buckmire R. Injection laryngoplasty for management of unilateral vocal fold paralysis. Curr Opin Otolaryngol Head Neck Surg. 2004;12(6):538–42.
30. Ryu CH, Kwon TK, Kim H, Kim HS, Park IS, Woo JH, et al. Guidelines for the management of unilateral vocal fold paralysis from the Korean Society of laryngology, phoniatrics and logopedics. Clin Exp Otorhinolaryngol. 2020;13(4):340–60.
31. Lee SW, Park KN, Oh SK, Jung CH, Mok JO, Kim CH. Long-term efficacy of primary intraoperative recurrent laryngeal nerve reinnervation in the management of thyroidectomy-related unilateral vocal fold paralysis. Acta Otolaryngol. 2014;134(11):1179–84.
32. Crumley RL. Unilateral recurrent laryngeal nerve paralysis. J Voice. 1994;8(1):79–83.
33. Lee SW, Park KN. A long-term comparative prospective study between reinnervation and injection laryngoplasty. Laryngoscope. 2018;128(8):1893–7.
34. Lee YJ, Lee SW. Ten-year outcomes of recurrent laryngeal nerve reinnervation for thyroidectomy-related unilateral vocal fold paralysis: a single-surgeon, prospective study. Am J Otolaryngol. 2024;45(3):104242.
35. Miyauchi A, Matsusaka K, Kihara M, Matsuzuka F, Hirai K, Yokozawa T, et al. The role of ansa-to-recurrent-laryngeal nerve anastomosis in operations for thyroid cancer. Eur J Surg. 1998;164(12):927–33.
36. Andrioli M, Valcavi R. Sonography of normal and abnormal thyroid and parathyroid glands. Front Horm Res. 2016;45:1–15.
37. Kiviniemi H, Vornanen T, Makela J. Prevention of complications of thyroid and parathyroid surgery. Duodecim; laaketieteellinen aikakauskirja. 2010;126(3):269–75.
38. Stefanou CK, Papathanakos G, Stefanou SK, Tepelenis K, Kitsouli A, Barbouti A, et al. Surgical tips and techniques to avoid complications of thyroid surgery. Innov Surg Sci. 2022;7(3–4):115–23.
39. Lukinovic J, Bilic M. Overview of thyroid surgery complications. Acta Clin Croat. 2020;59(Suppl 1):81–6.
40. Hicks G, George R, Sywak M. Short and long-term impact of parathyroid autotransplantation on parathyroid function after total thyroidectomy. Gland Surg. 2017;6(Suppl 1):S75–85.

Thyroid Surgery: Others

14

Dongbin Ahn and Bon Seok Koo

14.1 KQ 14.1. What Is the Appropriate Management When Unexpected Tracheal Injury Occurs During Thyroid Surgery?

Dongbin Ahn

To discuss management of unexpected tracheal injuries during thyroid surgery, it is necessary to understand the types of tracheal injuries that occur during thyroid surgery. Tracheal injuries can be classified based on the thickness (partial or full-layer injury) and circumference (window or segmental injury) of the trachea [1–3] (Table 14.1).

14.1.1 Partial-Layer Injury

Partial layer injury involves resection of the tracheal cartilage without extension into the tracheal lumen (no injury to the tracheal mucosa). This commonly results from tangential excision or tracheal shaving (Fig. 14.1). In this case, no additional surgical management is required to reconstruct the tracheal cartilage defect, provided that intact tracheal mucosa is confirmed in the surgical field [4, 5]. However, reinforcing coverage with fibrin sealant, with or without fibrin glue or other materials, is recommended to protect the injured tracheal wall and prevent inadvertent tearing of the tracheal mucosa due to strong coughing in the early postoperative period. In most cases, drain insertion is unnecessary because it is a partial layer injury that is not associated with air leakage. However, if the healing process is unfavorable because of possible air leakage during the operative period, a small negative-pressure drainage tube can be inserted for the early detection of air leakage.

> **Expert Opinion**
> For a partial tracheal wall defect, it is crucial to verify that the inner tracheal mucosa remains intact. To do this, deflate the balloon of the intubation tube, perform positive ventilation, and inspect for air leaks into the defect using a water leak test. If the mucosa is intact, apply a compression dressing and administer cough medicine

(continued)

D. Ahn (✉)
Department of Otolaryngology-Head and Neck Surgery, School of Medicine, Kyungpook National University, Daegu, Republic of Korea

B. S. Koo (✉)
Department of Otorhinolaryngology—Head and Neck Surgery, College of Medicine, Chungnam National University, Daejeon, Republic of Korea
e-mail: bskoo515@cnuh.co.kr

K.-J. Cho, J.-O. Park (eds.), *Management of Head and Neck Surgery Complications*,
https://doi.org/10.1007/978-981-96-1860-6_14

Table 14.1 Summary of management according to type of tracheal injury

	Partial-layer injury	Full-layer injury	
Subtype	–	Window injury	Segmental injury
Findings	Tracheal cartilage injury only without tracheal mucosa injury	Local and partial-circumferential defect	Wide and circumferential defect
Management	Reinforcing coverage with sealant materials	Primary closure or tracheostomy or tracheal fenestration (when primary closure is unavailable)	End-to-end anastomosis

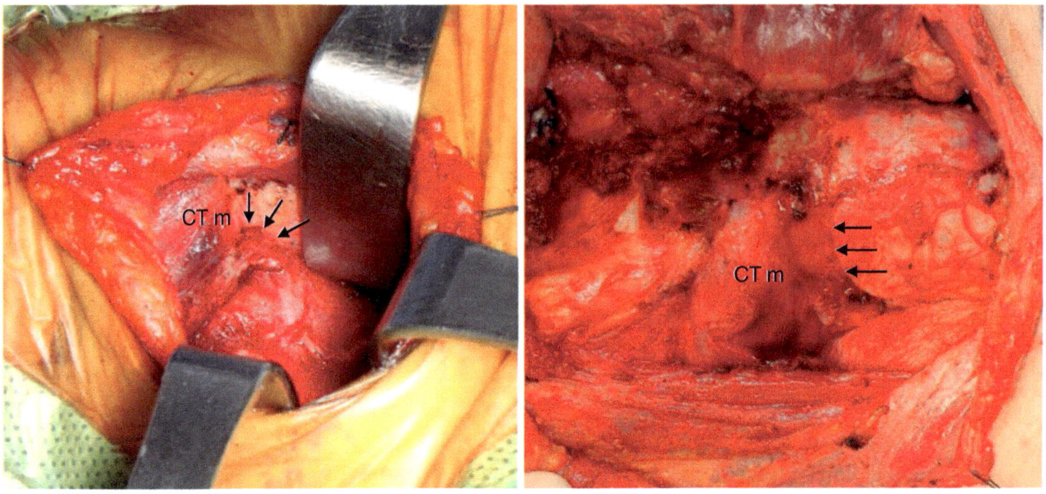

Fig. 14.1 Partial-layer injury of the trachea after thyroidectomy. Although the tracheal cartilage is partially resected (arrows), the intraluminal tracheal mucosa is not penetrated, maintaining the integrity of the tracheal lumen. CT, cricothyroid; m, muscle

over the defect area to prevent air leaks caused by coughing. Using positive pressure ventilation after balloon deflation is another method to assess the success of a tracheal repair. (Seung Won Lee)

Incidental tracheal perforation or laceration may occur during thyroid surgery, and it may be repaired immediately by simple suture and applying glue. (Phil-Sang Chung)

14.1.2 Full-Layer Injury

Full-layer trachea injuries are divided into window and segmental injuries according to the circumferential extent of the injury.

1) Window (wedge) injury
   A. Primary closure without tracheostomy
      This type of injury results from tracheal window resection and leads to localized defects in the tracheal wall. If the defect size is not extensive and both resection edges can be approximated, primary suturing is feasible, obviating the need for tracheostomy or tracheal fenestration [1, 2, 5]. The feasibility of primary closure of the trachea depends not only on the defect size but also on the defect shape because the trachea consists of cartilage that is hardly stretched. More specifically, defects with round or vertical axes rarely allow primary closure, whereas elliptical defects with transverse axes may permit primary closure. Therefore, a round defect can be transformed into an elliptical one

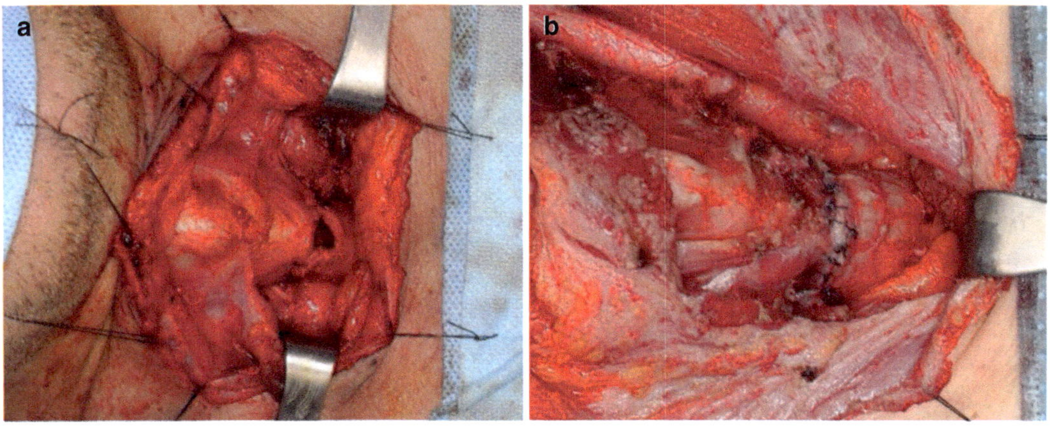

Fig. 14.2 Full-layer injury of trachea managed with primary closure. (**a**) A full-layer defect of the trachea is created after window resection of the trachea. (**b**) This defect can be managed with primary closure, particularly when the size is not extensive and the shape is elliptical along the transverse axis

by trimming the lateral margin of the round tracheal defect, leaving behind the posterior membranous wall of the trachea (Fig. 14.2). The technique is the same as the general suture technique of the trachea: an interrupted suture using 3-0 or 4-0 absorbable suture materials, such as Vicryl or polydioxanone (PDS), with a 5-mm distance between the stitches. Although some studies have advocated passing the suture through the submucosal plane to avoid injuring the intraluminal mucosa, this technical issue has a minimal impact on the tracheal wound healing process. The foremost technical point is anchoring one cartilage ring on each side during suturing to provide an adequate approximation of the trachea without tension and placing a suture knot outside the trachea to prevent granulation within the tracheal lumen. After primary closure, reinforcing coverage with fibrin sealant, with or without fibrin glue, is also helpful in preventing air leakage from closed sites.

B. Tracheostomy or tracheal fenestration

If the tracheal defect is full thickness with less than half of the tracheal circumference and primary closure is unavailable, tracheostomy or tracheal fenestration is a readily available option to manage tracheal defects. Simple tracheostomy by inserting a tracheostomy cannula is not recommended because the trachea is dissected from adjacent structures during thyroid cancer surgery, and a simple tracheostomy under this condition cannot ensure effective wound healing. Thus, tracheal fenestration that creates a tracheostoma by suturing the tracheal window wall to the skin of the cervical incision is preferred [1, 3, 6]. Although this technique offers several advantages, including a stable postoperative airway, reduced surgical complications, and less invasive surgery compared with tracheal end-to-end anastomosis, it also presents critical drawbacks, such as patient discomfort associated with prolonged maintenance of the tracheostoma and the need for second-stage surgery for tracheostoma closure. Stoma closure is usually performed using a local skin flap 3 months after the initial surgery, unless the patency of the airway is compromised during follow-up (Fig. 14.3).

Other than tracheal fenestration, a sternocleidomastoid (SCM) myoperiosteal flap can be used if single-stage reconstruction is needed. The clavicular head of the

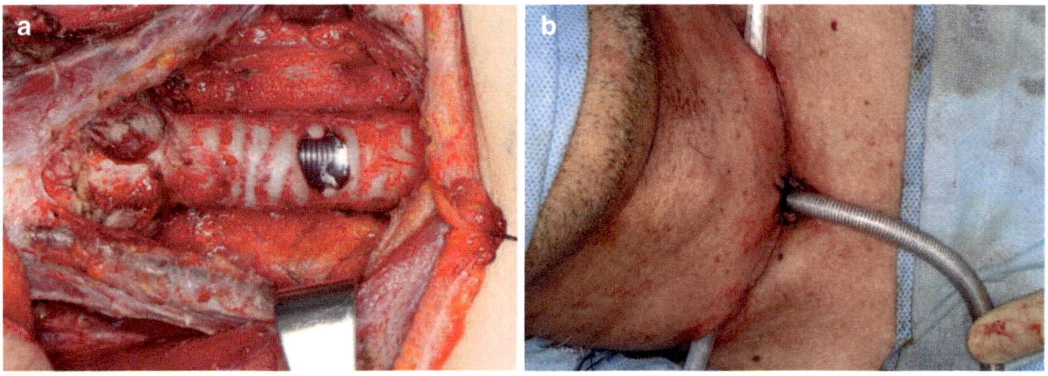

Fig. 14.3 Full-layer injury of the trachea managed with tracheal fenestration. (**a**) Full-layer injury of the trachea is created after window resection of the trachea. (**b**) Tracheal fenestration is performed by suturing the tracheal window wall to the skin of the cervical incision

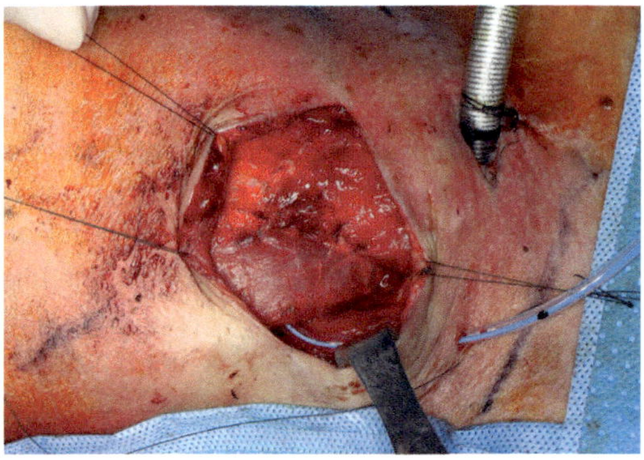

Fig. 14.4 Full-layer injury of the trachea managed with a sternocleidomastoid musculoperiosteal flap

SCM muscle, including the clavicular periosteum, is harvested from the clavicle and sutured to cover the tracheal defects. The myoperiosteal flap should be larger than the defective area. The SCM muscle is dissected to allow sufficient mobility of the flap to reach the defect without tension. With minimal dissection, the blood supply to the transverse cervical, superior thyroid, and occipital vessels (SCM) can be preserved to maintain vascularization (Fig. 14.4). Tracheostomy may be required in a separate neck incision for reconstruction of large defects [7].

2) Segmental (circumferential) injury

Unexpected cancer invasion requiring circumferential resection of the trachea is rarely encountered because most cases of tracheal invasion of such severity can be predicted through preoperative evaluation. Once the trachea is circumferentially resected, end-to-end anastomosis is the treatment of choice for reconstruction (Fig. 14.5) [1, 4, 8, 9]. Anastomosis is initiated from the posterior membranous trachea using 3-0 or 4-0 absorbable materials (Vicryl or PDS). The anastomosis then proceeds to the lateral and anterior tracheae by anchoring one cartilage ring to each tracheal side. The most critical principle for successful tracheal anastomosis is tension-free anastomosis; thus, supra- or infrahyoid release of the larynx is occasionally required along with appropriate finger dissection of the trachea in the superior mediastinum.

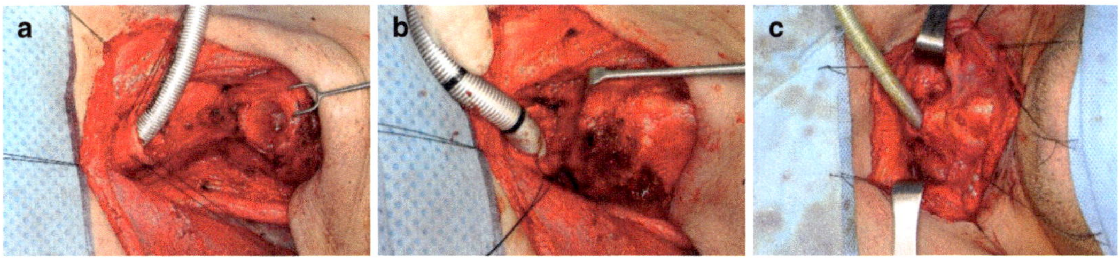

Fig. 14.5 Segmental injury of the trachea managed with end-to-end anastomosis. (**a**) The trachea is resected segmentally due to thyroid cancer invasion. (**b**) The anastomosis starts from the posterior membranous trachea and then (**c**) proceeds to the lateral and anterior tracheae

Expert Opinion

In advanced cases of thyroid cancer, tracheal invasion typically occurs laterally. When the invaded thyroid cancer is excised along with a portion of the trachea, 1–2 tracheal rings are usually left as lateral defects. Performing tracheal fenestration in this situation is akin to a lateral tracheotomy, facilitating easy postoperative airway management and offering safety benefits, such as a reduced risk of bilateral vocal fold paralysis, compared to tracheal resection with end-to-end anastomosis (TREE). Additionally, if the stoma from general fenestration is not too large, it often heals by secondary intention without requiring a stoma closure procedure. (Jeong-Soo Woo, Seung Won Lee)

TREE is typically performed by a head and neck surgeon rather than an endocrine surgeon. Often, it is accompanied by neck dissection, which provides a clear surgical field, making the technique itself relatively straightforward. However, the greatest challenge arises in cases requiring multiple TREEs, where there is a significant risk of unilateral recurrent laryngeal nerve (RLN) invasion. During TREE, it is crucial to preserve the function of the contralateral RLN. Any transient paresis of the contralateral RLN could result in bilateral vocal fold paralysis. (Seung Won Lee)

When closing a tracheal defect using a one-stage SCM myoperiosteal flap without fenestration, the periosteum attached to the clavicle of the SCM should be oriented inward toward the trachea to ensure an airtight seal. (Seung Won Lee)

Incidental tracheal perforation or laceration may occur during thyroid surgery, and it may be repaired immediately by simple suture and applying glue. (Phil-Sang Chung)

14.2 KQ 14.2. What Is the Appropriate Management When Unexpected Esophageal Injury Occurs During Thyroid Surgery?

Dongbin Ahn

To discuss the management of unexpected esophageal injuries during thyroid surgery, it is necessary to understand the characteristics of esophageal injuries in terms of depth (layer), circumference, and length.

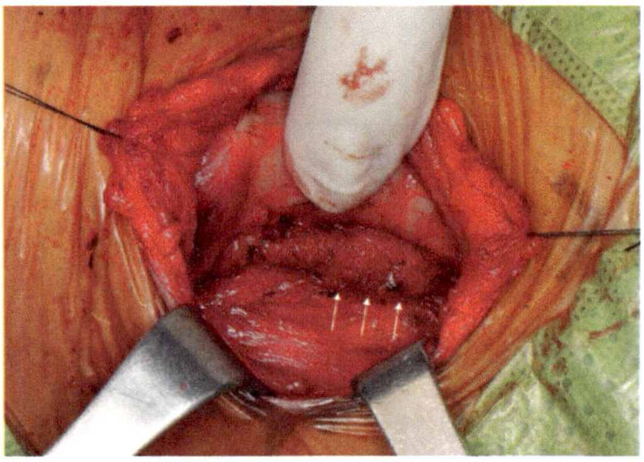

Fig. 14.6 Esophageal injury confined to the muscularis layer. After resection of the muscularis layer of the esophagus invaded by the tumor, an intact mucosa bulge (arrows) is identified

14.2.1 Injury Confined to the Muscularis Layer

Esophageal invasion by differentiated thyroid cancer is mostly confined to the muscularis layer without extension into the submucosa or mucosa because the esophageal mucosa is highly resistant to direct invasion [5, 10, 11]. Thus, most unexpected esophageal injuries resulting from the resection of locally advanced thyroid cancer are also confined to the muscularis. In such cases, no further management is required to reconstruct the resected muscularis of the esophagus [5, 8, 10, 11]. However, surgeons must ensure that the mucosa remains intact without tearing. An intact mucosal bulge should be identified after resection of the muscularis layer of the esophagus (Fig. 14.6). In addition, examination of esophageal integrity with an esophageal bougie or feeding tube placement facilitates precise inspection of mucosal injuries [4, 9–11]. If the mucosa is intact, patients maintain normal swallowing function postoperatively, and feeding tube insertion is unnecessary [11].

Expert Opinion

In cases of advanced thyroid cancer, partial resection of the esophagus can be performed without postoperative complications, provided the esophageal mucosa remains intact. Often, the trachea, recurrent laryngeal nerve, and a portion of the esophagus are simultaneously invaded. When the affected part of the esophagus is removed, there is a risk of perforation. To mitigate this risk, inserting an L tube during surgical anesthesia can be beneficial, as it provides an anatomical landmark for the esophagus, aiding in its palpation and reducing the likelihood of perforation. (Seung Won Lee)

The primary objective in repairing an esophageal injury should be to restore the anatomical structure as closely as possible to its pre-injury state, ensuring the integrity of the mucosa, submucosa, and muscle layers. The suture technique used for primary closure should mirror the pharyngeal mucosal repair method employed after total laryngectomy. This approach is particularly important to invert the inner esophageal mucosal layer into the lumen and align the sutured edges accurately. The extent of the injury and the presence of water-tight sutures can be assessed using the same technique as for tracheal injuries, by checking for air bubbles in saline. The success of the repair can be further confirmed through pharyngoesophagography performed 1 to 2 weeks later. (Jeong-Soo Woo)

14.2.2 Full-Thickness Injuries with Minor Mucosal Defect

Once a full-thickness defect is created after the excision of locally invasive thyroid cancer, the esophageal defect should be repaired using various methods depending on the extent of the defect. Esophageal invasion that is not detected or expected during preoperative evaluation is usually minor or non-extensive. Thus, primary closure is a widely available option, even in most cases of full-thickness esophageal injury (Fig. 14.7) [5, 8, 11]. If primary closure is planned, tension-free and watertight multilayer closure using 3-0 or 4-0 Vicryl suture materials

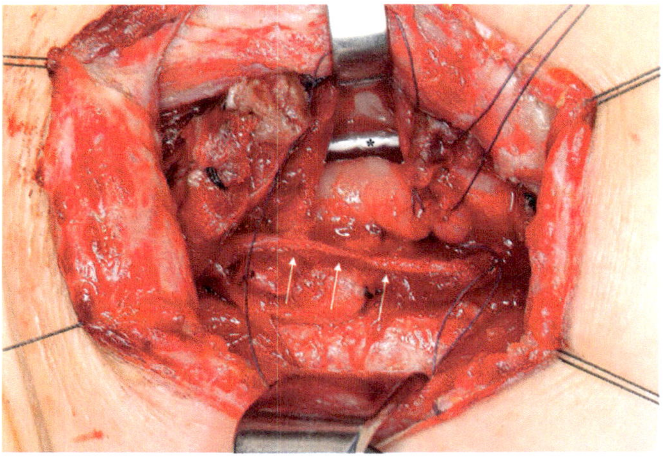

Fig. 14.7 Full-thickness esophageal injury. A full-thickness defect of the esophagus is created after excision of locally invasive thyroid cancer. The feeding tube (asterisk) is within the esophageal lumen, and the recurrent laryngeal nerve (arrows) is located beside the esophagus

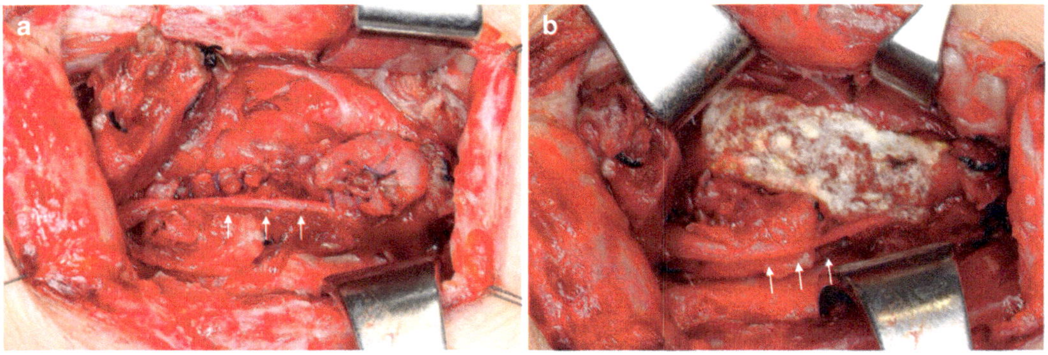

Fig. 14.8 Primary closure of the full-thickness esophageal injury. The esophagus is repaired by primary closure with interrupted suture using 4-0 Vicryl (**a**), and the closed site is covered with fibrin sealant (**b**). The recurrent laryngeal nerve (arrows) is seen beside the esophagus

is mandatory (Fig. 14.8a). After meticulous primary closure, reinforcing the coverage with fibrin sealant, with or without fibrin glue or other materials, is recommended (Fig. 14.8b). Moreover, additional reinforcement with a strap or sternocleidomastoid muscle flap can be used to supply sufficient blood flow to the repair site and promote healing, thereby preventing fistulas.

14.2.3 Full-Thickness Injuries with Segmental and Circumferential Esophageal Defects

Extensive full-thickness injuries to the esophagus during thyroid surgery that are undetected or unexpected during preoperative evaluation are rare. However, in the event of such cases, reconstruction using microvascular free tissue transfer of a fasciocutaneous flap or jejunum should be considered [4, 9–11]. The selection of the reconstruction technique depends on the surgical feasibility of each option and the experience of the reconstruction team [4, 9–11].

Expert Opinion
For small esophageal perforations, suturing is done in multiple layers, similar to the technique used in total laryngectomy. The key consideration during this process is to ensure a tension-free suture. A common reconstruction method for small esophageal defects involves using a pedicled flap from the strap muscles or sternocleidomastoid muscles. (Seung Won Lee)

14.3 KQ 14.3. What Are the Preventive Measures and Appropriate Treatments for Thyrotoxic Storm During Surgery for Graves' Disease?

Bon Seok Koo

Graves' disease (GD) is a common cause of hyperthyroidism. The treatment of Graves' disease aims to maintain normal thyroid function (euthyroid state) to minimize morbidity and mortality. These treatment goals can be achieved using antithyroid medications, radioactive iodine ablation, and surgery (subtotal or near-total thyroidectomy) (Fig. 14.9) [12]. Surgical treatment in patients with Graves' disease can be applied in the following cases: (1) when radioactive iodine ablation is not possible (during pregnancy or preparing for pregnancy) or when iodine uptake is poor and the therapeutic effect of radioactive iodine ablation is expected to be insignificant [12–14]; (2) when patients experience symptoms such as pain and dysphagia due to an enlarged thyroid [15]; and (3) in patients who require immediate surgical intervention for hyperthyroidism [12].

Expert Opinion
Currently, radioactive iodine therapy (RAI) is the most widely preferred treatment for Graves' disease in the United States, while in Korea, anti-thyroid medication is more commonly favored. However, the use of RAI is gradually increasing in Korea. For patients who have undergone RAI treatment, surgery for Graves' disease requires meticulous attention to prevent complications such as recurrent laryngeal nerve injury, postoperative hypothyroidism due to adhesions to surrounding tissues, and bleeding tendencies. (Seung Won Lee)

Many things need to be considered during thyroidectomy for Graves' disease to prevent intra- and postoperative bleeding and thyroid storm. Postoperative hematoma accompanying airway compromise is the most dangerous complication of thyroidectomy, and every thyroid surgeon and the supporting team should be aware of the emergency management. Postoperative scarring of the incision line may be minimized by appropriate skin incision and meticulous skin closure. (Phil-Sang Chung)

◆ Surgical treatment of patients with Graves' disease should be determined through adequate consultation and discussion with endocrinologists, nuclear medicine specialists, and patients.

Thyroid storm is a thyrotoxic disease that can occur in patients with hyperthyroidism, similar to Graves' disease. Thyroid storm clinically manifests as an excessive increase in circulating T3 and T4 levels [16]. Uncontrolled tachycardia, hypertension, and hyperthermia caused by thyroid storms can lead to poor outcomes. Therefore, if surgical treatment is selected for patients with Graves' disease, the euthyroid state must be maintained with antithyroidal drugs with or without β-adrenergic blockade before surgery. Furthermore, prior to surgery, the administration of potassium iodide (KI), a

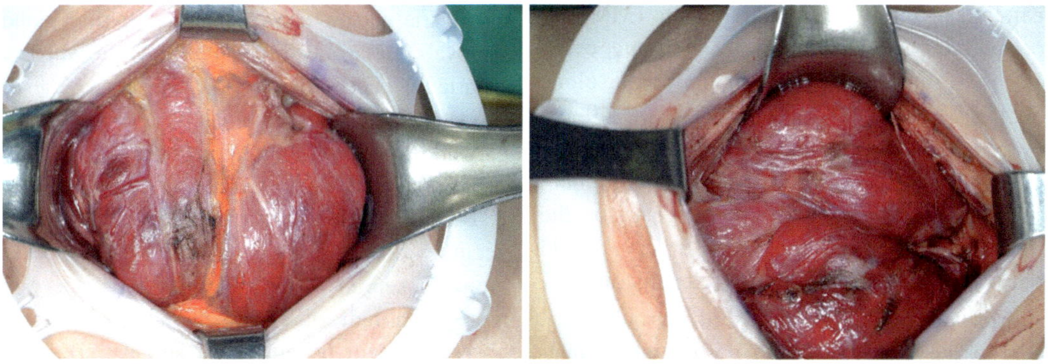

Fig. 14.9 Gross appearance during thyroid surgery in patients with Graves' disease (copyright Prof. Changmyeon Song)

Table 14.2 List of drugs and application methods before surgical treatment for Graves' disease

Saturated solution of potassium iodide	50 mg iodine per drop Mix 1–2 drops with water or orange juice thrice a day and administer for 10–14 days before surgery
Lugol's solution	8 mg iodine per drop 5–7 drops at a time, thrice a day
Vitamin D	Correction to normal values (vitamin D sufficiency: 30.1–100.0 ng/mL)

saturated solution of potassium iodide (SSKI), or Lugol's solution is recommended [17]. This regimen is also beneficial during thyroidectomy because it helps reduce thyroid blood flow, vascularization, and intraoperative blood loss [18, 19]. Additionally, to prevent hypocalcemia, which may occur after thyroid surgery, vitamin D levels should be measured before surgery and corrected if insufficient [20] (Table 14.2).

All preoperative treatments should be performed in close cooperation with the endocrinologist and carefully planned and performed before surgery.

> ◆ If surgery is planned as a treatment for Graves' disease, euthyroid status should be maintained before surgery, and preoperative treatment should be considered to minimize complications during surgery through a multidisciplinary team approach.

Patients with Graves' disease have enlarged thyroid glands. In addition, blood vessels are overdeveloped and relatively thin, and even minor surgical manipulations can cause bleeding. Therefore, accurate coagulation is required during dissection. Severe thyrotoxicosis, which can be triggered by anesthesia and thyroid gland manipulation, has a high mortality rate of approximately 10% [21]. Therefore, making precise skin incisions to ensure ample surgical margins and avoid excessive pressure on the thyroid gland is crucial. Furthermore, close communication and cooperation with anesthesiologists are essential to prepare for unexpected situations that may suddenly arise during surgery, including thyroid storms.

> ◆ To prevent a thyroid storm during thyroid surgery for Graves' disease, it is important to minimize thyroid manipulation by securing a wide surgical space. Close communication with the anesthesiologist during surgery is also essential.

If a thyroid storm occurs during surgery, vital signs are destabilized and accompanied by symptoms such as hyperpyrexia, tachycardia, and arrhythmia. It is necessary to objectively determine the severity of a storm based on the patient's biological signs and provide immediate treatment. Multimodal treatment, such as administration of intravenous methimazole (MMI) or propylthiouracil (PTU) (40 or 400 mg every 8 h), glucocorticoids (methylprednisolone 50 mg), or beta-blockers (propranolol 40 mg every 6 h), is required in such cases [20]. Due to the higher incidence and severity of complications associated with thyroid surgery for the treatment of Graves' disease, surgery should only be performed by experienced surgeons.

Considering the possibility of thyroid storm, appropriate observation and postoperative treatment are recommended [21]. In addition to closely monitoring the patient's vital signs, it is crucial to observe carefully for any signs of postoperative hemorrhage. Previously administered antithyroid drugs should be discontinued, along with appropriate weaning of the β-adrenergic blockade. Furthermore, appropriate calcium supplementation, with or without calcitriol, is recommended, guided by the measurement of serum calcium and intact parathyroid hormone levels [17].

◆ Following surgery, appropriate observation and treatment are required for a certain period in cooperation with an endocrinologist.

Expert Opinion
For surgeons with extensive experience in thyroid surgery, the most effective treatment for Graves' disease is surgery, with total thyroidectomy being the quickest and most efficient approach. (Jeong-Soo Woo)

14.4 KQ 14.4. How Should Postoperative Hematoma Be Managed, Particularly When Accompanied by Airway Compromise, After Thyroid Surgery?

Bon Seok Koo

Hematoma following thyroid surgery is a life-threatening complication that can result in airway compression, even with a small amount of bleeding in the narrow space left after thyroid gland removal [22]. Bleeding after thyroid surgery reportedly occurs between 0.45% and 4.2% of cases [23], and approximately one-quarter of patients experience an emergency due to airway compression caused by hematoma formation [24].

Bleeding after thyroid surgery most often occurs within 24 hours after surgery and is commonly observed within 6 hours after surgery in more than half of cases; therefore, intensive observation for 6 hours after surgery is necessary [22, 25]. When a hematoma causes airway compression, patients complain of pain, pressure sensation, respiratory distress, and anxiety. Physical examination may show swelling, ecchymosis, and oozing of the wound at the surgical site. However, in cases of airway compromise, the patient's condition can deteriorate rapidly without these physical findings. Consequently, if patients complain of symptoms, the possibility of hematoma formation should always be considered even if the aforementioned findings are absent.

◆ Bleeding after thyroid surgery is most prevalent within 6 hours after surgery. Therefore, if patients complain of specific symptoms such as pain/pressure sensation, respiratory distress, and anxiety within this period, close observation is recommended.

When a patient complains of the characteristic symptoms described above and bleeding is suspected based on physical findings, evaluation should be initiated along with essential treatment, considering the possibility of airway compression due to hematoma formation. While maintaining the patient in a head-up position of approximately 45°, it is essential to continuously monitor oxygen saturation and administer oxygen at a rate of 10 liters or more per minute [22]. In the case of airway compression due to hematoma, a senior surgeon should be notified, and intensive observation should be continued until the patient's symptoms stabilize. Where necessary, a flexible laryngoscope should be placed at the bedside for immediate airway evaluation. In addition, an airway intubation set and emergency box for hematoma evacuation should be prepared for immediate treatment. An emergency box for hematoma evacuation should also be prepared for immediate use in the ward [22].

Expert Opinion

If postoperative hematoma occurs after thyroid surgery, the surgeon must decide among close observation, emergency bedside hematoma removal, or returning to the operating room for bleeding control, depending on the patient's clinical symptoms. If tracheal compression from the hematoma progresses, the patient's breathing may worsen, potentially leading to respiratory arrest. Therefore, it is crucial to plan the appropriate intervention in advance. (Seung Won Lee)

◆ An emergency box for immediate hematoma evacuation should always be prepared and kept available near the patient. It is recommended to contain the following components:

(1) Artery clip
(2) Scalpel
(3) Scissors
(4) Forceps
(5) Sterile gauze and gloves
(6) Suction tip and suction tube

If respiratory distress persists during intensive observation, desaturation is confirmed even during oxygen supply, and prominent hematoma formation is confirmed on physical examination (notably swelling, ecchymosis, and wound oozing), immediate bedside hematoma removal should be performed. In anticipation of potential emergencies, such as cardiac arrest due to airway compromise, the emergency resuscitation team should be maintained on alert.

◆ Hematoma evacuation procedure after thyroid surgery (Fig. 14.10)

(1) Open the existing surgical incision using a scalpel. If it is sutured with a stapler, remove the staples quickly using a staple remover. If a skin bond is applied, rapidly remove a part of the bond and quickly open the incision using forceps. Opening the surgical site by one unit up to the subcutaneous sutures is preferable.
(2) Insert fingers into the surgical site and widen them to expand the space above the strap muscles. If a coagulated hematoma is visible, try dislodging it with your fingers. If the hematoma is actively bleeding, use suction and gauze to secure the view.
(3) If the strap muscle is sutured, use a scalpel to open the surgical site and expose the airway using the fingers.
(4) If the airway is secured, thoroughly cover the surgical site with sterilized gauze and move to the operating room for hemostasis.

Airway compression due to bleeding after thyroid surgery is a fatal complication; however, immediate and efficient treatment can help reduce the risk of death. Consequently, continuous preparation by forming a multidisciplinary team in advance is essential for the establishment of treatment protocols and for ongoing education.

The summary of the management protocol of hematoma after thyroid surgery is as follows (Fig. 14.11).

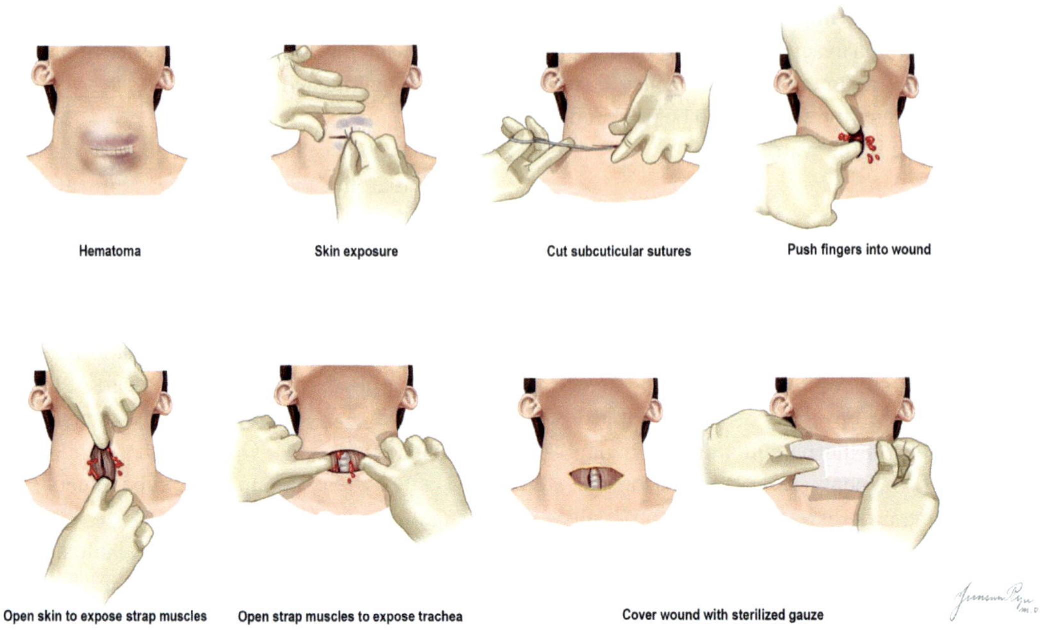

Fig. 14.10 Hematoma evacuation procedure

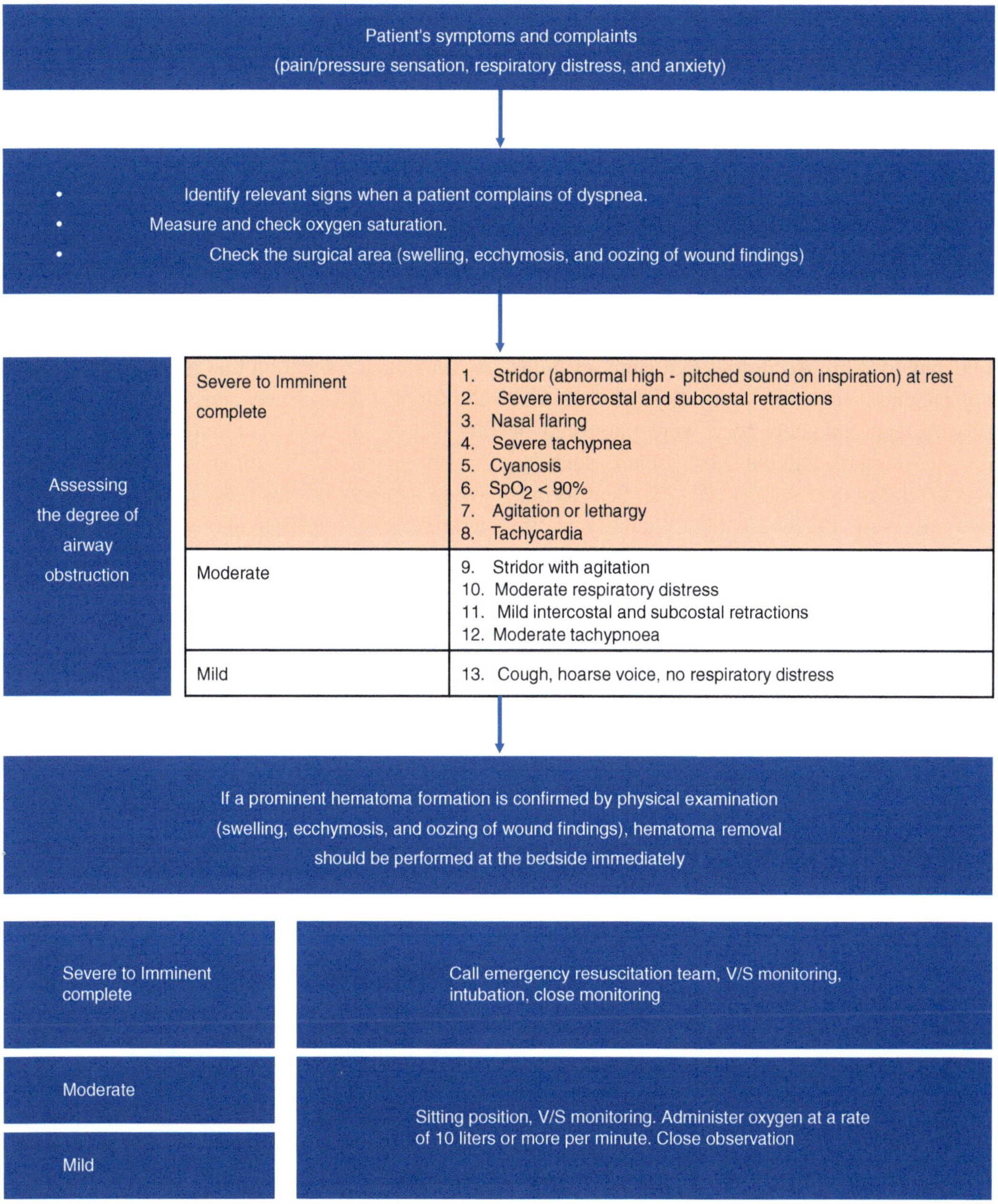

Fig. 14.11 Management protocol of hematoma after thyroid surgery

14.5 KQ 14.5. What Are the Appropriate Intraoperative and Postoperative Measures to Minimize Scarring After Thyroid Surgery?

Bon Seok Koo

Scar-related complications are the most common among the many long-term complications of thyroid surgery [26]. According to a study examining patients' views on morbidity after thyroid surgery, approximately 65% were interested in thyroid surgery without neck scars, such as robotic/endoscopic surgery [27, 28]. Scar formation adversely affects a patient's quality of life [29]. Therefore, when open thyroid surgery is performed, surgeons must focus on minimizing scarring.

Before appropriate treatment, during, or after surgery, it is necessary to provide patients with adequate information regarding scarring that may occur after thyroid surgery. This information should include details regarding the length of the incision made during the operation, which directly correlates with the eventual scar length at the site. Furthermore, patient history should clarify the possibility of scar-related complications (hypertrophic scarring and keloids). Patients with a history of severe scarring are more likely to experience poor scarring after surgery [30]. Furthermore, patients should be provided with adequate information about surgical techniques that minimize cervical scars or thyroid surgery techniques that do not cause cervical scars so that they can directly choose the surgical method.

◆ Before thyroid surgery, providing detailed information about the surgical method and scars that may occur after surgery is crucial. Additionally, by ascertaining whether there is a history of hypertrophic scars or keloids, the possibility of deep remaining scars can be identified in advance.

In conventional thyroidectomy, the following points should be considered when making an incision. First, an incision should be made by referring to Langer's line and the relaxed skin tension line, which minimizes skin tension after the incision (Fig. 14.12) [30]. The incision line that can reduce skin tension is usually in the horizontal direction of naturally occurring wrinkles on the neck and is as close to the sternal border as possible to a position where the surgical field of vision is not obstructed. If the deep natural crease is situated at a location that is not obstructed by the surgical field of view, it is an excellent option for making an incision at that location.

Mitigating the length of the incision line is recommended; however, excessive traction using a retractor to secure a field of view during surgery may damage the skin fibers and adversely influence scar formation. Therefore, it is crucial to design an incision of appropriate length to avoid excessive traction. The classic incision for conventional thyroidectomy ranges from 3.5 cm to 8.2 cm; in the case of open minimally invasive thyroidectomy, it is approximately 1.7 cm to 3.2 cm [31]. The length of the incision line does not significantly affect dissatisfaction with cosmetic outcomes that may occur because of postoperative scarring [30, 32].

◆ The incision line should be strategically planned along the horizontal direction of the natural neck crease to minimize skin tension. The incision length should be meticulously determined to the minimum length to prevent excessive traction during surgery.

When pulling the edge of the wound for skin suturing after surgery, a delicate instrument should be used to minimize the necessary traction and compression forces at the edge of the wound. Accordingly, the smallest suture is recommended to overcome wound tension adequately [30].

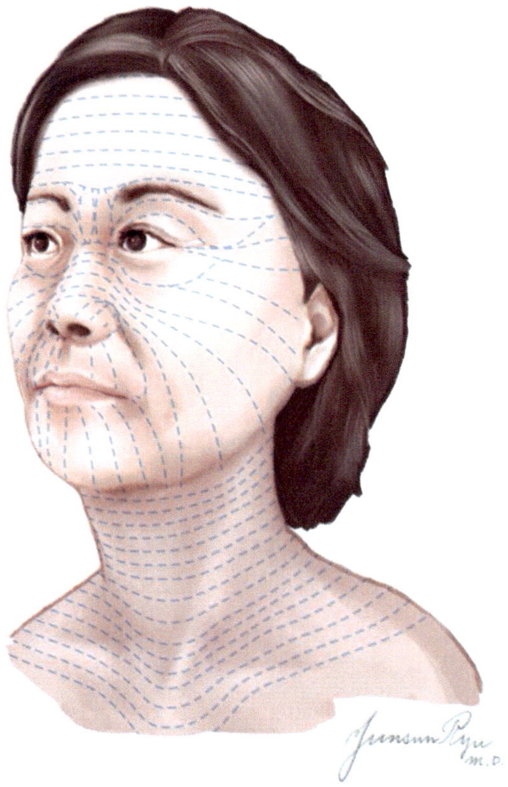

Fig. 14.12 Relaxed skin tension lines on the neck

Expert Opinion
A common mistake made by novice thyroid surgeons regarding scars is making an incision that is shorter than the ideal length, which leads to excessive traction and tissue damage during surgery. Additionally, overmanipulating the incision line epidermis with forceps can result in a short but hypertrophic scar. (Seung-Won Lee)

After surgery, the wound should be cleaned using a foam dressing to prevent infection. However, the use of antiseptics, such as alcohol or iodine, should be avoided, as they can aggravate scar formation owing to their cytotoxic action [30]. If sutures are used, they should be removed 5–7 days after surgery, and skin tape should be applied to minimize skin tension. In patients with a history of keloids and hypertrophic scar formation, silicone application, laser treatment, and Botox injections are reportedly effective and should be used appropriately [30, 33]. In a randomized study, surgical wound closure was followed by the injection of 50 U of Botox diluted in 1 mL of physiological saline into the platysmal muscle. After thyroidectomy, topical application of Botox to the wound area relieved muscle tension, reduced hypertrophic scar formation, and improved cosmetic outcomes [33]. As various silicone products are commercially available (silicone rubber, silicone sheets, and silicone tape), the choice of silicone can be tailored according to the patient's preference. The consistent use of silicone for approximately 3 or 4 months is recommended to achieve optimal efficacy.

After thyroid surgery, massaging the surgical region and performing neck exercises helps relieve scarring and prevent neck contractions. In areas of the wound with a low risk of infection, a small amount of moisturizer, such as vitamin E oil, cocoa butter, or scar cream, can be applied and rubbed gently in a circular motion using the fingertips. Cervical exercises can be performed 1 week after surgery by gradually increasing the number and intensity of exercises from a minimum of three to ten times for 2 weeks (Fig. 14.13).

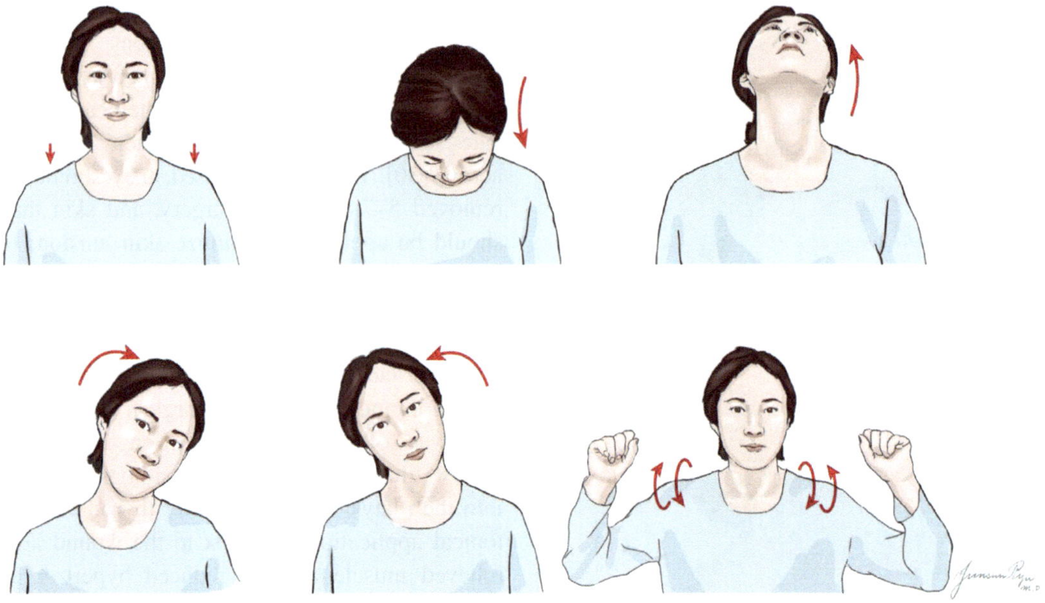

Fig. 14.13 Exercises for recovery after thyroid surgery

References

1. Matsumoto F, Ikeda K. Surgical management of tracheal invasion by well-differentiated thyroid cancer. Cancers (Basel). 2021;13(4):797.
2. Chernichenko N, Shaha AR. Role of tracheal resection in thyroid cancer. Curr Opin Oncol. 2012;24(1):29–34.
3. Honings J, Stephen AE, Marres HA, Gaissert HA. The management of thyroid carcinoma invading the larynx or trachea. Laryngoscope. 2010;120(4):682–9.
4. Shindo ML, Caruana SM, Kandil E, McCaffrey JC, Orloff LA, Porterfield JR, et al. Management of invasive well-differentiated thyroid cancer: an American Head and Neck Society consensus statement. AHNS consensus statement. Head Neck. 2014;36(10):1379–90.
5. Patel KN, Shaha AR. Locally advanced thyroid cancer. Curr Opin Otolaryngol Head Neck Surg. 2005;13(2):112–6.
6. Ito Y, Miyauchi A, Kihara M, Higashiyama T, Kobayashi K, Miya A. Airtight tracheocutaneostomy after window resection of the trachea for invasive papillary thyroid carcinoma: experience of 109 cases. World J Surg. 2014;38(3):660–6.
7. Xia X, Cai Y, Zhu X, Zhu Y, Shen L, Zhou Y, et al. Tracheal window resection and reconstruction via sternocleidomastoid flap for invasive thyroid carcinoma. Interact Cardiovasc Thorac Surg. 2021;33(6):899–904.
8. Kebebew E, Clark OH. Locally advanced differentiated thyroid cancer. Surg Oncol. 2003;12(2):91–9.
9. An SY, Kim KH. Surgical management of locally advanced thyroid cancer. Curr Opin Otolaryngol Head Neck Surg. 2010;18(2):119–23.
10. Price DL, Wong RJ, Randolph GW. Invasive thyroid cancer: management of the trachea and esophagus. Otolaryngol Clin North Am. 2008;41(6):1155–68.
11. McCaffrey JC. Aerodigestive tract invasion by well-differentiated thyroid carcinoma: diagnosis, management, prognosis, and biology. Laryngoscope. 2006;116(1):1–11.
12. Alsanea O, Clark OH. Treatment of Graves' disease: the advantages of surgery. Endocrinol Metab Clin North Am. 2000;29(2):321–37.
13. Goldstein R, Hart IR. Follow-up of solitary autonomous thyroid nodules treated with 131I. N Engl J Med. 1983;309(24):1473–6.
14. Klonecke A, Petersen MM, McDougall IR. Thyrotoxicosis with low thyroidal uptake of radioiodine. Semin Nucl Med. 1990;20(4):364–6.
15. Gittoes NJ, Franklyn JA. Hyperthyroidism. Current treatment guidelines. Drugs. 1998;55(4):543–53.
16. Satoh T, Isozaki O, Suzuki A, Wakino S, Iburi T, Tsuboi K, et al. 2016 Guidelines for the management of thyroid storm from The Japan Thyroid Association and Japan Endocrine Society (First edition). Endocr J. 2016;63(12):1025–64.
17. Ross DS, Burch HB, Cooper DS, Greenlee MC, Laurberg P, Maia AL, et al. 2016 American thyroid association guidelines for diagnosis and management

of hyperthyroidism and other causes of thyrotoxicosis. Thyroid. 2016;26(10):1343–421.
18. Erbil Y, Ozluk Y, Giris M, Salmaslioglu A, Issever H, Barbaros U, et al. Effect of Lugol solution on thyroid gland blood flow and microvessel density in the patients with Graves' disease. J Clin Endocrinol Metab. 2007;92(6):2182–9.
19. Ansaldo GL, Pretolesi F, Varaldo E, Meola C, Minuto M, Borgonovo G, et al. Doppler evaluation of intrathyroid arterial resistances during preoperative treatment with Lugol's iodide solution in patients with diffuse toxic goiter. J Am Coll Surg. 2000;191(6):607–12.
20. Kahaly GJ, Bartalena L, Hegedus L, Leenhardt L, Poppe K, Pearce SH. 2018 European thyroid association guideline for the management of graves' hyperthyroidism. Eur Thyroid J. 2018;7(4):167–86.
21. Reber A, Valenti L, Muller S. A patient with graves' disease scheduled for thyroidectomy with high risk for thyroid storm caused by severe medication nonadherence: anaesthetic and surgical considerations. Case Rep Anesthesiol. 2019;2019:4781902.
22. Iliff HA, El-Boghdadly K, Ahmad I, Davis J, Harris A, Khan S, et al. Management of haematoma after thyroid surgery: systematic review and multidisciplinary consensus guidelines from the Difficult Airway Society, the British Association of Endocrine and Thyroid Surgeons and the British Association of Otorhinolaryngology. Head and Neck Surgery. Anaesthesia. 2022;77(1):82–95.
23. Godballe C, Madsen AR, Pedersen HB, Sorensen CH, Pedersen U, Frisch T, et al. Post-thyroidectomy hemorrhage: a national study of patients treated at the Danish departments of ENT Head and Neck Surgery. Eur Arch Otorhinolaryngol. 2009;266(12):1945–52.
24. Farooq MS, Nouraei R, Kaddour H, Saharay M. Patterns, timing and consequences of post-thyroidectomy haemorrhage. Ann R Coll Surg Engl. 2017;99(1):60–2.
25. Lee HS, Lee BJ, Kim SW, Cha YW, Choi YS, Park YH, et al. Patterns of post-thyroidectomy hemorrhage. Clin Exp Otorhinolaryngol. 2009;2(2):72–7.
26. Arora A, Swords C, Garas G, Chaidas K, Prichard A, Budge J, et al. The perception of scar cosmesis following thyroid and parathyroid surgery: a prospective cohort study. Int J Surg. 2016;25:38–43.
27. Linos D, Kiriakopoulos A, Petralias A. Patient attitudes toward transaxillary robot-assisted thyroidectomy. World J Surg. 2013;37(8):1959–65.
28. Grover G, Sadler GP, Mihai R. Morbidity after thyroid surgery: patient perspective. Laryngoscope. 2013;123(9):2319–23.
29. Choi Y, Lee JH, Kim YH, Lee YS, Chang HS, Park CS, et al. Impact of postthyroidectomy scar on the quality of life of thyroid cancer patients. Ann Dermatol. 2014;26(6):693–9.
30. Son D, Harijan A. Overview of surgical scar prevention and management. J Korean Med Sci. 2014;29(6):751–7.
31. Dordea M, Aspinall SR. Short and long-term cosmesis of cervical thyroidectomy scars. Ann R Coll Surg Engl. 2016;98(1):11–7.
32. Toll EC, Loizou P, Davis CR, Porter GC, Pothier DD. Scars and satisfaction: do smaller scars improve patient-reported outcome? Eur Arch Otorhinolaryngol. 2012;269(1):309–13.
33. Bae DS, Koo DH, Kim JE, Cho JM, Park JO. Effect of botulinum toxin A on scar healing after thyroidectomy: a prospective double-blind randomized controlled trial. J Clin Med. 2020;9(3):868.

15 Endoscopic/Robotic Surgery-Associated Complications

Jun-Ook Park and Min Woo Park

15.1 KQ 15.1. How to Prevent and Manage Complications Associated with the Transoral Approach?

Jun-Ook Park

15.1.1 Selection of Appropriate Patients for Inexperienced Surgeons

A tumor in the right lobe of the thyroid is best managed by a right-handed surgeon. Less experienced surgeons are advised to select only patients with intrathyroidal tumors <1 cm in diameter in the right lower pole because visualization and manipulation of the superior pole can be challenging. Surgery may be difficult if the thyroid gland is large or if the patient has thyroiditis, which can cause bleeding. Additionally, rear enlargement of the tubercle of Zuckerkandl may obstruct the surgical view of the retrothyroid area, making it difficult to identify the recurrent laryngeal nerve.

Important factors to consider include:

◆ ***Patient selection for inexperienced surgeons***

Patients: Female patients without a prominent mandible or Adam's apple, who are not severely obese or very thin.

Tumor: Intrathyroidal tumor (<1 cm) in the right lower pole (for a right-handed surgeon).

Thyroid gland: A small gland with a small tubercle of Zuckerkandl and no pyramidal lobe.

Other considerations: No vascular anomaly, such as a retroesophageal subclavian artery.

Expert Opinion

Intrathyroidal tumors <1 cm in diameter are recommended for less experienced surgeons. However, even cases diagnosed as

(continued)

J.-O. Park (✉)
Department of Otolaryngology—Head and Neck Surgery, Seoul St. Mary's Hospital, The Catholic University, Seoul, Republic of Korea
e-mail: junook2000@catholic.ac.kr

M. W. Park (✉)
Department of Otolaryngology—Head and Neck Surgery, Kangdong Sacred Heart Hospital, Seoul, Republic of Korea
e-mail: subintern@kdh.or.kr

K.-J. Cho, J.-O. Park (eds.), *Management of Head and Neck Surgery Complications*,
https://doi.org/10.1007/978-981-96-1860-6_15

papillary thyroid microcarcinoma can be observed under active surveillance. It would be beneficial to include additional patient selection criteria and consider the tumor size threshold. While there are challenges with visualization and manipulation of the superior pole and the area surrounding the tubercle of Zuckerkandl, providing specific surgical techniques or tips can help to overcome these challenges. The surgeon's handedness may not be a primary criterion, as competence and confidence are more important factors. (Tsung-Lin Yang)

15.1.2 Preventing Mental Nerve Injury During Surgery

The mental nerve provides sensations to the lower lip, chin, and jaw. If a nerve is damaged during transoral thyroidectomy, numbness or tingling can develop in these areas.

15.1.2.1 Midline Oral Incision

A recent anatomical study by Yang et al. found that the safest zone for a midline oral incision is the trapezoid with a 3-cm baseline and a base angle of 50° [1]. This is considered safe because the medial branch of the mental nerve is usually absent in this region. However, small branches of the nerve lie between the mentalis muscle and the corner of the mouth, extending up to the corner. Surgeons should be cautious when approaching the lateral area of the lower lip to avoid damaging these small branches. Surgeons usually create a 2–2.5-cm incision in the center of the vestibule using a monopolar cautery device, typically 1–1.5 cm distant from the gingiva.

◆ ***The safest zone for midline oral incision***: A trapezoid with a 3-cm baseline and a base angle of 50° (Fig. 15.1).

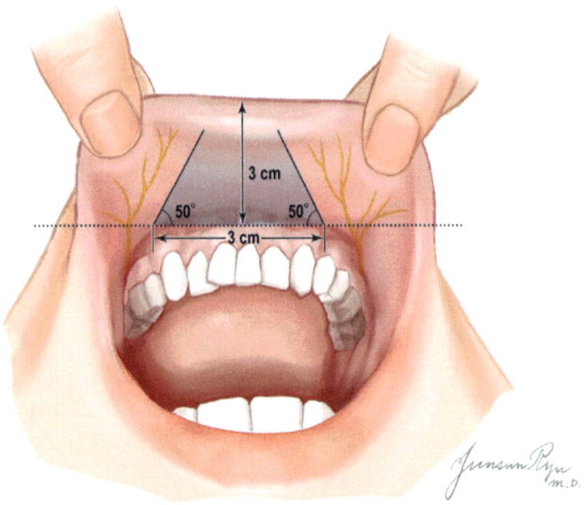

Fig. 15.1 The midline oral incision. To avoid injury to the mental nerve, a midline incision should be made in a trapezoid with a 3 cm baseline and a base angle of 50°

15.1.2.2 Lateral Incision

◆ ***The safest zone for the two lateral incisions***: The mental nerve exits the mandible through the mental foramen and courses along the anterior surface of the mandible, then branches into smaller nerves that supply sensation to the lower lip and chin. The mental foramen is usually located between the lower first and second premolars. To avoid injury to the mental nerve, lateral incisions should be created in more posterior regions (Fig. 15.2).

To prevent damage to the mental nerve, a 5-mm lateral incision may be made on the buccal mucosa near the second premolar, approximately 1.5–2 cm distant from the gingivobuccal fold. Depending on the surgical system used, a 5-mm cannula (for endoscopic surgery) or an 8-mm cannula (for da Vinci Xi surgery) can be inserted through the incision to access the surgical site while minimizing the risk of nerve damage.

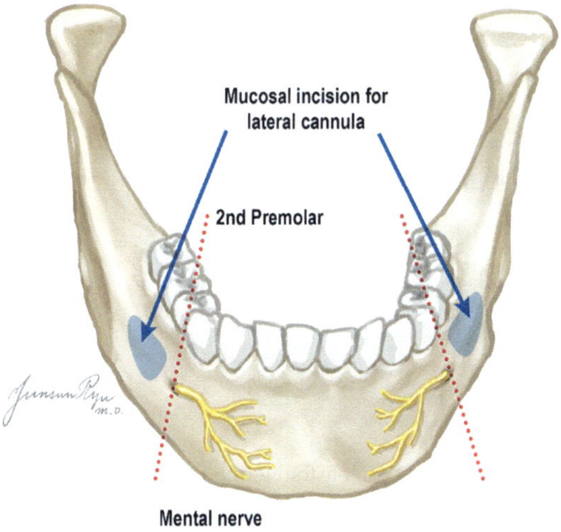

Fig. 15.2 Two lateral oral incisions. To avoid injury to the mental nerve, both lateral incisions in the buccal mucosa should be created posteriorly near the second premolar

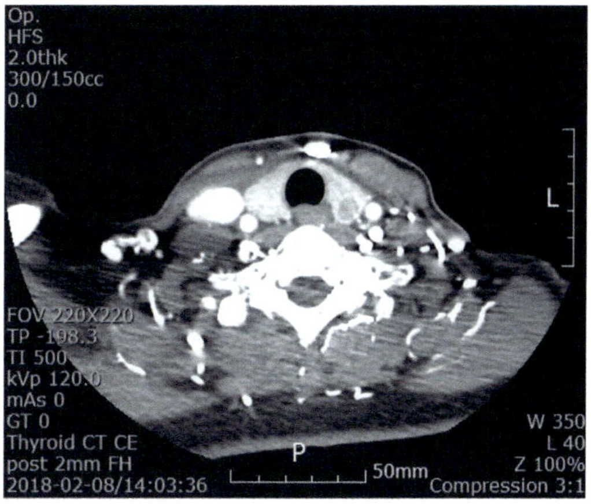

Fig. 15.3 Scan demonstrating the importance of avoiding injury to the large, anterior jugular vein located in the midline when creating a working space

15.1.3 Prevention of CO_2 Embolism During Surgery

The risk of CO_2 embolism during robotic or endoscopic surgery is considerably low (approximately 0.001%) [2]. However, if embolism occurs, its consequences may be serious. During transoral endoscopic or robotic thyroidectomy, a working space is created by artificially expanding the neck spaces that do not naturally lie along the fascial plane of the neck. This differs from endoscopic abdominal surgery, which is performed within the normal abdominal cavity. During the creation of the working space using blunt instruments, several small blood vessels can be damaged, increasing the risk of CO_2 entering the circulatory system via damaged veins, arteries, or microvasculature and potentially creating blockages in the right atrium or pulmonary artery [3, 4].

To reduce the risk of CO_2 embolism during transoral thyroid surgery:

1) Minimizing the risk of vascular damage. Before surgery, always check the neck computed tomography and identify the locations of larger vessels, such as the anterior jugular vein. Use blunt instruments, such as a Hegar uterine dilator, to create a working space and gently rotate the dilator to expand the space. Initially, create a minimum working space, and subsequently insert the endoscope and widen the space while visually checking for safety. If the large anterior jugular vein lies at the midline, care should be taken to avoid damaging the vein when separating the strap muscles (Fig. 15.3).
2) Reduce CO_2 injection pressure/flow rate. Hold the initial CO_2 pressure below 6 mmHg and, during surgery, at approximately 3–4 mmHg at a flow rate of 12–15 L/min, depending on the surgical system utilized.
3) Monitor end-tidal CO_2 ($ETCO_2$) levels. Such measurements sensitively and non-invasively detect CO_2 embolisms, and $ETCO_2$ levels may increase or decrease. A temporary increase indicates an increase in dissolved CO_2 in the blood, and a rapid decrease indicates that the embolism blocks some of the pulmonary vasculature [5]. Close collaboration between anesthesiologists and surgeons is recommended. It is important to monitor the $ETCO_2$ level continuously and maintain it below 40 mmHg.
4) Use a self-retaining retractor instead of CO_2. Recently, several authors have reported successful transoral surgery in the absence of gas insufflation using a self-retaining retractor. The detailed procedures have been published [6–8].

◆ ***Preventing CO_2 embolism during surgery***

1) Minimize the risk of vascular damage when creating the working space
2) Reduce the CO_2 injection pressure/flow rate (not exceeding a pressure of 6 mmHg at a flow rate of 12–15 L/min)
3) Monitor the end-tidal carbon dioxide ($ETCO_2$) level (maintain below 40 mmHg)
4) Use a self-retaining retractor rather than CO_2

Expert Opinion

Management of carbon dioxide embolism during surgery:

1. Stop operation immediately if vital signs are compromised
2. Prevent further gas entry
   2.1. Discontinue carbon dioxide insufflation
   2.2. Discontinue nitrous oxide and ventilate with 100% O_2
   2.3. Left lateral decubitus position
3. Adequate hydration
4. Central venous catheterization: aspiration of carbon dioxide
5. Resuscitation (Myung-Chul Lee)

Mentioning the use of a self-retaining retractor is valuable. Using this technique, the surgery will be performed in a gasless manner, which requires different surgical techniques. Therefore, detailed descriptions or listing these techniques in a different paragraph or section would be beneficial. (Tsung-Lin Yang)

15.1.4 Management of Wound Infection

The transoral approach involves an incision within the oral cavity, which is a cleanly contaminated rather than a clean wound. Particularly, if a vestibular abscess is present or oral hygiene is poor, infection can occur despite the use of antibiotics. Wound infections can also be caused by contamination when aspirating a seroma (Fig. 15.4).

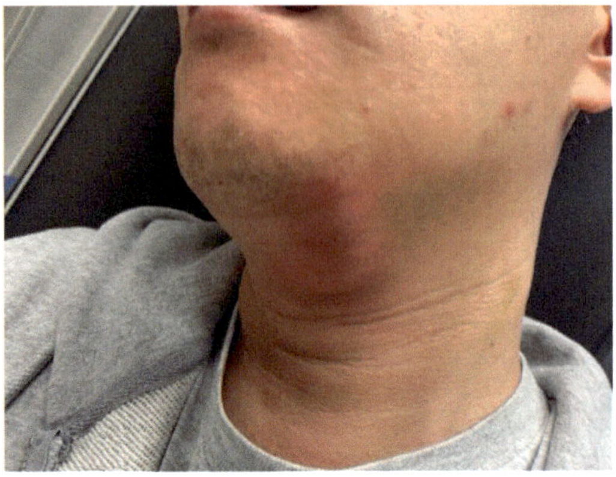

Fig. 15.4 Scan demonstrating the importance of avoiding injury to the large anterior jugular vein located at the midline when creating a working space

◆ ***To prevent wound infection***

1) Thoroughly decontaminate the oral cavity with saline and povidone-iodine before surgery.
2) After surgery, irrigate the working space thoroughly and suture the oral mucosa in a watertight manner.
3) It has not been conclusively established whether prophylactic antibiotics are necessary.

If wound infection does occur:

◆ ***To manage wound infection***

1) Administer antibiotics
2) Aspirate the area with erythema and swelling and check for pus
3) If there is no improvement after adequate pus drainage and antibiotic use, consider creating a small incision (1–2 mm) to drain the area, perform irrigation, and administer antibiotics

Expert Opinion
The transoral approach correctly identifies the procedure as a clean-contaminated wound. There is a risk associated with poor oral hygiene, but specific recommendations for preoperative oral care or assessment protocols are not provided. The suggestion to use saline and povidone-iodine for oral cavity decontamination is appropriate. However, providing a detailed protocol, including specific concentration and volume recommendations for these solutions, would be useful. The importance of thorough irrigation and watertight suturing is mentioned. Providing more detailed techniques or tips for achieving these outcomes would improve the guidance. (Tsung-Lin Yang)

15.2 KQ 15.2. How to Prevent and Manage Complications Related to the Transaxillary Approach? (Traction Injury, Axillary Skin Flap Perforation, etc.)

Min Woo Park

Endoscopic or robotic thyroid surgery using a transaxillary approach is one of the most popular scarless approaches. Concerning feasibility, safety, and cosmesis, current evidence supports transaxillary robotic or endoscopic thyroidectomy as a feasible and safe approach. Importantly, this approach is cosmetically superior to open surgery [9–11]. Although wide subcutaneous dissection and long operative times increase postoperative chest pain, literature has consistently shown that improvement in pain and paresthesia following transaxillary thyroid surgery is superior to that following conventional open surgery [11].

◆ Wide subcutaneous dissection and a long operative time can increase postoperative chest pain and paresthesia following transaxillary thyroid surgery.

15.2.1 Complications

Complications that may occur after transaxillary thyroid surgery can be classified into thyroidectomy- and technique-related types [12]. The prevention of thyroidectomy-related complications will be discussed in other chapters, while the prevention of technique-related complications will be discussed below.

1) Thyroidectomy-related complications

    Transient hypoparathyroidism is the most common complication of transaxillary thyroid surgery after total thyroidectomy [11, 13]. Most patients with transient hypoparathyroidism recover normal serum calcium levels and are relieved of hypocalcemic symptoms within two months of surgery. Intraoperative recurrent laryngeal nerve injuries can occur, most of which involve temporary paralysis. Moreover, transient hoarseness generally resolves within 2–3 months. Furthermore, some patients may experience postoperative bleeding. Delayed postoperative tracheal perforations have also been reported.

Expert Opinion
The transaxillary approach provides the same view as open thyroidectomy and preserves the parathyroid glands and recurrent laryngeal nerve, but it relies heavily on the surgeon's experience. Understanding anatomy and dissection planes is crucial, as incorrect dissection can lead to fibrotic bands, requiring open surgery and diminishing the benefits of minimally invasive techniques. (Seung-Won Lee)

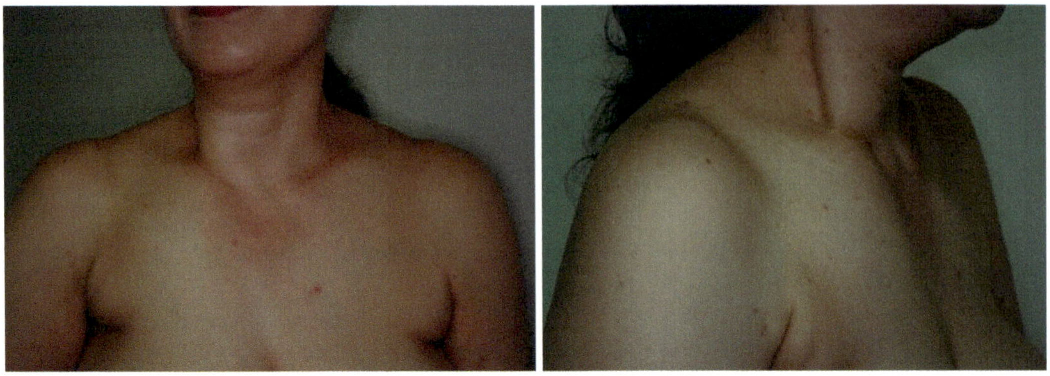

Fig. 15.5 Sternocleidomastoid muscle fibrosis and seroma in the chest area (copyright Prof. Myung-Chul Lee)

2) Technique-related complications

Technique-related complications associated with the transaxillary approach include axillary skin flap perforation and transient brachial nerve paralysis. Transient brachial nerve paralysis can occur due to hyperextension of the arm on the lesioned side. Most patients recover spontaneously within two months. However, some patients develop arm lymphedema, which can be resolved with physical therapy and conservative management. Most patients reported dysesthesia over the working space that lasted approximately one month, which subsequently decreased over time. Resolution within 3 months is expected [12, 14, 15].

Postoperative seroma or hematoma can form in the transaxillary flap area due to extensive subcutaneous dissection from the axilla to the neck. Most seromas can be treated with repeated aspiration and compressive dressings. Additionally, because the surgical approach involves the sternocleidomastoid muscle, a fibrotic band can form in the muscle postoperatively (Fig. 15.5). Local steroid injections may be helpful in the presence of fibrotic bands.

Solutions:

1. Minimize surgical time.
2. Release the rigid retractor every 1–2 hours during prolonged surgeries.
3. Use negative pressure drainage for seromas or hematomas and apply broad chest compression with devices like a Surgibra.
4. Begin chest and neck stretching one month post-surgery. (Myung-Chul Lee)

A thorough understanding of the dissection plane's anatomy is crucial. Dissecting along an incorrect plane or using excessive manipulation can lead to the formation of fibrotic bands resulting from abnormal wound healing of the sternocleidomastoid muscle. These bands can be both cosmetically and functionally undesirable, necessitating fibrotic band lysis through an open approach when symptoms are severe. In such cases, the benefits of endoscopic or robotic surgery are significantly diminished. (Seung-Won Lee)

Expert Opinion

This procedure has a broader scope than anterior thyroidectomy, with longer operation times and the use of a rigid retractor system, which can damage muscles or subcutaneous tissue.

◆ The complications of transaxillary thyroid surgery can be divided into thyroidectomy- and technique-related types. The technique-related complications of concern are axillary skin flap perforation and transient brachial nerve paralysis.

15.2.2 Prevention of Technical Complications

1) Brachial plexus injury

Brachial plexus nerve injury is relatively rare, with a reported incidence of 0.1%. However, if this occurs, it can negatively affect the patient's quality of life. Therefore, caution should be exercised in this regard.

The simplest way to prevent brachial plexus injury is to avoid raising the patient's arm excessively during surgery. Brachial plexus paralysis is associated with excessive elevation of the affected arm. Unlike other surgical methods, the transaxillary surgical approach is performed through the axilla while the affected arm is elevated. Therefore, the arm must be raised to create a working space on the chest. However, excessive pulling can cause traction on the brachial plexus, leading to injury. Notably, such injuries are generally temporary, and most patients recover within 2–3 months. However, the prevention of injury is crucial. To prevent injury, the arm should be raised until gentle pressure is felt without tight traction (Fig. 15.6). If brachial plexus paralysis occurs permanently, no treatment is available. Therefore, prevention is of paramount importance.

◆ To prevent brachial plexus injury, it is necessary to raise the arm only until the point where gentle pressure is felt without tight traction.

Expert Opinion

Regarding the prevention of brachial plexus injury, it would be beneficial to provide context that compares this injury to other surgical complications and how it varies with different types of arm positions. Since it has never happened in our practice, it may be important to learn from these rare cases, especially those with incomplete recovery. While it is mentioned that most patients recover within 2–3 months, it would be useful to address whether rehabilitation is needed during these periods. In addition to avoiding raising the arm excessively high, suggesting specific guidelines or metrics for safe arm positioning could be beneficial. Additionally, discussing whether the use of specific arm supports would be beneficial could be valuable. (Tsung-Lin Yang)

2) Skin flap perforation

Perforation of the skin flap can occur during elevation. Accurate identification of the proper surgical plane is crucial to avoid creating holes in the skin flap during elevation. Once the precise surgical plane is identified, it is important to lift the flap while performing appropriate retraction [16] (Fig. 15.7).

Transitioning from the chest to the neck can be challenging because of the curved nature of the clavicle, which may hinder effective retraction. If retraction is unsuccessful,

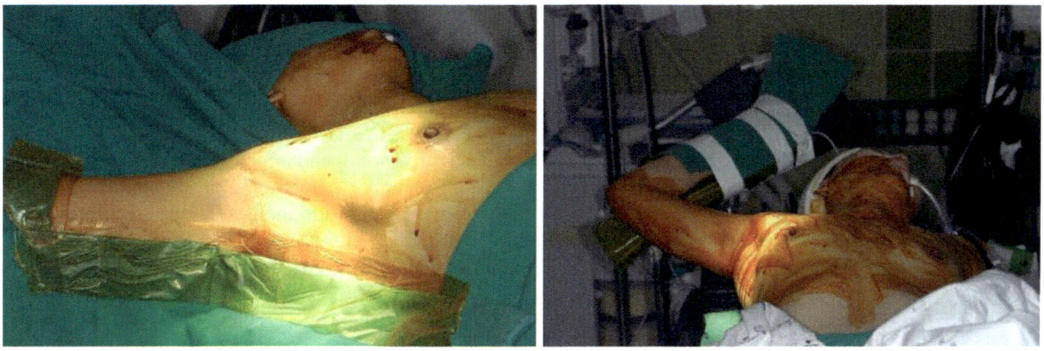

Fig. 15.6 Arm position for the prevention of brachial plexus injury

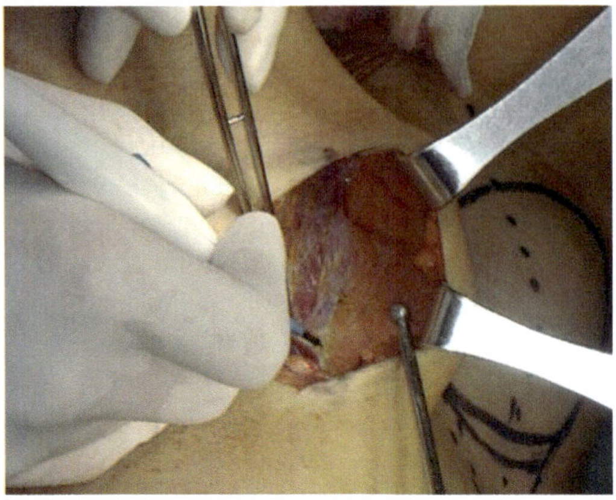

Fig. 15.7 Flap elevation: In the chest area, flap dissection is performed above the pectoralis major muscle. In the neck area, it is performed under the platysma muscle

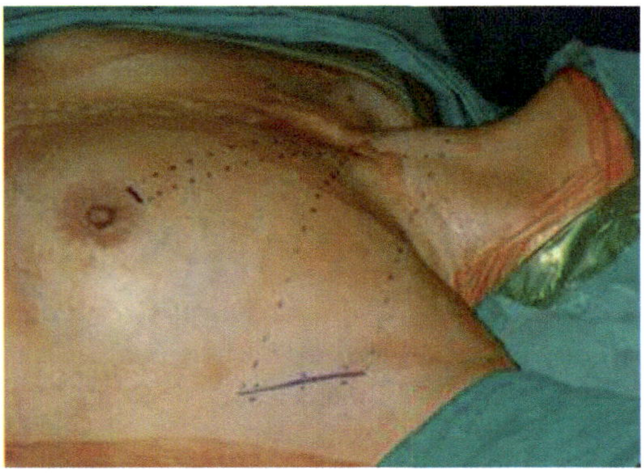

Fig. 15.8 Skin areas at risk of perforation: transition point from the chest to the neck (during flap elevation) and contralateral thyroid skin area (during surgery)

there is a risk of violating the surgical plane, leading to flap perforation in this area (Fig. 15.8).

In the event of flap perforation, the affected area should be marginally excised, and primary sutures should be applied to ensure proper healing.

◆ To avoid creating holes in the skin flap during elevation, it is crucial to accurately identify the proper surgical plane. In the event of flap perforation, the affected area should be marginally excised, and primary sutures should be applied to ensure proper healing.

Expert Opinion

Regarding skin flap perforation, it is also rare and has not happened in our practice. Identifying the proper surgical plane, particularly at the clavicle transition zone, lacks specific techniques or methods. Detailing anatomical landmarks or tools that can aid in this process would be beneficial. Referring to specific figures is good practice, but ensuring these illustrations clearly demonstrate the concepts and techniques is important. Specifying the application of specific types of retractors or techniques to minimize the risk of flap perforation is crucial. (Tsung-Lin Yang)

Skin perforation is most likely to occur in the level V area, where the chest transitions to the neck. Preventing this requires cadaver dissection training and a solid understanding of anatomy. (Seung-Won Lee)

References

1. Yang HM, Shin KJ, Min J, Woo SH. Anatomical study of gasless transoral thyroidectomy and clinical application. Surg Endosc. 2020;34(8):3414–23.
2. Bonjer HJ, Hazebroek EJ, Kazemier G, Giuffrida MC, Meijer WS, Lange JF. Open versus closed establishment of pneumoperitoneum in laparoscopic surgery. Br J Surg. 1997;84(5):599–602.
3. Kim CS, Liu J, Kwon JY, Shin SK, Kim KJ. Venous air embolism during surgery, especially cesarean delivery. J Korean Med Sci. 2008;23(5):753–61.
4. Magrina JF. Complications of laparoscopic surgery. Clin Obstet Gynecol. 2002;45(2):469–80.
5. Park EY, Kwon JY, Kim KJ. Carbon dioxide embolism during laparoscopic surgery. Yonsei Med J. 2012;53(3):459–66.
6. Park JO, Park YJ, Kim MR, Sun DI, Kim MS, Koh YW. Gasless transoral endoscopic thyroidectomy vestibular approach (gasless TOETVA). Surg Endosc. 2019;33(9):3034–9.
7. Park JO, Lee DH, Kim MR, Kim SY, Han JH, Sun DI. Transoral endoscopic thyroidectomy using a self-retaining retractor as an alternative to carbon dioxide gas insufflation: a comparative analysis of 131 cases. Oral Oncol. 2021;121:105463.
8. Park YM, Kim DH, Moon YM, Lim JY, Choi EC, Kim SH, et al. Gasless transoral robotic thyroidectomy using the DaVinci SP system: feasibility, safety, and operative technique. Oral Oncol. 2019;95:136–42.

9. Aidan P, Arora A, Lorincz B, Tolley N, Garas G. Robotic thyroid surgery: current perspectives and future considerations. ORL J Otorhinolaryngol Relat Spec. 2018;80(3–4):186–94.
10. Kim MJ, Nam KH, Lee SG, Choi JB, Kim TH, Lee CR, et al. Yonsei experience of 5000 gasless transaxillary robotic thyroidectomies. World J Surg. 2018;42(2):393–401.
11. Lee YM, Yi O, Sung TY, Chung KW, Yoon JH, Hong SJ. Surgical outcomes of robotic thyroid surgery using a double incision gasless transaxillary approach: analysis of 400 cases treated by the same surgeon. Head Neck. 2014;36(10):1413–9.
12. Aidan P, Pickburn H, Monpeyssen H, Boccara G. Indications for the gasless transaxillary robotic approach to thyroid surgery: experience of forty-seven procedures at the American Hospital of Paris. Eur Thyroid J. 2013;2(2):102–9.
13. Stang MT, Yip L, Wharry L, Bartlett DL, McCoy KL, Carty SE. Gasless transaxillary endoscopic thyroidectomy with robotic assistance: a high-volume experience in North America. Thyroid. 2018;28(12):1655–61.
14. Cong R, Li X, Ouyang H, Xue W, Zhang Z, Xia F. Gasless, endoscopic trans-axillary thyroid surgery: our series of the first 51 human cases. World J Surg Oncol. 2022;20(1):9.
15. Sun B, Li P, Cong R, Zhou D, Zhang Z, Xia F, et al. Gasless endoscopic transaxillary thyroid surgery: CUSUM analysis of a single surgeon's experience from 105 preliminary procedures. Surg Endosc. 2022;36(11):8270–9.
16. Piccoli M, Mullineris B, Santi D, Gozzo D. Advances in robotic transaxillary thyroidectomy in Europe. Curr Surg Rep. 2017;5(8):17.

Part VII

Reconstructive Surgery

16 Flap Monitoring and Management of Failing Free Flap

Jun-Ook Park

16.1 KQ 16.1. What Are the Practical Methods for Postoperative Monitoring of a Free Flap?

Jun-Ook Park

Monitoring free flaps in the head and neck region presents various challenges compared with similar flaps in other body regions. Conventional methods for postoperative flap monitoring include assessment of color, temperature, capillary refill, and pinprick tests. Additional tools such as handheld and implantable Dopplers, as well as near-infrared spectroscopy (NIRS), can supplement conventional methods. Optimal monitoring methods for patients undergoing flap surgery should be safe, rapid, consistent, reliable, recordable, and cost effective. Although several monitoring methods have been developed and clinically evaluated, a consensus on the best approach is yet to be reached. The flap salvage rate is useful for evaluating monitoring effectiveness, whereas the false-positive rate can be used to compare different monitoring methods. Large-scale studies have demonstrated comparable flap success rates (97–99%) and salvage rates (ca. 80%) among different monitoring systems [1]. Re-exploration following free flap surgery typically occurs within 24 h, with the initial 6 h being the period of greatest re-exploration frequency.

◆ Flap monitoring should be performed hourly during the initial 24 h following surgery, followed by monitoring every 2 h for the next 48 h.

Expert Opinion
In older patients, age-related morphological variations (e.g., wrinkled epidermis, reduced vascularization, dehydration) may hamper the early detection of flap failure. (Young Hoon Joo)

Although it is ideal for surgeons to perform postoperative flap monitoring, this is not always possible. In many instances, monitoring is performed by residents or intensive care unit nurses. Therefore, adequate training of these individuals is essential to ensure effective com-

Supplementary Information The online version contains supplementary material available at https://doi.org/10.1007/978-981-96-1860-6_16.

J.-O. Park (✉)
Department of Otolaryngology—Head and Neck Surgery, Seoul St. Mary's Hospital, The Catholic University, Seoul, Republic of Korea
e-mail: junook2000@catholic.ac.kr

K.-J. Cho, J.-O. Park (eds.), *Management of Head and Neck Surgery Complications*,
https://doi.org/10.1007/978-981-96-1860-6_16

munication of the flap's condition to the surgeon. Smartphone photography has emerged as a popular tool for communicating flap status and alerting surgeons, with a reported accuracy rate of approximately 94% [2]. However, comparing flap colors over time can be difficult because of differences in lighting conditions, locations, and the time at which photos are taken.

◆ Smartphone photography can be a valuable tool for communicating flap status, provided that residents or nurses can take consistent and reliable photos. Therefore, establishing institutional standards for camera settings, lighting, distance to an object, and other relevant factors is important.

The simplest way to evaluate flap viability is to assess its color, swelling, temperature, and capillary refill.

Color, swelling, temperature, and capillary refill

◆ ***Healthy flap:*** appears pink, has minimal swelling, and is warm. Capillary refill is the time taken for blood to reach a compressed area, which typically takes 2–3 s.

◆ ***Congested flap:*** appears blue and swollen, with a capillary refill <2 s (Fig. 16.1a).

◆ ***Ischemic flap:*** appears pale, cold to touch, and has a capillary refill >3 s (Fig. 16.1b).

The pinprick test involves pricking the flap with a needle (25–30 gauge) and watching for bleeding. This test is particularly useful when evaluations based on color, temperature, and capillary refill are inconclusive. The test should be performed at a distance from the vessels to prevent unintentional vessel injury.

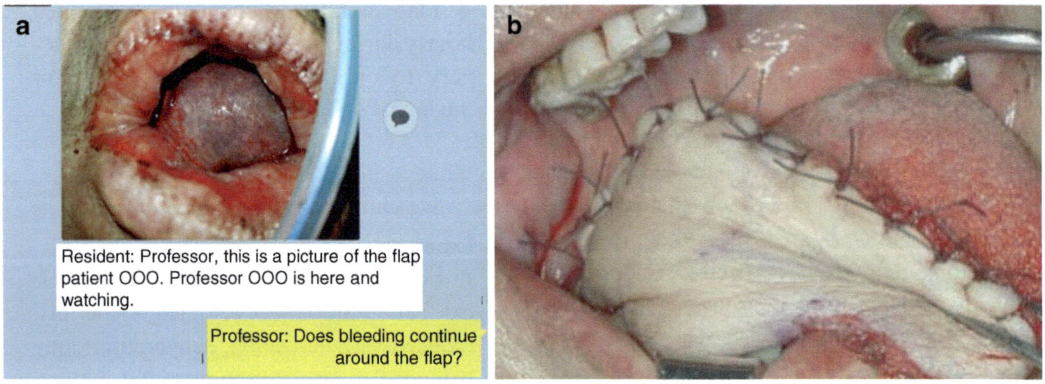

Fig. 16.1 Flap color. (**a**) The left panel shows a blue and swollen flap caused by venous congestion in a reconstructed tongue cancer patient. Residents photographed the flap and used an online communication channel to share its status and related information with surgeons. (**b**) The right panel shows a pale flap caused by arterial insufficiency, resulting in an ischemic flap in another patient with tongue reconstruction due to cancer

Pinprick test

◆ ***Healthy flap***: A bright red bleed appears a few seconds after the flap is pricked with the needle (Video 16.1; pinprick test in a healthy flap).

◆ ***Congested flap:*** A dark or black bleed appears immediately after the flap is pricked with the needle.

◆ ***Ischemic flaps***: Little or no blood flow out after the flap is pricked with the needle.

Expert Opinion

When a large flap is sutured into a narrow space, a temporary congestion might occur with dark bleeding in the pinprick test. (Man-Ki Chung)

Handheld Doppler (Video 16.2; Arterial sound in handheld Doppler) is commonly used as a supplementary method to conventional flap monitoring. However, no studies have evaluated this as a standalone technique [3].

Handheld Doppler

The Doppler signal may not always be distinguishable in all flaps, and even if detected, it can be difficult to differentiate it from the surrounding vessels. Therefore, using Doppler in conjunction with conventional flap monitoring methods is recommended for a more accurate diagnosis.

Implantable Doppler is a monitoring technique that involves attaching a 20-MHz ultrasound probe to the venous pedicle, which is connected to an external monitor using an electrode. However, false-positive rates of 5–20% have been reported. A study comparing the salvage rates of implantable Doppler and conventional methods reported salvage rates of 81% and 60%, respectively [4]. Near-infrared spectroscopy (NIRS) is a noninvasive technique that uses an externally secured probe to deliver near-infrared light to tissues. It measures hemoglobin and oxygen content through selective light absorption by hemoglobin. According to a systematic review, the false-positive rate for NIRS was 0%. Furthermore, compared to conventional monitoring, the salvage rates for free flaps monitored with NIRS were 85% and 48%, respectively [5]. NIRS does not require active monitoring by personnel, as alarms are set for specific concentrations of oxygenated and deoxygenated hemoglobin, as well as tissue oxygen saturation. However, NIRS can only be used for flaps that are not buried at depths >20 mm.

16.2 KQ 16.2. What Are the Strategies for Managing a Compromised Free Flap?

Jun-Ook Park

◆ **Algorithm for the management of a compromised free flap**

An algorithm for the management of a compromised free flap is shown in Fig. 16.2 [6].

(1) Conduct flap monitoring using conventional methods (color, temperature, capillary refill, and pinprick test) in combination with a handheld Doppler. *(Refer to KQ 16.1 for more information).*
(2) Perform immediate re-exploration in the presence of any indications of flap compromise during monitoring to confirm the presence of a thrombus within the pedicle.
(3) In the absence of evidence of pedicle thrombosis, assess other potential causes of compromised blood flow, such as kinking of the pedicle (Video 16.3; compromised blood flow due to kinking of the pedicle), compression from a hematoma or other sources, or tension. If a specific cause is identified, appropriate measures should be taken to address it and restore blood flow.

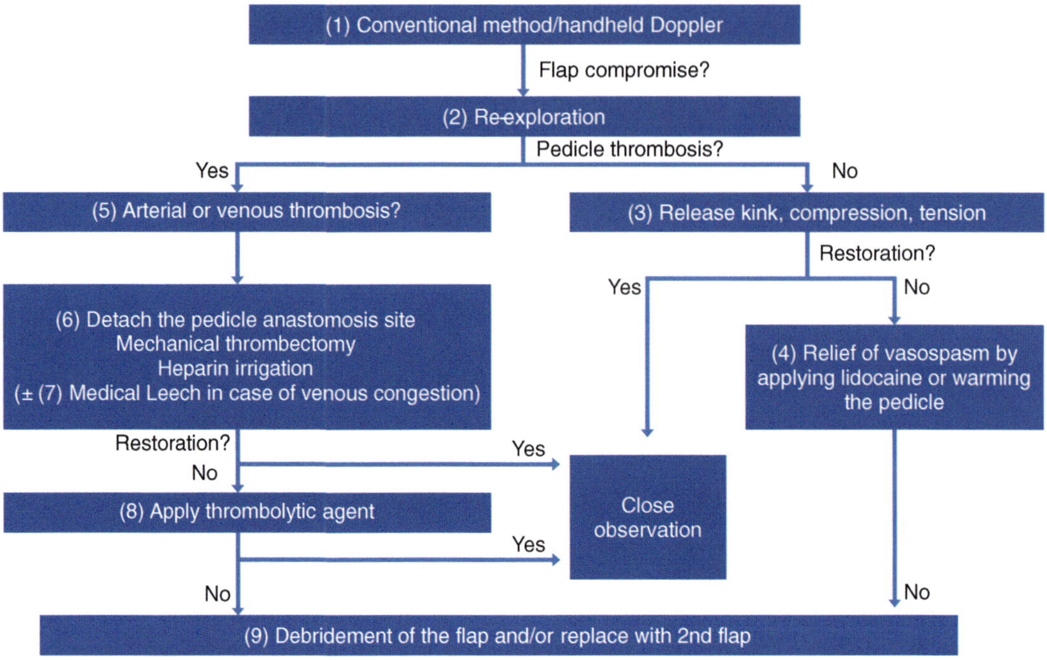

Fig. 16.2 Algorithm for management of compromised free flap

(4) If blood flow does not improve despite correction of potential causes, warming the pedicle using warm saline irrigation or warm saline-soaked gauze can help relieve vasospasm. Lidocaine can also be applied to affected areas to aid vasodilation.

(5) If evidence of thrombosis is found within the pedicle, determine whether arterial or venous thrombosis is involved.

(6) If thrombosis is confirmed, the anastomosis site of the affected pedicle must be detached, and mechanical thrombectomy using Jeweler forceps should be performed to remove the thrombus. Next, heparin irrigation should ensure adequate anticoagulation within the vessel (Fig. 16.3).

(7) Medical leeches can treat venous congestion intraoperatively or postoperatively. *Hirudo medicinalis*, a commonly used medical leech, secretes anticoagulant and antiplatelet substances. The leech has a large posterior sucker for attachment and crawling and a small mobile head containing three jaws in a triradiate configuration that must be directed to the desired site (Fig. 16.4). Before using medical leeches, the following preparation is necessary:

① Perform complete blood count and coagulation studies.

② Block the oropharynx to prevent the leech from migrating to the distal aerodigestive tract.

③ Place one leech per 3 cm^2 and prick the flap skin with a 20-gauge needle to position the leech at the desired feeding site.

④ Change to a new leech every 2 h and discontinue when sufficient restoration of flap color has been achieved. Antibiotics should be administered 24 h after use, and the detached leech should be immersed in 70% ethanol.

⑤ Irrigate with normal saline or other solutions after leech detachment and blood clot removal.

Medical leech use is contraindicated in patients who are immunocompromised,

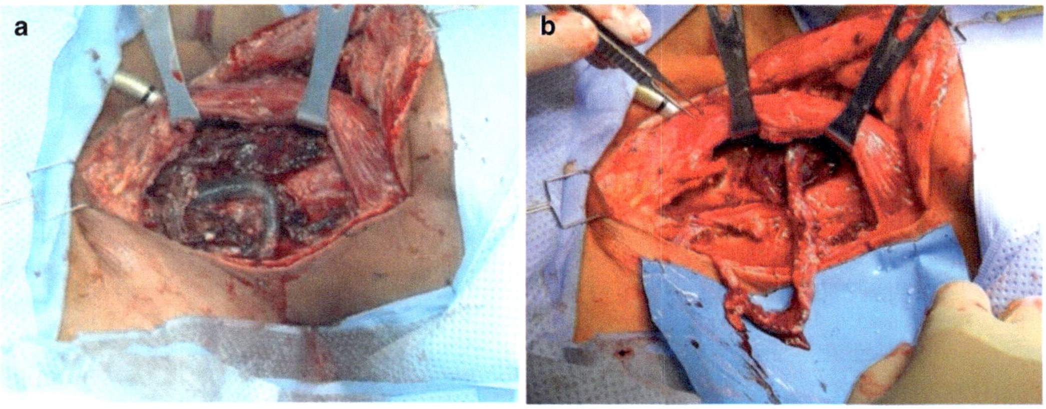

Fig. 16.3 Venous congestion. (**a**) The left panel shows a thrombus occupying the pedicle, causing venous congestion. (**b**) The right panel shows successful drainage of venous blood through the venous pedicle following thrombectomy and heparin irrigation

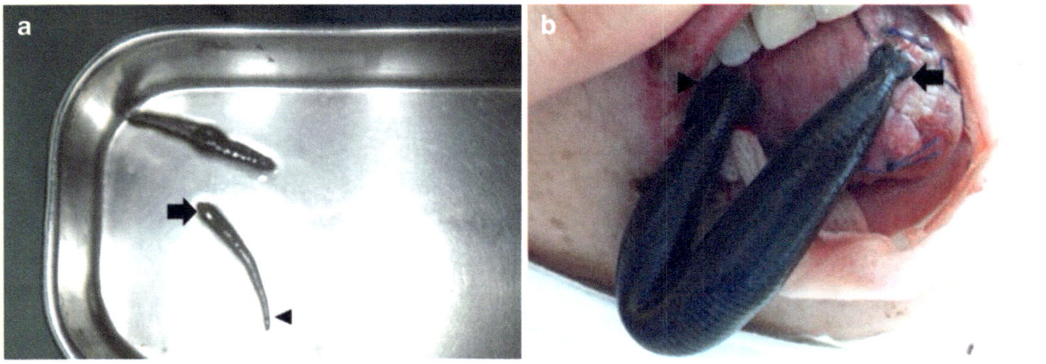

Fig. 16.4 (**a**) The left panel displays the preparation of a medical leech, (**b**) whereas the right panel shows the application of a medical leech in the oral cavity to salvage the failing flap. The head of the leech is indicated by the arrowhead, and the posterior sucker is represented by the arrow

refuse blood transfusions or leech therapy, have arterial insufficiency, are at risk of anaphylaxis, or have mental health issues.

(8) If reperfusion is not achieved after thrombectomy and heparin irrigation, thrombolytic agents such as urokinase can be administered [7]. A continuous infusion of urokinase (100,000–200,000 IU) mixed with normal saline (10–20 mL) can be administered into the arterial pedicle through a butterfly needle while maintaining external venous drainage via a detached venous anastomosis site to prevent systemic circulation (Fig. 16.5). Although higher doses of urokinase can be more effective, exceeding 500,000 IU per

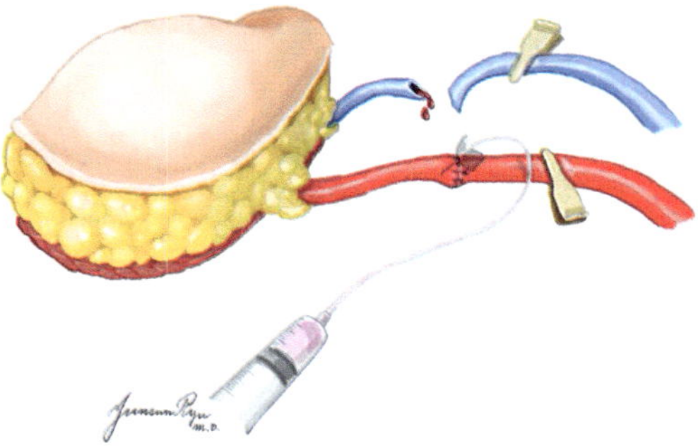

Fig. 16.5 Administration of a continuous infusion of urokinase mixed with normal saline into the arterial pedicle through a butterfly needle while maintaining external venous drainage via a detached venous anastomosis site to prevent systemic circulation

day can increase the risk of systemic side effects, such as intracranial hemorrhage and hematochezia. Thrombolysis can be observed, leading to bleeding or fluid mixed with urokinase at the flap margin, followed by transparent fluid drainage through the venous pedicle. Urokinase infusion is stopped once venous drainage is observed at a sufficient rate and has continued for 15 min.

(9) If reperfusion is unsuccessful despite all of these procedures, flap debridement or replacement with a second flap may be necessary.

Expert Opinion

Local mucosal flaps, such as the facial artery musculo-mucosal flap, tends to have a temporary congestion for several days before stabilization of venous drainage. During that critical period, medical leeches can help to relieve severe venous congestion. (Man-Ki Chung)

References

1. Chae MP, Rozen WM, Whitaker IS, Chubb D, Grinsell D, Ashton MW, et al. Current evidence for postoperative monitoring of microvascular free flaps: a systematic review. Ann Plast Surg. 2015;74(5):621–32.
2. Engel H, Huang JJ, Tsao CK, Lin CY, Chou PY, Brey EM, et al. Remote real-time monitoring of free flaps via smartphone photography and 3G wireless Internet: a prospective study evidencing diagnostic accuracy. Microsurgery. 2011;31(8):589–95.
3. Moubayed SP, Mourad M, Urken ML. What are the optimal monitoring techniques in head and neck microvascular reconstruction? ORL J Otorhinolaryngol Relat Spec. 2016;78(5):241–4.
4. Poder TG, Fortier PH. Implantable Doppler in monitoring free flaps: a cost-effectiveness analysis based on a systematic review of the literature. Eur Ann Otorhinolaryngol Head Neck Dis. 2013;130(2):79–85.
5. Chen Y, Shen Z, Shao Z, Yu P, Wu J. Free flap monitoring using near-infrared spectroscopy: a systemic review. Ann Plast Surg. 2016;76(5):590–7.
6. Chang EI, Hanasono MM, Butler CE. Management of unfavorable outcomes in head and neck free flap reconstruction: experience-based lessons from the MD Anderson Cancer Center. Clin Plast Surg. 2016;43(4):653–67.
7. Kim JH, Yoon S, Kwon H, Oh DY, Jun YJ, Moon SH. Safe and effective thrombolysis in free flap salvage: intra-arterial urokinase infusion. PLoS One. 2023;18(3):e0282908.

Vascular Issues During Flap Reconstruction

17

Eun-Jae Chung and Chung Man Ki

17.1 KQ 17.1. What Do We Do When the Length of the Vascular Pedicle Is Insufficient to Reach the Available Recipient Vessels?

Eun-Jae Chung

Free flaps have resulted in innovative changes in head and neck cancer surgery. However, this is not universally applicable. Regardless of how successfully a free flap is applied, if an artery or vein cannot be secured for anastomosis, the free flap that is difficult to perform is considered inefficient. Even if arteries and veins for anastomosis are secured with difficulty, failure to connect them to the flap pedicle, or achieving anastomosis after exceeding the ischemic time of the free flap, or if the vascular condition, despite being obtained with difficulty, is unfavorable and results in flap failure, it can impose a significant burden not only on the patient but also on the medical team.

Therefore, for successful free flap surgery, planning for the optimal flap that can achieve the required functional and aesthetic goals at the recipient site, as well as strategizing on securing the optimal artery and vein at the recipient site and ensuring smooth alignment of the flap pedicle with the secured artery and vein, is essential [2]. Meticulous planning from the preoperative stage is highly important for maximizing the success rate of free-flap surgeries.

Securing the appropriate vasculature at the recipient site is important when performing salvage surgery in areas that have previously undergone surgery and radiation therapy due to tumor recurrence [3]. This is also crucial in surgeries for midface lesions, such as sinonasal malignancies, which in most cases require a long pedicle.

This chapter focuses on describing the author's approach to conducting the surgery successfully when vasculature at the recipient site is inadequate during free-flap procedures.

Supplementary Information The online version contains supplementary material available at https://doi.org/10.1007/978-981-96-1860-6_17.

E.-J. Chung (✉)
Department of Otorhinolaryngology–Head and Neck Surgery, Seoul National University Hospital, Seoul National University College of Medicine, Seoul, Republic of Korea
e-mail: voicechung@snu.ac.kr

C. Man Ki (✉)
Department of Otorhinolaryngology—Head and Neck Surgery, School of Medicine, Samsung Medical Center, Sungkyunkwan University, Seoul, Republic of Korea

K.-J. Cho, J.-O. Park (eds.), *Management of Head and Neck Surgery Complications*,
https://doi.org/10.1007/978-981-96-1860-6_17

◆ Securing the appropriate vasculature at the recipient site is important when performing salvage surgery in areas previously treated with surgery and radiation therapy due to tumor recurrence. This is equally vital in surgeries for midface lesions, such as sinonasal malignancy, where a long pedicle is often required.

17.1.1 Preoperative Considerations

Encountering a complex situation during surgery without careful preparation increases the risk of free-flap failure due to incorrect judgment or surgical techniques. Therefore, meticulous preparation is required, involving image simulation prior to surgery. This includes selecting the appropriate flap, planning its insertion, positioning the pedicle in the right direction, and preparing the recipient vessel for anastomosis. In the case of salvage surgery, particularly for in-field recurrence following a previous surgery, a careful review of past surgical records and enhanced computed tomography scans is essential.

Furthermore, in cases where securing suitable vessels in salvage surgery patients is highly likely to be challenging, the patient's age, overall health, tumor stage, and life expectancy should be considered when planning the surgery. In such situations, it may be necessary to establish a surgical plan using a pedicled flap instead of a free flap [5]. Additionally, during surgical preparation, the possibility of using a pedicled flap must be considered, and this information should be communicated to the patient and their caregivers.

While various clinical scenarios may arise in salvage surgeries, particularly those involving bone reconstruction or reconstruction of the palate, sinonasal area, or other midface sections, the pedicle may be insufficient to facilitate direct anastomosis to the recipient vessel in some cases [6]. Therefore, it is imperative to recognize that in cases where the pedicle cannot reach the recipient vessel, vein grafting may be necessary, emphasizing the importance of thorough preparation for various scenarios. In the author's practice, when such situations are anticipated, the author also prepares the saved forearm for potential vein grafting, enabling immediate use of the cephalic vein.

Pedicle length varies depending on the type of free flap used. For example, in the case of a radial forearm free flap, the pedicle can be secured for a prolonged time when it is obtained proximal to the point where the cephalic vein and vena comitantes merge. Similarly, in the case of a latissimus dorsi free flap, a substantial additional length can be obtained by harvesting a large amount of muscle, making it useful in vessel-depleted neck conditions.

◆ It is necessary to prepare meticulously by conducting thorough image simulations before surgery. This includes selecting the appropriate flap, planning its insertion, positioning the pedicle in the right direction, and preparing the recipient vessel for anastomosis.

◆ It is imperative to be aware that in cases where the pedicle cannot reach the recipient vessel, a vein graft may be necessary.

17.1.2 Intraoperative Considerations

17.1.2.1 Arterial Considerations

Regarding arteries, the author prefers to use branches of the external carotid artery that were not utilized or areas that were not dissected in previous surgeries. The author secures the lingual artery, which is not commonly used in the initial surgery. Alternatively, in the case of the facial artery, the digastric muscle is incised and the facial artery is secured up to its origin from the stump of the external carotid artery. If securing the facial, lingual, and superior thyroid arteries proves challenging, we may also consider using the transverse cervical artery or, when necessary, the internal mammary artery. The author prefers to trace the external artery further distally to the lingual artery, ligating it more distally, and separating it below the hypoglossal nerve.

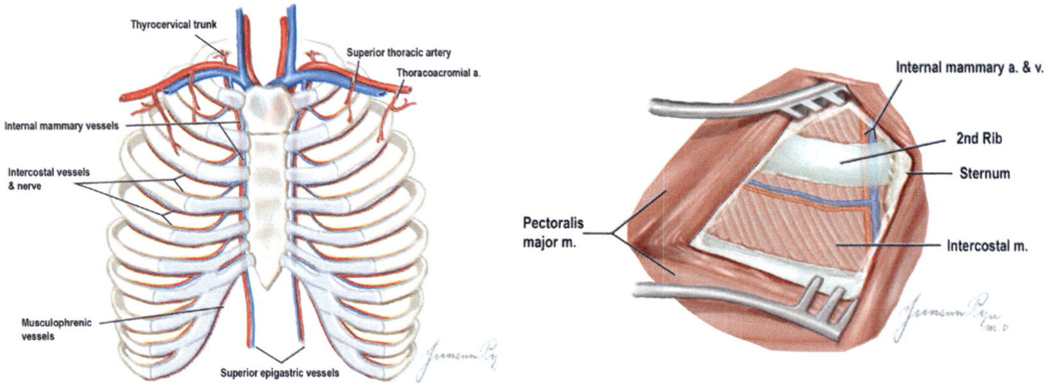

Fig. 17.1 Surgical anatomy of the internal mammary vessels for the vessel-depleted neck. a, artery; v, vein; m, muscle

Subsequently, we can perform anastomosis at the branch origin from the external carotid artery in the mid-neck, analogous to the process in the end-to-side anastomosis technique (Video 17.1).

The internal mammary artery is secured by partially removing the second rib from the medial side (Fig. 17.1) [1]. After opening the pectoralis major muscle on the chest and confirming the second rib, a portion of the rib is removed from the medial side. Subsequently, the perichondrium at the base should be opened to access the internal mammary artery and vein, which runs vertically.

Expert Opinion
The author notes that it is not necessary to remove the 2nd rib to use the internal mammary artery; it can be passed below the 2nd rib, which provides sufficient length. This approach is particularly useful in radial forearm free flaps with a long vascular pedicle. (Min-Sik Kim)

If anastomosis with the pedicle remains impossible using these methods, vein graft interposition should be performed [4]. Vein grafts are typically created using the external jugular or cephalic veins. In cases where vein grafting also needs to be performed for the arteries, the likelihood that interpositional vein grafts will be required for vein anastomosis is great. Therefore, ischemic time will inevitably be prolonged in such situations.

Expert Opinion
As a last option, an end-to-side anastomosis to the internal carotid artery (ICA) can be used with a caution of preserving and not damaging the intima of the ICA. (Man Ki Chung)

Expert Opinion
Our preference for arterial anastomoses is the saphenous vein, because it is thicker and often multiple vein grafts are required (for both the artery and vein) in such cases. (Gia Gill and Antoine Eskander)

Expert Opinion
The author states that in most cases, when the flap is placed in the appropriate position, an end-to-side anastomosis to the internal jugular vein is easier and more effective than an end-to-end anastomosis as an interposition graft. (Min-Sik Kim)

17.1.2.2 Venous Considerations

The possibility that veins may not be available for salvage surgery must be considered. The threshold for the interposition graft of the vein is lower than that of the artery. The author prefers to obtain a long cephalic vein graft and perform end-to-side anastomosis as an interpositional graft to the internal jugular vein (Video 17.2) if an appropriate vein is unavailable. A critical concern is ensuring optimal arterial coverage, even after providing an interposition graft for a vein.

Expert Opinion

In cases where the pedicle cannot reach the recipient vessel, the vein for graft in the same field of neck dissection, such as the facial vein or external jugular vein, can be used. (Min-Sik Kim)

◆ Regarding arteries, the author prefers to use branches of the external carotid artery, which were unutilized or areas not dissected in previous surgeries.

◆ In cases where securing the facial, lingual, and superior thyroid arteries proves challenging, we may also consider using the transverse cervical artery or, when necessary, the internal mammary artery. The author performs anastomosis at the origin of the external carotid artery branches, employing an approach similar to the end-to-side anastomosis technique.

17.2 KQ 17.2. How to Handle Mismatched Donor and Recipient Arteries?

Eun-Jae Chung

The donor artery of the free flap and the main branches of the external carotid artery on the recipient side, such as the facial and superior thyroid arteries, typically exhibit similar sizes, facilitating surgery without major complications [7]. However, as described in the previous chapter, limitations may arise regarding the availability of arteries and veins in salvage surgery cases, particularly among patients who have previously undergone free-flap surgery.

Expert Opinion

Identifying and preparing recipient vessels for anastomosis before raising the free flap, measuring the donor vessel length from the defect site, and securing side branches during flap elevation are essential steps for managing potential vessel mismatches. (Chung-Hwan Baek)

In the case of a discrepancy in the donor and recipient vessel sizes, the primary approach is to predict the mismatch while minimizing the potential discrepancy [8]. In particular, significant arterial size mismatch can lead directly to graft failure. Therefore, proper preparation to ensure appropriate blood vessel and pedicle geometry through simulation before surgery is important [9]. In some cases, modifying the plan from free flap to pedicle flap may be advisable. For veins, the author prefers end-to-side anastomosis to the internal jugular vein. If deemed necessary, the author prefers vein grafting to ensure successful end-to-side anastomosis to the internal jugular vein.

Various techniques are used to resolve discrepancies in vessel diameter. In the case of veins, anastomosis is possible even if the difference is large. However, anastomosis is still feasible with a diameter mismatch of approximately 2:1 for arteries. The basic approach to compensate for this mismatch is to dilate the vessel gently using a dilator. Endothelial damage is critical for the arteries, and thus, it is crucial to perform it as gently as possible.

Expert Opinion
Over-preparing and over-dilating arteries before anastomosis should be avoided to prevent delayed pseudoaneurysm and vessel rupture; necessary dilation should be done carefully. (Gia Gill and Antoine Eskander)

In the case of veins, dilating the lumen with a dilator often helps to overcome a significant portion of the mismatch [11]. In case of a size mismatch, cutting the smaller vessel obliquely and using double clamps on both sides can be helpful to overcome the mismatch (Fig. 17.2).

Expert Opinion
When using a vein coupler, the sufficient size should be selected to avoid a bottleneck of venous flow. (Chung-Hwan Baek)

In case of a mismatch in the vessel diameter, it is important to consider the direction of blood flow, particularly in arteries. When blood flows from a smaller-diameter vessel to a larger one (i.e., where the recipient vessel is smaller and the donor vessel is larger), the risk of thrombus formation decreases. Conversely, in the reverse scenario (where the recipient vessel is larger and the donor vessel is smaller), turbulence in the flow can occur, thereby also increasing the risk of thrombus formation.

Expert Opinion
Before venous anastomosis, the donor vein's return flow should be checked. If venous return is inadequate, the arterial anastomosis site should be reviewed. Venous anastomosis should connect the tributary to the main vein, using a recipient vein of sufficient size and proper positioning to prevent congestion. (Chung-Hwan Baek)

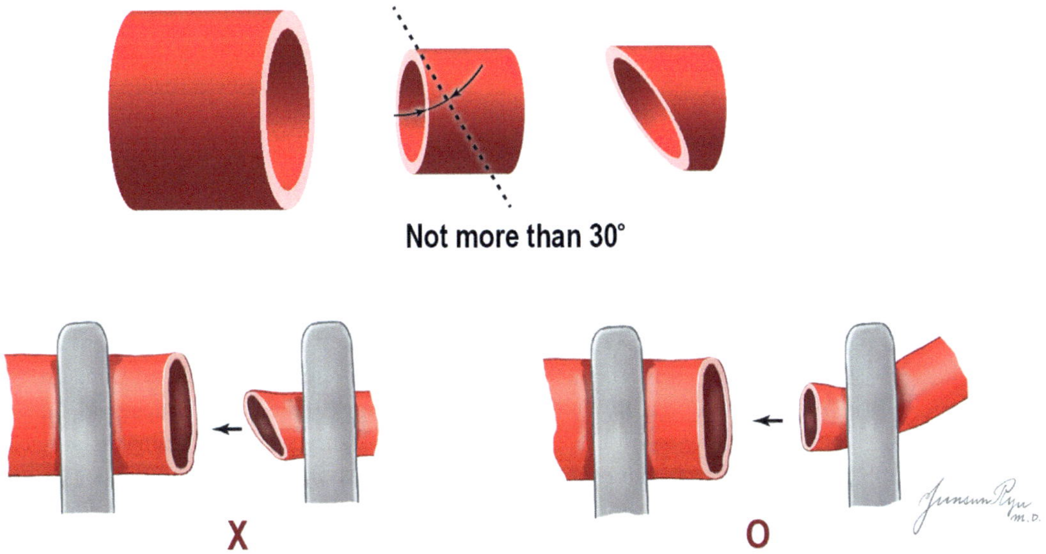

Fig. 17.2 Basic technique to compensate for the mismatch discrepancies in vessel diameter. Cutting the smaller vessel obliquely can be helpful to overcome mismatch

When resolving vessel size mismatching proves difficult or inappropriate with the use of standard methods, an end-to-side anastomosis approach is employed. Use of end-to-side anastomosis on the internal jugular vein, or alternatively, on vessels such as the external jugular or facial vein, is considered an option for veins [10]. For arteries, the author prefers to perform anastomosis to the origin of the external carotid artery branches, similar to the end-to-side approach (Video 17.3).

Expert Opinion

When the thickness of the donor and recipient vessel walls differ, the thicker vessel should be pierced radially with a needle to ensure proper alignment with the thinner vessel, and the suture intervals should be wider for the thicker vessel than for the thinner one. (Young Hoon Joo)

When an interposition vein graft is necessary, even for an artery, vein graft interposition is almost always required. Therefore, anticipating and preparing for such situations is essential to avoid panic and confusion when they suddenly occur.

◆ An anastomosis can be feasible with a diameter mismatch of approximately 2:1 for arteries.

◆ The basic approach to compensate for the mismatch is to dilate the vessel gently using a dilator. Endothelial damage would be critical for arteries, and thus it is crucial to perform the procedure as gently as possible.

◆ If the recipient vessel is larger and the donor vessel is smaller, turbulence in the flow can occur, thereby increasing the risk of thrombus formation.

◆ When resolving vessel size mismatching proves difficult or inappropriate with conventional methods, an end-to-side anastomosis approach is employed.

17.3 KQ 17.3. What Should Be Done When the Recipient Artery Has an Unhealthy Intima or an Atherosclerotic Plaque?

Chung Man Ki

In microvascular surgery, the selection of an appropriate recipient artery is crucial for the success of free-flap reconstructive surgery. The most common cause of microvascular anastomotic failure is vein-related issues. However, through early detection and exploration, thrombus removal, addressing vein kinking, or external compression, the likelihood of resolution is high. Nevertheless, in cases of arterial insufficiency, the risk of flap failure remains significant, even with exploration, and it is sometimes necessary to locate and suture another healthy recipient artery as an alternative. The initial selection of an appropriate recipient artery for vascular anastomosis is paramount for achieving success in microvascular surgery [12].

◆ Arterial insufficiency is a rare cause of microvascular failure. However, when it does happen, it is more difficult to solve than a venous problem. Locating another healthy artery and anastomosing it to the donor artery are worth considering.

To determine the appropriate recipient artery, it is essential to refer to patient history and preoperative imaging studies. If a patient has undergone previous surgeries, consulting the surgical records is necessary because of potential limitations, such as the availability of vessels for selection. Furthermore, CT scans or ultrasonography can provide valuable insights into the condition of the cervical vasculature and highlight possible complications, such as atherosclerosis.

The criteria for an ideal recipient artery include minimal size mismatch compared to the donor-side artery and an appropriate distance between the recipient and donor vessels to allow tension-free anastomosis [13]. The recipient artery must also exhibit expansile pulsation visible under a microscope. During arterial sectioning and observation, high-pressure spurting of arterial flow must be monitored, and the absence of atherosclerotic plaques or an unhealthy intimal flap is paramount for success. A cross-sectional incision or small puncture of the sidewall of the artery is required to assess the presence of plaque or an unhealthy intimal flap within the vessel. This was followed by continuous irrigation with a heparinized saline solution to prevent vessel wall collapse. Continuous irrigation with 2% lidocaine also helps prevent arterial spasms.

◆ The appropriate recipient artery needs to show visible expansile pulsation with spurting blood flow from a transected lumen. Also, size mismatch and distance between the vessels must also be considered.

The most problematic condition is the presence of an atherosclerotic plaque or an unhealthy intimal layer in the recipient artery. Atherosclerotic plaques or unhealthy intimal flaps can induce turbulence in blood flow or serve as intrinsic coagulation factors, thereby increasing the risk of thrombosis. These conditions increase the probability of flap failure by disrupting blood flow dynamics and increasing the propensity for thrombotic events.

The possible strategies for different situations are depicted in Fig. 17.3.

Situation 1: Proximal exploration

If a significant plaque or an unhealthy intimal flap is identified within the recipient vessel, it is advisable to select a different recipient vessel, preferably one that is plaque-free and has a clean intimal surface. At a location near the initially chosen recipient artery, gradual and cautious removal of the plaque or unhealthy intimal flap should be performed, progressing towards the proximal area until a clean area is achieved. This study aimed to uncover a clean, plaque-free area with healthy intima to ensure a suitable recipient site for subsequent anastomosis. When a more ideal recipient artery (plaque-free with a healthy intimal flap) is located and secured by proximal exploration, anastomosis with the donor artery can be performed.

◆ Proximal dissection of the recipient artery is required to locate and ensure a clean area without plaques or an unhealthy intimal flap.

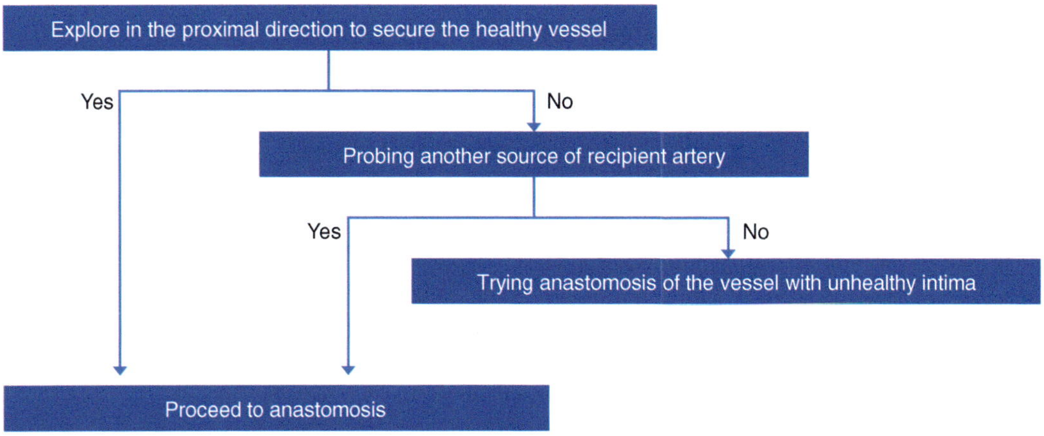

Fig. 17.3 Algorithm for addressing unhealthy intima or atherosclerotic plaque in the recipient artery during surgical procedures

Situation 2: Probing for another recipient artery

Commonly used recipient arteries in the cervical region include the facial and superior thyroidal arteries. However, in cases where their use is precluded by the presence of a plaque or an unhealthy intimal flap, alternative external carotid artery branches, such as the transverse cervical artery or superficial temporal artery, should be considered. If employing an external carotid artery branch is challenging, using the external carotid artery as a recipient vessel is a viable option.

Expert Opinion
Surgeons may perform a longitudinal cut to remove plaques and secure a clear anastomotic margin. In severe cases, especially with recipient arteries, it may be necessary to cut to the external carotid artery or use it for anastomosis. Gentle techniques are recommended to avoid intimal separation, and vein grafts can be helpful for atraumatic anastomosis. (Chung-Hwan Baek)

In this scenario, owing to the potential size mismatch between the donor and external carotid arteries, achieving end-to-end anastomosis could be challenging. Therefore, an end-to-side anastomosis, created in a similar way to a vein anastomosis, may be a suitable method. Using tools such as bulldog vascular clamps, the blood flow within the external carotid artery was temporarily halted, followed by the creation of an appropriately sized hole on the vessel sidewall. During this process, careful inspection of the hole is imperative to ensure the absence of plaque or an unhealthy intimal flap, both above and below the external carotid artery.

When performing end-to-side artery anastomosis, it is crucial to account for the stiffer and less flexible nature of arterial vessel walls compared to veins. Hence, the selection of an appropriate suture size is of paramount importance. In addition, excessive tension during suturing may cause bleeding around the bite site. Meticulous adjustment of the length and pressure of the sutures on both sides of the vessel walls is paramount for successful hemostasis.

◆ When branches of the external carotid artery are not suitable, an end-to-side anastomosis with the external carotid artery can be an alternative option. Care must be taken not to apply excessive pressure during suturing.

Situation 3: Anastomosis of the vessel with a plaque or unhealthy intimal flap

If a plaque is present but is not expected to pose an issue during vascular suturing, a cautious attempt at suturing can be considered. During this process, the selection of appropriately sized clamps is crucial for preventing excessive tension, which may lead to plaque fractures or damage to the inner vessel walls. Typically, a dilator is used to expand the vessel lumen prior to arterial suturing. However, in the presence of plaques or an unhealthy intimal flap, it is advisable to abstain from this step to avoid further damage to the vessel wall.

To minimize vessel wall damage during suturing, a round needle and the smallest available suture size should be used [14]. Interrupted sutures were preferred over continuous sutures. Interrupted sutures allow precise suturing with a comprehensive assessment of the internal condition of the vessel after each suture placement, offering advantages in terms of accuracy and opportunities for detailed inspection. Moreover, as the needle passes through the vessel wall, moving it from the inner to the outer side while preventing plaque dislodgement or additional intimal flap damage is recommended.

Expert Opinion
In cases of severe diabetes, where vessels are very fragile and prone to tearing, the techniques mentioned above—using double needles for gentle intraluminal-to-extraluminal suturing with minimal force—can also be highly beneficial. (Min-Sik Kim)

Expert Opinion
Using a strong clamp can cause atherosclerotic plaques to rupture by impacting the vessel wall, so an appropriate clamp must be applied. (Young Hoon Joo)

In cases where both the recipient and donor vessels exhibit plaques or an unhealthy intimal flap, the use of double needles for simultaneous intraluminal-to-extraluminal suturing can be highly beneficial [15]. Furthermore, excessive pressure on the sutures should be avoided. Gentle suturing with minimal force is essential to prevent tearing of the fragile vessel wall, plaque breakage, or an unhealthy intimal flap within the vessel lumen.

Expert Opinion
Dilation of calcified vessels can cause cracks in the intima, either circumferentially or partially. If there is enough vessel length, trimming can be attempted, but intimal calcification often persists. In such cases, after anastomosis, a small muscle patch may be used to manage leaks. (Gia Gill and Antoine Eskander)

◆ In case of a minimal plaque or minimal damage to the intimal flap within a recipient artery, meticulous anastomosis can be performed. The key is to minimize vessel wall damage during suturing.

17.4 KQ 17.4. What Should Be Done When Anterolateral Thigh Perforators Are Small, Absent, or Injured?

Chung Man Ki

The anterolateral thigh (ALT) flap receives blood from the septocutaneous or musculocutaneous perforator arteries originating from the descending branch of the lateral circumflex femoral artery (LCFA). According to previous studies, over 80% of cases are of the musculocutaneous type, whereas approximately 20% are of the septocutaneous type. Additionally, there are rare instances in which perforators arise from the transverse branch rather than from the descending branch of the LCFA [12, 16].

Anatomically, the descending branch of the LCFA descends along the intermuscular septum between the rectus femoris and vastus lateralis muscles. The perforators from the descending branch exit at a midpoint approximately within a circle of 3 cm radius along a line connecting the anterior superior iliac spine and the superior lateral border of the patella. In some cases, the descending branch of the LCFA bifurcates into the medial and lateral subbranches upon exiting (Video 17.4).

Septocutaneous perforators emerge through the fascia between the rectus femoris and vastus lateralis muscles to supply the skin. In contrast, musculocutaneous perforators traverse the vastus lateralis muscle, giving rise to multiple intermuscular branches before exiting the skin.

The success of detecting suitable perforators in anterolateral thigh (ALT) free flap raising depends on various factors, including the surgeon's experience, patient anatomy, and imaging techniques used. Although ALT flaps are generally considered reliable and versatile, there is always the possibility of unsuitable perforators not being detected during preoperative planning or intraoperative exploration. In approximately 2% of cases, no skin-supplying perforators exist or are too small in diameter to be suitable for supplying the surgical flap.

Thorough preoperative assessment and planning are essential. Imaging techniques such as Doppler ultrasound, CT angiography, and magnetic resonance angiography have been used to identify perforators, including their size, location, and course. This can help predict potential complications and facilitate the planning of an appropriate surgical approach.

Although a lack of suitable perforators is a possibility, this is not frequent. This risk is further reduced when the procedures are performed by experienced surgical teams. Surgeons often use a range of strategies and backup plans to handle unexpected situations and ensure the best possible outcomes for patients. Several strategies can be considered when managing small, absent, or injured perforators using ALT-free flaps.

These steps are shown in Fig. 17.4.

17.4.1 Strategy 1

Exploring adjacent perforators: If the primary perforator is small, absent, or injured, nearby perforators within the same anatomical zone should be explored. The anterolateral thigh region typically contains multiple perforators that can be used as alternatives [17]. It is feasible to reliably identify perforators throughout the thigh region and is not limited to the vastus lateralis muscle. A freestyle perforator flap can be designed according to the location of the perforators. When perforators in the lateral thigh are weak and sparse, those in the anteromedial or median thigh regions are relatively healthy and reliable. The identification and utilization of a healthy adjacent perforator can salvage the flap. Preoperative CT angiography of the lower extremities and the use of an intraoperative handheld Doppler probe can be helpful.

Expert Opinion

The handheld Doppler and pre-operative imaging are not always reliable for identifying perforator vessels in anterolateral thigh flap procedures, as they may pick up incorrect signals or fail to detect smaller perforators. Pre-operative CT has low sensitivity, so it is rarely used. (Gia Gill and Antoine Eskander)

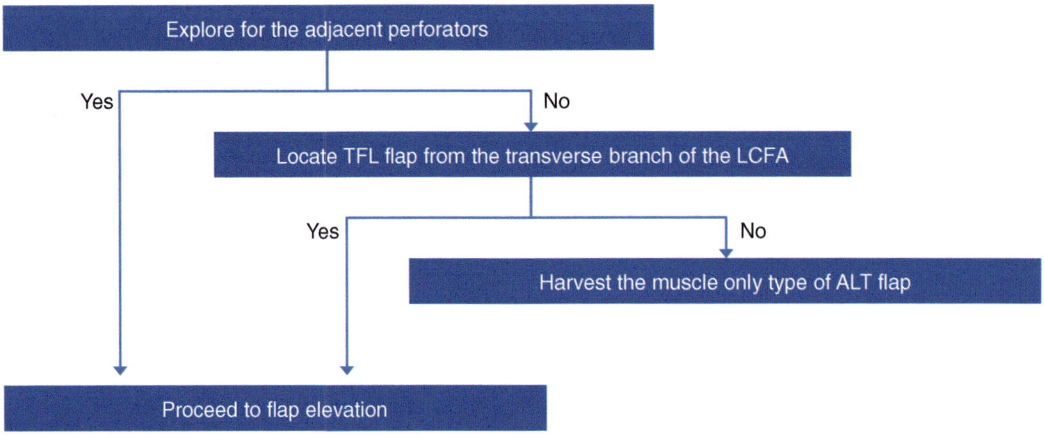

Fig. 17.4 Algorithm for managing small, absent, or injured anterolateral thigh perforators. TFL, tensor fasciae lata; LCFA, lateral circumflex femoral artery; ALT, anterolateral thigh

17.4.2 Strategy 2

If an appropriate perforator supplying the skin paddle cannot be identified around the vastus lateralis muscle, an alternative approach is to confirm the lateral circumflex femoral vessel and locate the vessel supplying the tensor fasciae latae [18]. This allows for the harvesting of the tensor fasciae latae (TFL) free flap. The TFL flap is supplied by perforators from the transverse branch of the LCFA. Thus, the pedicle may be shorter than that of the ALT free flap. The TFL flap has a reliable and consistent skin territory with minimal vascular variation. Hence, if perforators for the ALT-free flap are unreliable, the TFL-free flap could be a good alternative.

Expert Opinion

Adding fascia lata or intact vastus lateralis fascia over the muscle flap aids in epithelial regeneration and prevents myositis. However, the blood supply to the fascia lata must be checked before dividing the ALT vascular pedicle. If skin reconstruction is necessary, a skin graft from the compromised ALT flap can be applied over the muscle layer. (Chung-Hwan Baek)

17.4.3 Strategy 3

When perforators that extend to the skin are not identified under loupes or a microscope, a myocutaneous ALT free flap incorporating a part of the vastus lateralis muscle and the overlying skin can be raised. However, it can only be harvested if the blood supply to the skin is well preserved by unidentified but undamaged perforators. Sutures between the muscle and skin paddle can prevent shearing forces, thus protecting the small perforators. Myocutaneous ALT-free flaps are bulky and lack pliability. Therefore, careful trimming is necessary before flap insertion into the defect. If perforator viability is uncertain, a muscle-only ALT free flap supplied by the main branch of the LCFA is an option. Depending on the characteristics of the defect, skin grafting over the muscle surface or healing by secondary intention may be considered.

17.4.4 Strategy 4

If suitable perforators cannot be identified and a backup plan is not feasible, preparation and exploration of the contralateral thigh should also be considered. Alternatively, another reconstruction option could be chosen.

Every case is unique, and the approach depends on various factors, including the patient's condition, the extent of perforator compromise, and available resources. Careful planning and adaptability during surgery are key to successfully managing small, absent, or injured perforators during ALT free flap procedures.

References

1. Jacobson AS, Smith M, Urken ML. Internal mammary artery and vein as recipient vessels in head and neck reconstruction. JAMA Otolaryngol Head Neck Surg. 2013;139(6):623–8.
2. Kushida-Contreras BH, Manrique OJ, Gaxiola-García MA. Head and neck reconstruction of the vessel-depleted neck: a systematic review of the literature. Ann Surg Oncol. 2021;28(5):2882–95.
3. Breik O, Praveen P, Parmar S. The vessel-depleted neck in head and neck microvascular reconstruction: extreme solutions for extreme situations. Curr Opin Otolaryngol Head Neck Surg. 2020;28(2):129–35.
4. Wong KK, Higgins KM, Enepekides D. Microvascular reconstruction in the vessel-depleted neck. J Curr Opin Otolaryngol Head Neck Surg. 2010;18(4):223–6.
5. Correia C, Wang W, Vincent AG, Chan D, Ducic Y. Regional salvage flap options in head and neck reconstruction. Semin Plast Surg. 2020;34(4):293–8.
6. Dalgorf D, Higgins K. Reconstruction of the midface and maxilla. Curr Opin Otolaryngol Head Neck Surg. 2008;16(4):303–11.
7. Raja Sabapathy S. Chapter 9: Vessels. In: Wei F-C, Mardini S, editors. Flaps and reconstructive surgery. Edinburgh: Saunders; 2009. p. 80–92.
8. Rickard RF, McPhaden AR, Hudson DA. Healing of two microarterial anastomoses with diameter mismatch. J Surg Res. 2014;191(1):239–49.
9. Turker T, Tsai TM, Thirkannad S. Size discrepancy in vessels during microvascular anastomosis: two techniques to overcome this problem. Hand Surg. 2012;17(3):413–7.

10. Tsai YT, Lin TS. The suitability of end-to-side microvascular anastomosis in free flap transfer for limb reconstruction. Ann Plast Surg. 2012;68(2):171–4.
11. Suri MP, Ahmad QG, Yadav PS. Managing venous discrepancy: simple method. J Reconstr Microsurg. 2009;25(8):497–9.
12. Mardini S, Wei FC. Flaps and reconstructive surgery. New York: Elsevier; 2009.
13. MacDonald JD. Learning to perform microvascular anastomosis. Skull Base. 2005;15(3):229–40.
14. Pafitanis G, Kyprianou K, Chen HC. Microvascular anastomosis in atherosclerotic vessels: technical challenges and recommendations. J Plast Reconstr Aesthet Surg. 2021;74(7):1633–701.
15. Miyamoto S, Okazaki M, Takushima A, et al. Versatility of a posterior-wall-first anastomotic technique using a shortthread double-needle microsuture for atherosclerotic arterial anastomosis. Microsurgery. 2008;28:505–8.
16. Zaretski A, Wei FC, Lin CH, Cheng MH, Tsao CK, Wallace CG. Anterolateral thigh perforator flaps in head and neck reconstruction. Semin Plast Surg. 2006;20(2):64–72.
17. Lee SS, Hong JW, Lee WJ, Yun IS. Perforating patterns of cutaneous perforator vessels in anterolateral thigh flaps for head and neck reconstruction and clinical outcomes. Arch Craniofac Surg. 2022;23(2):64–70.
18. Akhtar MS, Khurram MF, Khan AH. Versatility of pedicled tensor fascia lata flap: a useful and reliable technique for reconstruction of different anatomical districts. Plast Surg Int. 2014;2014:846082.

18 Miscellaneous Issues

Yoo Seob Shin

18.1 KQ 18.1. What Are the Tips for Reducing Esthetic Defects of the Forearm After Radial Forearm Free Flap Harvesting?

Yoo Seob Shin

The radial forearm free flap (RFFF) is a markedly reliable flap used for various head and neck reconstructions. The RFFF has several advantages, including its thin and pliable nature, with a long, large vessel caliber, and a constant pedicle. However, obvious donor-site morbidity may be a clinical conundrum. The donor site for RFFF has obvious esthetic deformities, including excessive scarring and hyperpigmentation in conspicuous areas. In addition, failure of the skin graft can lead to exposure of the tendons underneath. Therefore, considerable effort and caution may be needed to ameliorate donor-site morbidity associated with harvesting of an RFFF.

> ◆ Flap harvesting should be performed with meticulous suprafascial dissection, preserving the paratenons.

The suprafascial dissection technique with a meshed skin graft is generally accepted as a better method than subfascial dissection for enhanced functional, cosmetic, and tendon exposure outcomes [1].

When dissecting the fibrous tissue underneath the forearm fascia, the enveloping paratenon of the forearm muscle tendons should be carefully preserved to create a favorable wound bed for subsequent skin grafting. Extensive handling and abrasive oversewing of the adjacent muscle bellies should be avoided.

Approximating the flexor carpi radialis and brachioradialis muscles might be helpful in minimizing tendon exposure because these could provide a more sufficient wound bed for skin graft survival than achieved with bare tendons [2]. Undermining and approximating the marginal skin flap toward the donor-site defect and locating the margin at the wound bed to encourage coverage of the undermined space are useful techniques. If the paratenon is inadequate for full tendon coverage, surgeons can use the adjacent flexor carpi ulnaris for complete wound bed coverage.

Y. S. Shin (✉)
Department of Otolaryngology, School of Medicine, Ajou University, Suwon, Republic of Korea
e-mail: ysshinmd@ajou.ac.kr

K.-J. Cho, J.-O. Park (eds.), *Management of Head and Neck Surgery Complications*,
https://doi.org/10.1007/978-981-96-1860-6_18

Expert Opinion
De-epithelialized radial forearm flaps offer easier suturing, but may cause more contracture, particularly when repairing mobile areas, such as the tongue. (Chung-Hwan Baek)

◆ Closure of the donor site can be achieved using various techniques.

Regarding using a meshed or sheet skin graft in cases where primary closure cannot be performed for an RFFF donor-site defect, various surgical techniques have been applied to expedite wound healing and achieve a better cosmetic outcome.

Skin Grafts
◆ ***Split-thickness skin graft***: To prevent the formation of secondary donor-site defects, one option is to consider harvesting a split-thickness skin graft (STSG) directly from the RFFF for closure of its donor site.
◆ ***Full-thickness skin graft:*** A full-thickness skin graft (FTSG) may provide a better esthetic outcome than that achieved with an STSG, although the difference might be marginal. In contrast to STSG donor sites, opting for primary closure at the secondary donor site reduces morbidity.
◆ ***Allogenic graft***: Allogenic grafts often entail a prolonged wound-healing period. However, this approach mitigates additional donor-site morbidity while yielding similar esthetic and functional outcomes.

FTSG and STSG showed the same short- and long-term outcomes in the repair of RFFF donor sites in a previous study [3]. In other investigations, FTSG showed better esthetic results in RFFF donor-site closure than did STSG, although these differences were marginal. FTSG exhibits advantages, such as better healing results, and less tendon exposure, and wound breakdown. Furthermore, secondary donor-site morbidity at the groin or abdominal wall might be reduced because the skin-harvested site can be closed primarily, whereas STSG donor sites need to heal secondarily.

AlloDerm is a structurally intact, decellularized human cadaveric dermis that can be used as a substitute for STSG or FTSG. This does not necessarily leave secondary defects for skin harvesting; however, the healing process may be prolonged, particularly in specific groups of patients.

Expert Opinion
A 12/1000-inch split-thickness graft is commonly used for faster healing, while a 14/1000-inch graft is used to reduce contracture. Full-thickness grafts require careful defatting for better uptake. (Chung-Hwan Baek)

Direct Closure or Local Flap
◆ ***Direct closure:*** Primary closure should be prioritized whenever possible, particularly for defects <2–3 cm in size.
◆ ***Local flaps:*** Several local flap techniques, including Z-plasty, V-Y plasty, and a bilobed flap could be applied based on the size of the defect and elasticity of surrounding tissue.

Primary closure of the radial forearm flap donor site is generally considered the best option but is only applicable to small or narrow wounds. In defects exceeding 2–3 cm in size, depending on the patient's tissue elasticity, primary closure cannot be achieved without additional special approaches.

Expert Opinion
In clinical practice, direct closure of donor defects is uncommon unless the defect is very small and located proximally. (Chung-Hwan Baek)

Several transpositional fasciocutaneous flap techniques have been adapted for RFFF closure. These local flap techniques avoid secondary donor-site morbidity and provide esthetically favorable wound closure [4]. The Z-plasty closure technique can be used for RFFF donor-site closure. A Z-shaped incision can generate two triangular skin paddles that are reunited after transposition, effectively elongating the forearm tissue and facilitating defect coverage. However, its application for defects exceeding 4 × 6 cm has not been reported [5].

Expert Opinion
The ulnar artery perforator-based islanded V-Y flap closure can achieve closure of defects up to 4 cm. (Min-Sik Kim)

Another plausible local flap technique for RFFF donor-site closure is a transpositional ulnar fasciocutaneous flap with a V-Y advancement technique in the proximal forearm [6]. The original donor-site defect is closed using a V-shaped flap and an ulnar artery-based fasciocutaneous flap (Fig. 18.1). This procedure may eliminate the need for a skin graft, minimize donor-site morbidity, and improve esthetic outcomes. The use of a bilobed transposition flap based on the ulnar artery has distinct advantages over other conventional approaches for donor-site closure [7]. The bilobed flap should be designed with both large and small lobes. After RFFF harvesting, the bilobed flaps should be rotated, as the large lobe is located to cover the RFFF donor defect, whereas the remaining small lobe is used to cover the large lobe defect (Fig. 18.2). This could be a feasible alternative for closing RFFF donor-site defects measuring ≤5 cm.

- Preoperative prediction of donor-site wound problems might be helpful in selecting the manner of donor-site wound closure.

Some studies have evaluated postoperative wound healing and graft failure, with particular emphasis on the impact of obesity, diabetes, peripheral vascular disease, cardiac problems, and smoking on postoperative wound healing. These clinical characteristics can be checked based on clinical history, body mass index, body

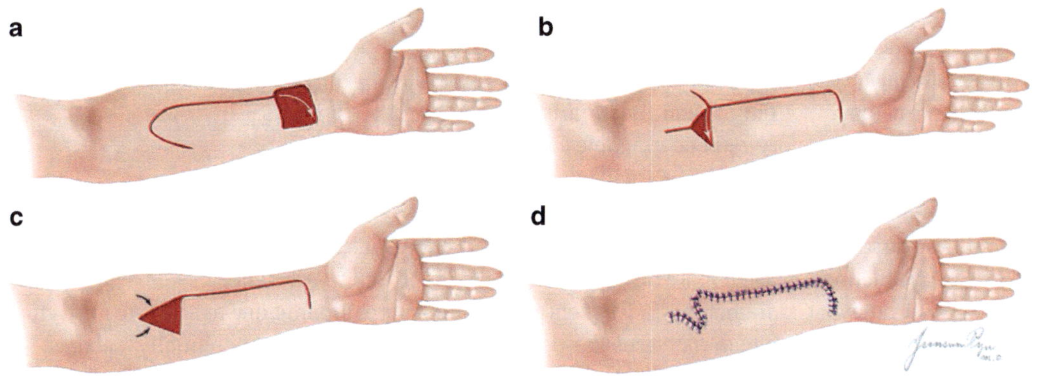

Fig. 18.1 Modified V–Y plasty. (**a**) Rotation/advancement of the ulnar-based flap. (**b**) Attempted proximal closure by V–Y advancement. (**c**) Incorporation of "Z-plasty." (**d**) Closure following transposition of flaps

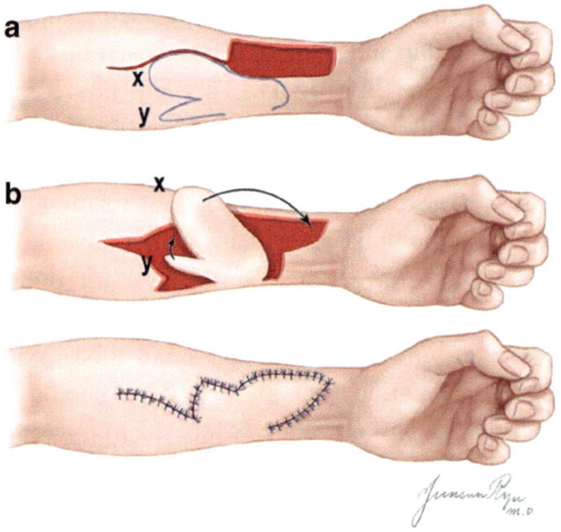

Fig. 18.2 Bilobed flap technique. (**a**) x: a large lobe for radial forearm free flap (RFFF) defect, y: a small lobe for large lobe defect. (**b**) Transposition of the flaps; the RFFF donor-site defect is covered with the large lobe, and the small lobe is for the large lobe defect

weight, or waist–hip ratio. As these unfavorable clinical factors are significantly correlated with negative esthetic outcomes, surgeons should carefully consider surgical method selection and postoperative care [8].

18.2 KQ 18.2. How to Prevent and Manage Ectropion Following Flap Reconstruction for Maxillectomy Defects

Yoo Seob Shin

The reconstruction of the lower orbital rim can provide adequate structural support to the orbital contents to maintain not only visual function but also to provide satisfactory esthetic outcomes for facial symmetry. Reconstruction of total maxillectomy defects remains one of the most challenging clinical hurdles in the head and neck region. These reconstructions are even more difficult considering that adjuvant radiotherapy is frequently required for these cases, which increases the risk of fibrosis, deterioration of function, and adverse esthetic outcomes, including diplopia, ectropion, enophthalmos, and lagophthalmos.

Preserving a Pretarsal Portion of Orbicularis Muscle

◆ To prevent ectropion, the pretarsal portion of the orbicularis muscle should be preserved for maintenance of proper lower lid tonus.

◆ Modifications of the Weber–Ferguson incision are other plausible options. Transconjunctival, midfacial degloving with a transconjunctival–retrocaruncular approach or infraorbital rim osteotomy should be considered.

Postoperative ectropion may be attributed to scar changes in the anterior lamella of the inferior eyelid. Ectropion is one of the most common deformities encountered by surgeons using the subciliary approach. Many investigations have shown that skin-only subciliary dissection might be associated with a significantly increased incidence of postoperative ectropion (42%), whereas the skin–muscle stepwise flap-dissection technique significantly ameliorates the development of both transient and permanent ectropion. A subciliary incision via stepwise dissection should be applied to preserve the muscle strip, avoiding excessive scarring of the lower eyelid, and eventually preventing loss of muscle tonus and ectropion (Fig. 18.3).

Expert Opinion

When performing a total maxillectomy, it is best to avoid subciliary incisions to prevent postoperative lower eyelid ectropion. (Chung-Hwan Baek)

Patients undergoing maxillectomy via a standard approach may be at risk of developing lower eyelid malpositioning due to scarring and lymphedema, which may be potentially enhanced by adjuvant radiotherapy. Therefore, modifications of the Weber–Ferguson approach are advisable as follows: transconjunctival instead of subciliar

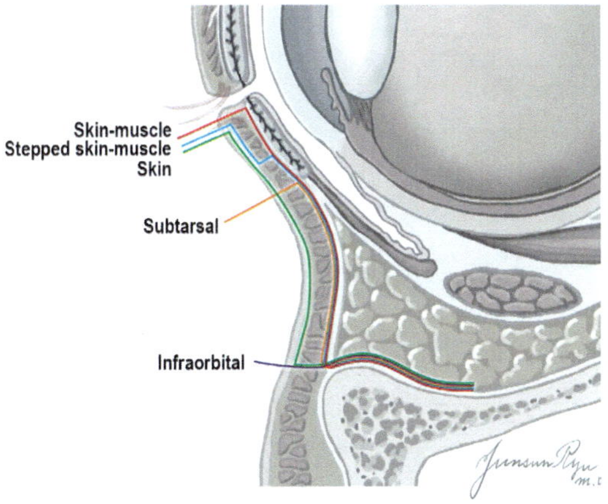

Fig. 18.3 Stepped skin-muscle subciliary incision

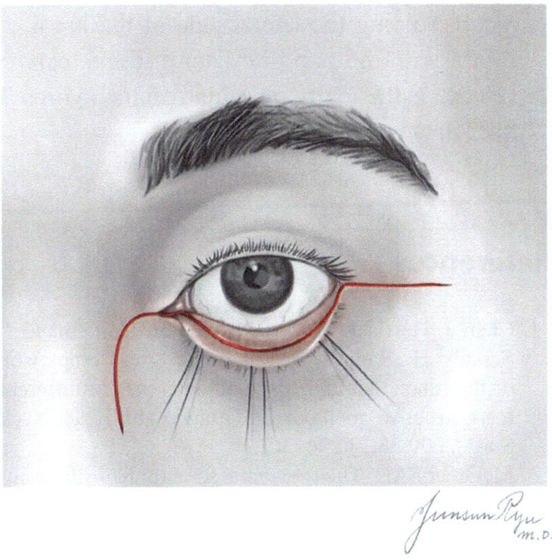

Fig. 18.4 Stepped skin-muscle subciliary incision

incisions, midfacial degloving with a transconjunctival retrocaruncular approach, and infraorbital rim osteotomy. To improve functional and esthetic results in the medial canthal region, another helpful modification of a standard incision is a modified lateral rhinotomy approach (Fig. 18.4).

Expert Opinion
With advancements in surgical tools, most maxillectomies can now be performed using a Weber–Ferguson incision with Lynch extension, minimizing the risk of ectropion. (Chung-Hwan Baek)

Proper Reconstruction of the Infraorbital Rim

◆ The infraorbital rim provides strong structural support to the lower eyelid and eyeball, and its accurate positioning might be needed to avoid the development of ectropion.

◆ ***A vascularized bone flap*** could provide stability to the infra-orbital framework and reduce the development of secondary complications.

Expert Opinion
An infraorbital extension incision can be used instead, but it may cause prolonged eyelid and conjunctival edema. (Chung-Hwan Baek)

Postoperative ectropion is the most common complication after maxillectomy, occurring in approximately 40% of patients, regardless of the reconstructive technique used [9]. Ectropion not only deteriorates esthetic outcomes but also has a negative functional impact in terms of the development of exposure keratitis, conjunctivitis, epiphora, and eventually a decrease in visual acuity. Various reconstruction techniques have been used to provide stable and solid structural support

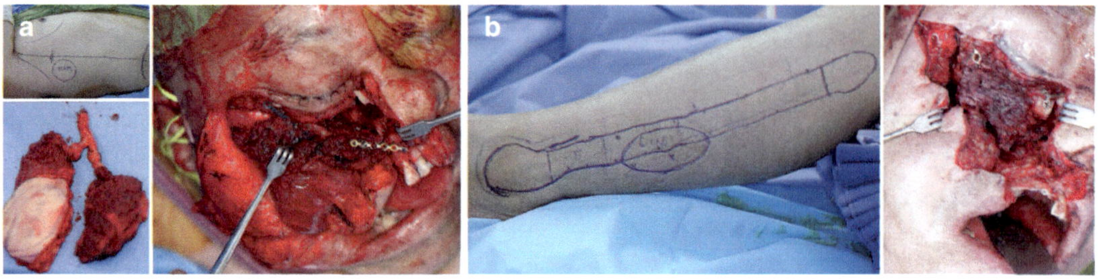

Fig. 18.5 Infraorbital rim reconstruction with a bone-containing free flap. (**a**) Scapula free flap. (**b**) Fibula free flap

to the orbital contents after removal of the inferior orbital rim. Bone-containing free flaps, such as fibular, iliac crest, costal, or scapular free flaps, have frequently been used because of their better resistance to bone resorption than achieved with simple bone grafts (Fig. 18.5). A bone-free flap can also be used to reconstruct the bony maxillary arch for dental rehabilitation [10].

Alloplastic implants, particularly titanium meshes, can also be utilized. Despite promising early esthetic and functional results, the long-term risks of material exposure and implant-related infections are much more significant than those associated with autologous grafts, considering the frequent use of adjuvant radiotherapy.

Another option for reconstructing the inferior orbital wall is the use of fascia lata strips. The fascia lata strip has advantages in terms of ease and rapidity of harvesting, as well as a lower risk of donor-site morbidity and long-term complications. However, esthetic and functional outcomes may not be satisfactory in patients without bony repair of the infraorbital rim [11].

In conclusion, compared with non-vascularized tissue or soft tissue used for orbital floor reconstruction after maxillectomy, rigid bone-free flaps or alloplastic implants combined with free flaps should be chosen for better postoperative ophthalmologic, functional, and esthetic outcomes.

Expert Opinion

Using the fascia lata of the anterolateral thigh free flap and the medial vastus medialis fascia to support the remaining bone structure beneath the orbit securely, while reconstructing the lateral side of the nasal cavity with the opposite lateral fascia, can achieve esthetically pleasing results. (Min-Sik Kim)

References

1. Chau J, Harris J, Nesbitt P, Allen H, Guillemaud J, Seikaly H. Radial forearm donor site: comparison of the functional and cosmetic outcomes of different reconstructive methods. J Otolaryngol Head Neck Surg. 2009;38(2):294–301.
2. McGregor AD. The free radial forearm flap--the management of the secondary defect. Br J Plast Surg. 1987;40(1):83–5.
3. Sidebottom AJ, Stevens L, Moore M, Magennis P, Devine JC, Brown JS, et al. Repair of the radial free flap donor site with full or partial thickness skin grafts: a prospective randomised controlled trial. Int J Oral Maxillofac Surg. 2000;29(3):194–7.
4. Antes G, Sauerland S, Seiler CM. Evidence-based medicine--from best research evidence to a better surgical practice and health care. Langenbecks Arch Surg. 2006;391(2):61–7.

5. Hui KC, Zhang F, Lineaweaver WC. Z-plasty closure of the donor defect of the radial forearm free flap. J Reconstr Microsurg. 1999;15(1):19–21.
6. Bardsley AF, Soutar DS, Elliot D, Batchelor AG. Reducing morbidity in the radial forearm flap donor site. Plast Reconstr Surg. 1990;86(2):287–92. discussion 93-4.
7. Hsieh CH, Kuo YR, Yao SF, Liang CC, Jeng SF. Primary closure of radial forearm flap donor defects with a bilobed flap based on the fasciocutaneous perforator of the ulnar artery. Plast Reconstr Surg. 2004;113(5):1355–60.
8. Wilson JA, Clark JJ. Obesity: impediment to postsurgical wound healing. Adv Skin Wound Care. 2004;17(8):426–35.
9. Sweeney AR, Walker B, Bhrany AD, Chang SH, Jian-Amadi A. Ophthalmic changes following maxillectomy with or without postoperative radiation therapy. J Craniofac Surg. 2019;30(5):1448–51.
10. Dugast S, Longis J, Anquetil M, Piot B, Corre P, Huon JF, et al. Reconstruction techniques of the orbit after Brown class III maxillectomy: a systematic review. Head Neck. 2023;45(6):1581–93.
11. Joo YH, Cho KJ, Park JO, Kim MS. Usefulness of the anterolateral thigh flap with vascularized fascia lata for reconstruction of orbital floor and nasal surface after total maxillectomy. Laryngoscope. 2013;123(9):2125–s30.

Part VIII

Specific Consideration

19 Postoperative Carotid Blow-out

Jeong-Seok Choi, Kangmin Kim, Sang-Yeon Kim, and Jeongkye Hwang

19.1 KQ 19.1. What Are the Urgent Procedures to Be Implemented When Carotid Blow-Out Occurs?

Jeong-Seok Choi

The content on carotid blow-out is divided into three chapters as follows (Fig. 19.1).

Carotid blow-out is a common complication in patients with advanced head and neck cancer, often occurring due to radiation-induced necrosis, recurrent tumors, and delayed wound healing. Carotid blow-out events can be classified into three categories: threatening, impending, and acute. Threatening carotid blow-out is diagnosed based on clinical observations, such as visible carotid artery exposure or evidence of arterial wall damage, along with radiological signs of necrosis of the surrounding artery. Impending carotid blow-out involves temporary bleeding episodes that typically resolve naturally or can be managed using packing or pressure. Sentinel hemorrhage is associated with pseudoaneurysms, which can lead to vascular rupture due to the lack of structural support in the pseudoaneurysm walls, making the rupture unpredictable. An acute carotid blow-out signifies uncontrolled, non-self-limiting bleeding that requires immediate intervention and poses a severe threat to life. Managing massive bleeding from an acute carotid blow-out is a formidable challenge for the medical team. Initial management involves identifying the underlying cause, along with implementing strategies for effectively controlling life-threatening bleeding, and addressing potential complications that may affect overall survival [1].

J.-S. Choi (✉)
Department of Otolaryngology—Head and Neck Surgery, Inha University Hospital, Inha University College of Medicine, Incheon, Republic of Korea
e-mail: jschoi@inha.ac.kr

K. Kim (✉)
Department of Neurosurgery, Seoul National University Hospital, Seoul National University College of Medicine, Seoul, South Korea
e-mail: quintus@snu.ac.kr

S.-Y. Kim (✉)
Department of Otolaryngology—Head and Neck Surgery, Seoul St. Mary's Hospital, College of Medicine, The Catholic University of Korea, Seoul, Republic of Korea
e-mail: ksyent@catholic.ac.kr

J. Hwang
Department of Vascular & Transplant Surgery, Department of Surgery, Eunpyeong St. Mary's Hospital, College of Medicine, The Catholic University of Korea, Seoul, Republic of Korea
e-mail: jjungyong@catholic.ac.kr

K.-J. Cho, J.-O. Park (eds.), *Management of Head and Neck Surgery Complications*,
https://doi.org/10.1007/978-981-96-1860-6_19

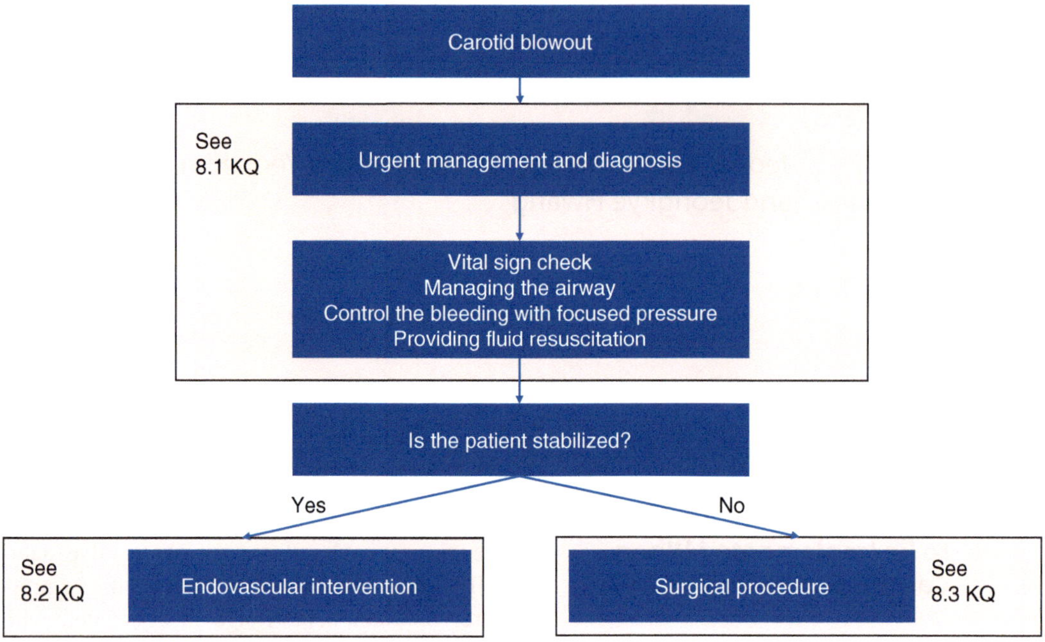

Fig. 19.1 Algorithm for management of carotid blow-out

> **Expert Opinion**
> It is important to identify patients at risk of carotid blow-out. These include patients with an exposed carotid artery, an open wound near the carotid artery, a pharyngocutaneous fistula with an exposed carotid artery, and those with a sentinel bleed. (David Eisele)
>
> Carotid blow-out is closely associated not only with tumor infiltration, but also with prior treatments, such as radiation therapy; underlying conditions, like diabetes; and concurrent nutrient deficiency. (Yuh S Jung)

The diagnosis of carotid blow-out relies on a combination of physical and radiological assessments to detect visible bleeding from the exposed arteries or sentinel hemorrhage. When the patient's hemodynamic status is stable, the initial evaluation begins with a comprehensive medical history, including inquiries about prior carotid blow-out instances and cancer history and treatment. General examinations should encompass a thorough assessment of the head and neck, upper respiratory endoscopy, and comprehensive neurological evaluation. Furthermore, laboratory tests are recommended to assess parameters such as anemia, thrombocytopenia, and coagulation abnormalities. Radiological imaging remains a crucial component of the diagnostic process. If the carotid artery exposure is not directly visible in a neck wound, contrast-enhanced computed tomography (CT) can be highly valuable. It can reveal the presence of a tumor or an air interface with the carotid artery, identifying the location and extent of exposure. After stabilizing the patient, angiography is performed to assess both carotid arteries. This evaluation checks for bleeding sites, aneurysmal dilation, and completeness of cerebral circulation. Furthermore, it looks for any signs of tumor blush, indicating the bleeding site. Combining angiography and CT scan findings can help pinpoint the potential location. CT angiography is the preferred imaging method because of its high accuracy in diagnosing impending or acute carotid blow-out, providing critical insights into necrosis, pseudoaneurysms, or contrast material leakage detection (Fig. 19.2) [2, 3].

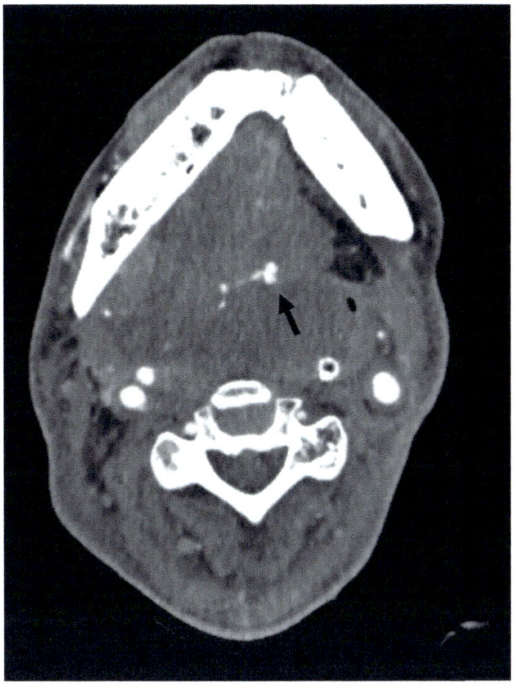

Fig. 19.2 Computed tomography image showing extravasation of contrast from the lingual artery (arrow)

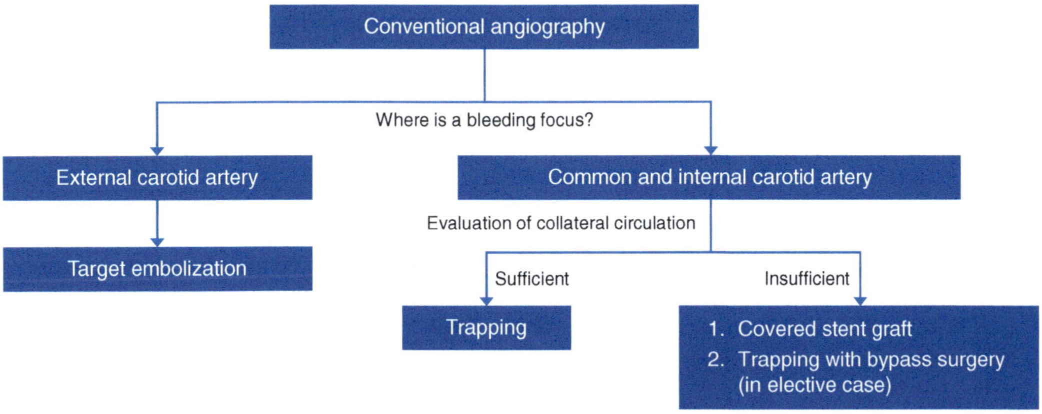

Fig. 19.3 Algorithm for endovascular treatment of carotid blow-out

In the event of a carotid blow-out, if you are alone, call for help and wear protective gear. The most critical step is ensuring that the patient is not left unattended. Request immediate medical assistance for suspected cardiac arrest. If the emergency kit is not nearby, ask someone to retrieve it while you begin resuscitation assessment.

Expert Opinion

Patients at risk of blow-out should be quickly admitted to or transferred to an intensive care unit (ICU) for close monitoring. The ICU team should be informed of the concerns and the overall plan of care. The patient should be closely monitored,

(continued)

both physiologically and neurologically. Blood pressure should be controlled, and the patient should be on bed rest with the head of the bed elevated. Two intravenous access sites should be placed and maintained. A type and cross order for blood transfusion should be in place, with two units of packed red blood cells readily available. An ambu bag and continuous suction devices should be kept in the ICU room. The following operating room instrument sets should also be in the room: basic neck set, vascular set, and tracheostomy set. Once the patient is stabilized in the ICU, a timely management plan should be developed with head and neck surgery, reconstructive surgery, and vascular surgery, as indicated. (David Eisele)

Even if the carotid artery cannot be directly visualized, immediate action should be taken with CT angiography or, if necessary, an interventional procedure. Delays in action and decision-making can significantly increase mortality rates. (Yuh S Jung)

Essentials for the Emergency Kit

◆ Airway management equipment (suction, intubation, and tracheostomy)

◆ Intravenous supplies (cannulae, syringes, and fluids)

◆ Personal protective gear (gloves, aprons, and goggles)

◆ Medications (intravenous midazolam)

◆ Sterile dressings and waste disposal items

The top priorities are airway control, bleeding management through pressure application, and fluid resuscitation facilitated by establishing large-bore venous access. It is crucial to protect the patient's airway and prevent blood contamination when using an endotracheal tube with a cuff. Hemodynamic support, which may include the administration of blood products, may be necessary for patients with hemodynamic instability. If patients do not respond to resuscitation with blood products, vasoconstrictors may be required to maintain organ perfusion. Patients with a history of carotid blow-out may develop carotid artery dysfunction, potentially resulting in arrhythmias, and should be continuously monitored for cardiac function. Local packing techniques may be considered if the patient is hemodynamically stable and experiences sentinel bleeding. However, in cases of massive bleeding and unstable patient conditions, direct pressure can be applied to the bleeding site until the source of arterial bleeding can be identified. Handling neck wounds beyond applying pressure for hemorrhage control requires caution.

Expert Opinion

If a carotid blow-out occurs before definitive management, emergency measures should be initiated immediately. A code should be initiated, and direct digital pressure applied to the site of hemorrhage. Adequate airway patency must be ensured. Fluid resuscitation and blood transfusion should be initiated as indicated. The patient should then be prepared for emergency transfer to the operating room or interventional radiology suite to control the source of the hemorrhage. (David Eisele)

If possible, an emergency blood test, including hemoglobin levels, should be conducted and blood supplies should be secured in advance to ensure immediate resuscitation if needed. (Yuh S Jung)

◆ The initial approach should prioritize resuscitating and stabilizing the patient, which involves managing the airway, controlling bleeding with focused pressure, and providing fluid resuscitation.

◆ Simply placing multiple dressings over the bleeding site is inadequate and inappro-

(continued)

priate. Instead, it is advisable to use a gloved finger to apply focused pressure directly on the hemorrhage site, temporarily controlling the bleeding until definitive treatment can be administered.

◆ This stabilization phase enables accurate diagnostic angiography and subsequent endovascular treatment. In cases where interventional radiology procedures are unavailable or proven unsuccessful, emergency surgical intervention becomes necessary.

Expert Opinion

The patient and family members should be reassured and offered emotional support. (David Eisele)

In the context of carotid blow-out, it is crucial to inform patients and their families about the severe and potentially fatal nature of this condition, in advance. (Yuh S Jung)

After confirming a carotid blow-out, a multidisciplinary approach encompassing carotid artery surgery, interventional radiology, and vascular surgery is essential to reduce the risk of acute arterial bleeding. Further diagnostic and therapeutic interventions should only be considered after the patient has stabilized from a cardiac and respiratory perspective. These fundamental principles have significantly reduced the incidence of cardiac and neurological ischemic events. Previously, definitive management of carotid blow-out involved emergent ligation or re-exploration; however, due to the high complication and mortality rates associated with this approach, it has been replaced by endovascular procedures. These procedures can be broadly categorized as vascular sacrifices performed via stenting and embolization. Endovascular reconstruction management with stent placement for immediate hemostasis is reasonable, but may not yield favorable long-term results due to delayed complications. In an impending or life-threatening carotid blow-out, an open and compassionate discussion should be had with the patient and their family.

The most successful strategy for managing carotid blow-out is to intervene proactively before rupture occurs to prevent this catastrophic event. Swift initial resuscitation and prompt identification of the source of bleeding, followed by immediate intervention, are critical components for managing massive bleeding events. Employing comprehensive management strategies can lead to successful patient survival and can achieve hemostasis [4, 5].

Expert Opinion

Endovascular procedures are now considered the standard treatment, with surgical intervention used as a secondary option if endovascular treatment is not feasible. (Yuh S Jung)

Management of Carotid Blow-out

◆ If alone, call for help, wear protective gear, and do not leave the patient alone to minimize distress. Request a cardiac arrest call for urgent medical support. If the emergency box is not nearby, have someone retrieve it while you start the resuscitation assessment.

◆Check for airway blockages caused by bleeding in the mouth or throat. In tracheostomy patients, inflate the cuff, inspect for blockages, and use suction to clear blood or clots. For skilled personnel, tracheal intubation is an option for securing the airway.

◆The patient's respiratory rate may increase due to anxiety and shock. Hemorrhage can lead to hypoxia or aspiration, further worsening respiratory distress.

◆Assess hemodynamics with vital signs and capillary refill. Gain IV access, urgently extract blood samples, and initiate an IV for fluid replacement. Consider blood

(continued)

transfusion. Apply pressure to the bleeding sites and consider packing around the endotracheal tube for hemostasis. Inotropic agents are administered to patients who continue to experience persistent shock (systolic blood pressure <90 mmHg or diastolic blood pressure <60 mmHg) despite receiving significant fluid resuscitation.

◆ Closely monitor consciousness as hypovolemia and hypoxia can result in reduced awareness, confusion, and agitation. Consider using intravenous midazolam for anxiety relief.

◆ Once the patient is hemodynamically stable, promptly refer them for further definitive treatment. Adequate planning should have already assessed the patient's suitability for surgical or endovascular procedures and established the most efficient referral route.

◆ Relocate patients to a side room to reduce disturbance to others and create more space for patient care. Critical care in the intensive care unit should be provided according to the patient's condition and clinical evaluations. Ensure that an easily accessible emergency equipment box is prepared without causing additional distress to the patient.

19.2 KQ 19.2. What Are the Radiological Interventions for Managing Carotid Blow-Outs?

Kangmin Kim

(1) Reconstructive approach

Targeted embolization can be considered if a branch of the external carotid artery is the focus of bleeding. After placing the *microcatheter as close to the bleeding focus as possible, the target artery can be occluded using embolic material* (Fig. 19.4). Glue (n-butyl cyanoacrylate), polyvinyl alcohol particles, onyx, or coils can be used as embolic materials. The bleeding focus itself must be occluded; if only proximal occlusion of the target artery is performed, bleeding may recur because of collateral anastomosis of the external carotid artery. Importantly, dangerous anastomoses between the external and internal carotid arteries may cause cerebral infarction due to embolism. Therefore, the presence of dangerous anastomoses should be confirmed using superselective angiography.

Covered stent grafting should be considered in cases of massive bleeding caused by damage to the internal or common carotid artery. A covered stent graft is a balloon-mounted metal stent covered with a polytetrafluoroethylene (PTFE) membrane. As shown here, a covered stent graft was placed in the bleeding focus, and the balloon was inflated to adhere the stent graft to the arterial wall (Fig. 19.5). Recurrent bleeding can occur if a gap exists between the arterial wall and the stent graft, known as an "endoleak." Good wall apposition of the covered stent graft is important to prevent endoleaks. Additionally, repeated balloon angioplasties should be performed during the procedure, if necessary.

(2) Deconstructive approach

The deconstructive approach involves occlusion of the damaged carotid artery. This process is referred to as "trapping" and is the best management strategy for bleeding recurrence (Fig. 19.6). However, trapping carries the risk of cerebral infarction. Therefore, it is contraindicated in patients with carotid blow-out and should only be performed in inevitable cases. Before trapping, complete angiography must be performed to evaluate the collateral circulation. Due to the risk of cerebral infarction after trapping, cooperation with a neurosurgeon is essential for post-trapping management.

(3) Elective endovascular treatment

As the life expectancy of patients with head and neck cancer increases, damaged carotid arteries are more frequently detected on CT or

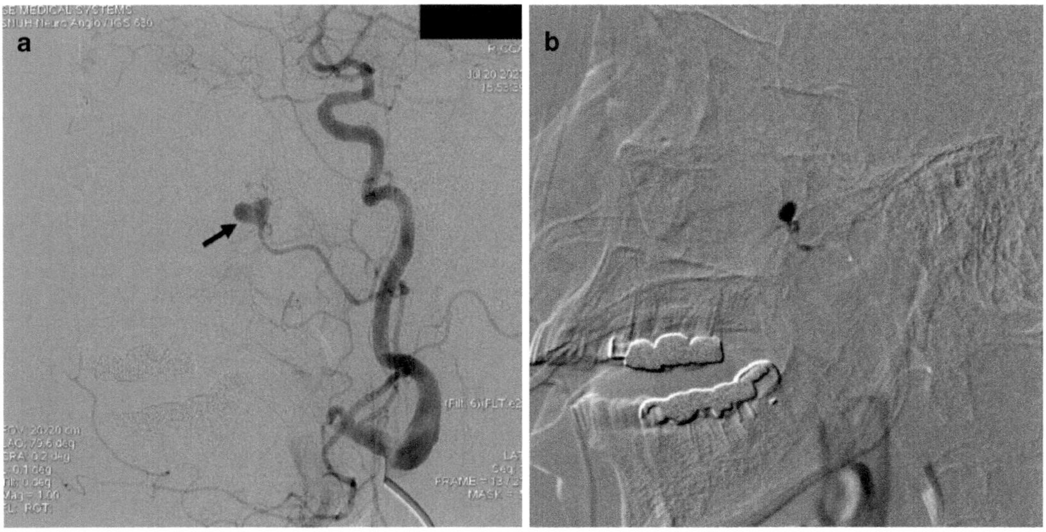

Fig. 19.4 (**a**) Bleeding from the internal maxillary artery (arrow). (**b**) Embolization using glue (n-butyl cyanoacrylate)

MRI before carotid blow-out occurs. If a carotid blow-out is judged as impending and the patient's cancer is cured, elective endovascular treatment of the damaged carotid artery should be considered. First, a balloon occlusion test must be performed. If collateral circulation is deemed sufficient, carotid artery trapping should be performed. If collateral circulation is insufficient, carotid artery trapping after extracranial-intracranial bypass surgery is recommended (Fig. 19.7).

(4) Considerations for head and neck surgeons

Endovascular treatment is an effective and rapid method for carotid blow-outs. Neurological complications rarely occur in cases of targeted embolization of the external carotid artery. However, endovascular treatment of the internal and common carotid arteries carries the risk of neurological complications.

Trapping is the most definitive endovascular treatment for carotid blow-out. However, even if sufficient collateral circulation is confirmed through angiography in an emergency situation or if the balloon test for occlusion is passed in an elective case, it does not guarantee that there are no neurological complications after trapping. It is well known that there is a risk of cerebral infarction, even if a balloon test for occlusion is performed [6]. Moreover, there is a risk of distal thromboembolism due to retrograde flow in the distal segment of the trapped carotid artery.

> **Expert Opinion**
> If the angiography demonstrates an abnormality of the common carotid artery or the internal carotid artery, a balloon occlusion test of the vessel is typically performed. If the balloon occlusion test confirms sufficient collateral cerebral perfusion, embolization of the vessel can be undertaken with a low risk of stroke. Post-embolization hypotension must be avoided. (David Eisele)

Carotid artery trapping after extracranial-intracranial bypass surgery may be considered in the following situations: (1) stable vital signs, (2) no evidence of head and neck cancer recurrence, and (3) insufficient collateral flow on conventional angiography and balloon tests for occlusion. Carotid artery trapping after

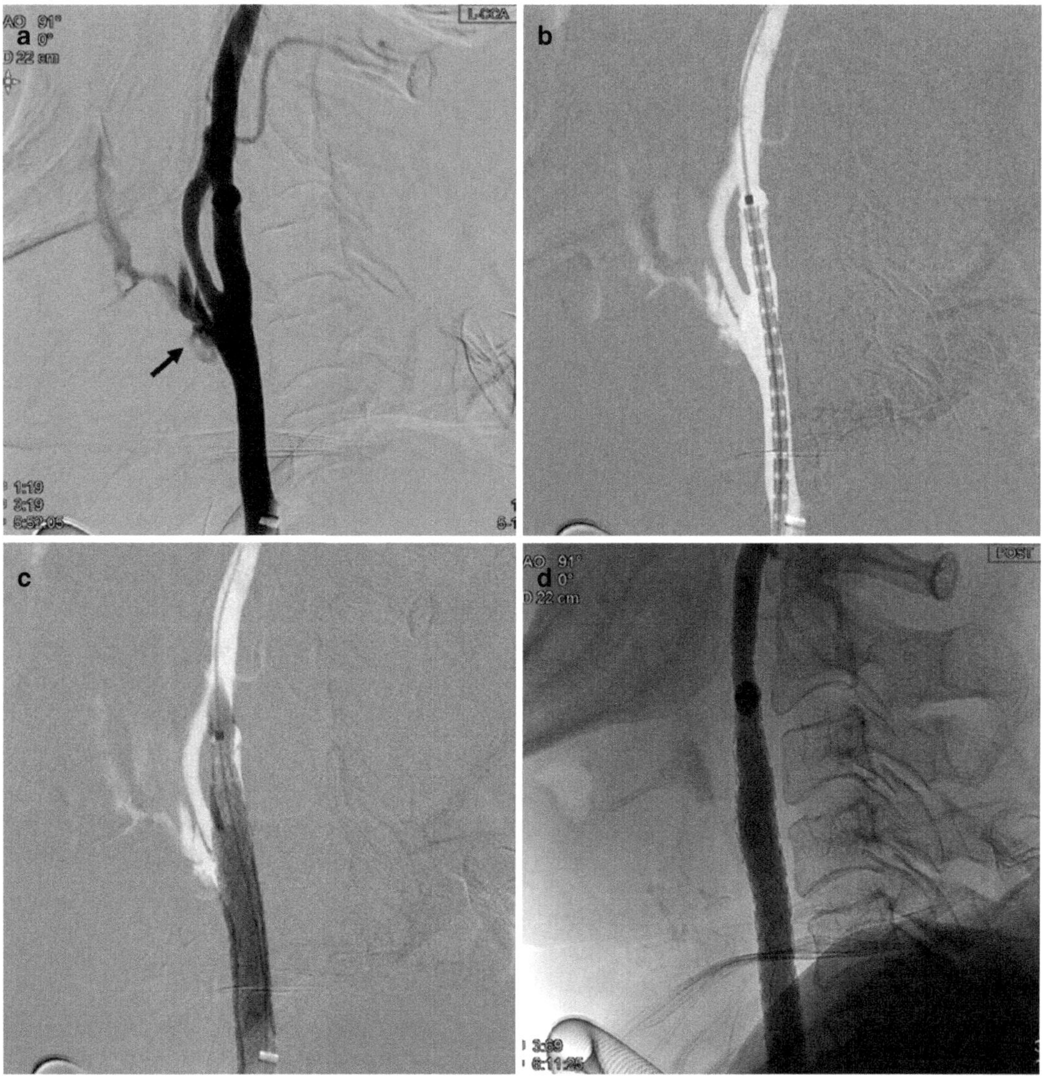

Fig. 19.5 (**a**) Massive bleeding from the common carotid artery (arrow). (**b**, **c**) Covered stent graft is placed and deployed in the carotid artery. (**d**) Carotid blow-out is successfully treated

extracranial–intracranial bypass surgery is the safest method. However, this procedure is difficult to perform in emergencies involving massive bleeding. In emergencies, carotid artery trapping is only possible in some patients [7].

Therefore, reconstructive treatment with covered stent grafts is preferred. However, this method has significant drawbacks [8, 9]. First, covered stent grafts are highly thrombogenic and require antiplatelet medications [9]. However, antiplatelet agents cannot be administered before endovascular treatment when massive bleeding is caused by carotid blow-out. Therefore, the risk of thromboembolism is high until after the procedure, following the administration of antiplatelet agents. Additionally, when covered stent grafts are used in small vessels, such as the petrous segment of the internal carotid artery, the risk of in-stent thrombosis is high even with the use of antiplatelet agents.

Second, if there is a gap between the covered stent graft and the arterial wall, rebleeding may occur due to endoleaks. A large case study reported a higher risk of rebleeding with covered

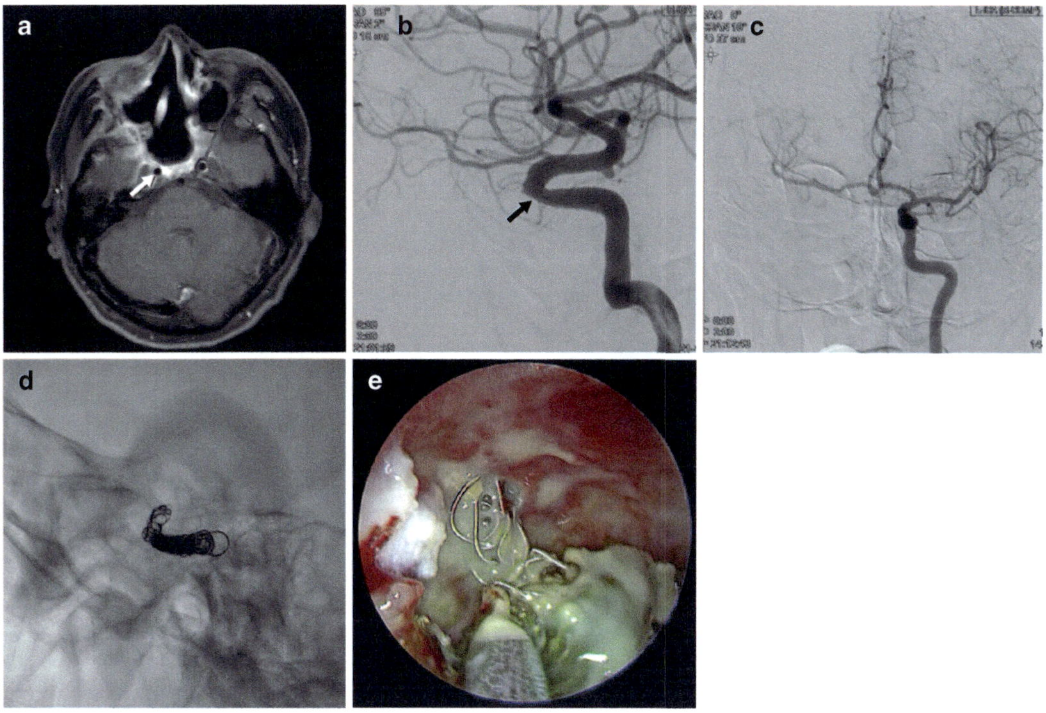

Fig. 19.6 (**a**) The patient has recurrent and massive oral bleeding. Magnetic resonance image shows osteoradionecrosis around the right cavernous internal carotid artery (white arrow). (**b**) Angiography shows the narrowed lumen of the internal carotid artery due to inflammation (black arrow). (**c**) Abundant collateral flow from the left internal carotid artery. (**d**) Trapping of the cavernous internal carotid artery. (**e**) Follow-up endoscopy with the coil mass exposed in the necrotic cavity due to osteoradionecrosis progression. However, no further bleeding events occurred

stent grafts than with trapping [10]. Therefore, regular follow-up is necessary to confirm the presence of endoleaks. If the endoleak does not resolve, carotid artery trapping should also be considered.

Expert Opinion
After the endovascular control of the carotid artery hemorrhage, reconstructive surgery can then be performed to achieve vessel coverage with vascularized tissue, as indicated. (David Eisele)

Key Points
(1) There are two methods for endovascular treatment of a carotid blow-out: a reconstructive approach and a deconstructive approach.
(2) Target embolization of the external carotid artery is considered to be relatively safe, with a low risk of neurological complications.
(3) Trapping of the internal and common carotid arteries is a definitive solution with demonstrated long-term outcomes. However, it carries the risk of neurological complications. Thus,

(continued)

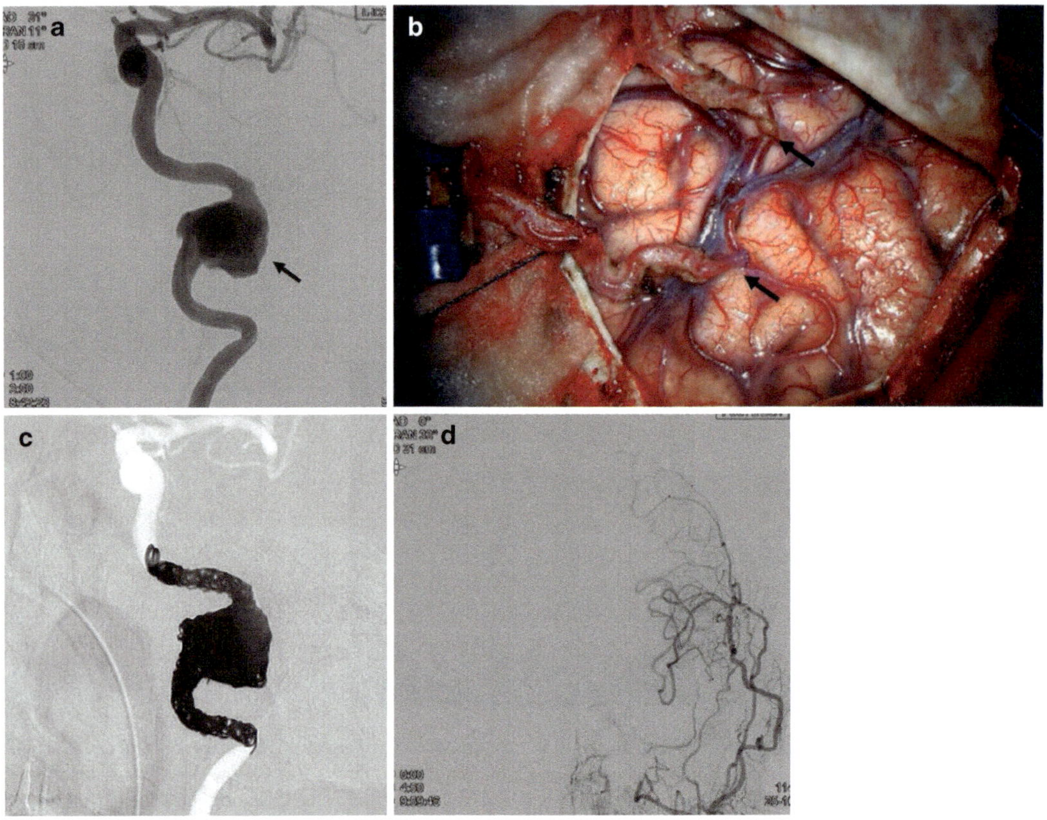

Fig. 19.7 (**a**) Angiography showing the large fusiform aneurysm (arrow) caused by osteoradionecrosis. (**b**) Extracranial-intracranial bypass surgery (arrows) in a patient with insufficient collateral flow. (**c**) Trapping of the internal carotid artery. (**d**) Cerebral blood flow is maintained by bypass after trapping the internal carotid artery

bypass surgery should be considered together with trapping if necessary.

(4) Although a covered stent graft is an ideal reconstructive treatment, it has relatively low durability and a high stent-induced thromboembolic risk. Therefore, long-term antiplatelet agents must be used.

19.3 KQ 19.3. What Are the Surgical Procedures for Managing Carotid Blow-Outs?

Sang-Yeon Kim and Jeongkye Hwang

Patients who are at low risk and have only carotid exposure can be initially monitored using localized wound care, concurrently preparing for possible procedures to cover the exposed vessel. Conversely, high-risk patients with a significant history of sentinel bleeding should be further assessed once their medical condition has stabilized. This evaluation must encompass establishing wide intravenous access, providing fluid resuscitation, ensuring airway security, and arranging for blood type determination and compatibility in cases of rebleeding.

Expert Opinion

Early detection of potential carotid blow-out and prompt surgical intervention are key and confers a significantly improved prognosis compared to delayed treatment at the time of manifestation of blow-out. (David Eisele)

If sentinel bleeding is suspected, promptly perform computed tomography angiography or other necessary studies to identify the bleeding site and initiate appropriate treatment, without delay. (Yuh S Jung)

Before the 1980s, surgical intervention involving repair or ligation of the artery was the standard of care [13]. However, surgical ligation of the carotid artery for carotid blow-out results in a high mortality rate (40%) and significantly increases the occurrence of major neurological complications (60%) [11]. Over the last few years, the use of endovascular interventions has brought about a profound transformation in the management of carotid blow-outs, resulting in a substantial reduction in both mortality and the occurrence of neurological complications.

The outcomes and morbidity associated with surgical intervention, including neurological complications, wound-healing issues, and even the risk of re-bleeding, are considerably more significant due to the challenges inherent in performing surgery and administering anesthesia in an unstable patient, particularly when dealing with a wound infiltrated by a tumor and infection. Surgical intervention aimed at carotid artery ligation should be considered a last resort if interventional angiography cannot be performed (Fig. 19.8). If such an intervention is necessary, the patient must first be fully stabilized, with adequate blood replacement readily available and administered. Furthermore, the artery should be ligated (rather than repaired) and covered with vascularized tissue in areas where the wall is healthy. The wound must be appropriately debrided, and any fistula should be externalized.

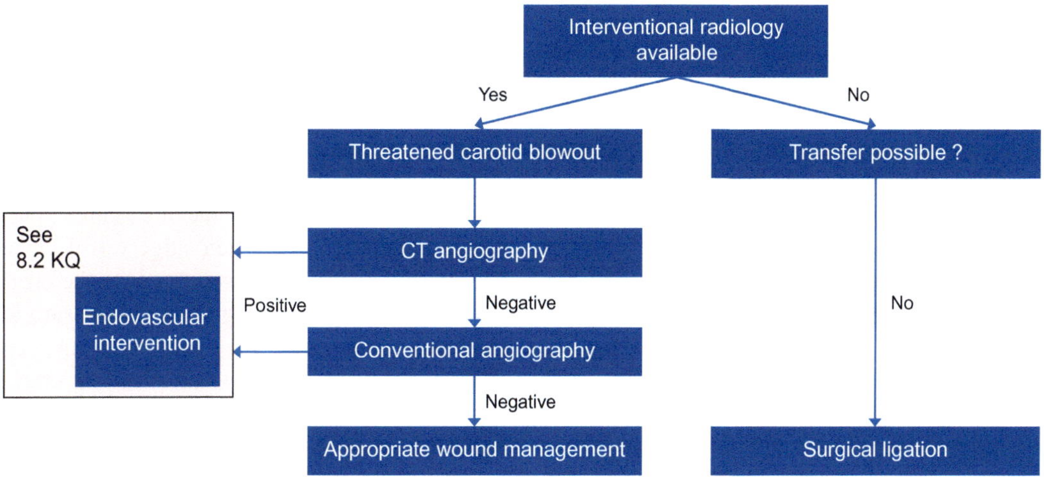

Fig. 19.8. Algorithm for surgical management of carotid blow-out. CT, computed tomography

◆ Primary role of surgery in the acute management of carotid blow-out

① Carotid artery ligation
② Carotid artery bypass
③ Closure of a mucocutaneous fistula
④ Vascularized tissue coverage of the involved carotid artery
⑤ Neck exploration to ascertain whether a recurrent tumor is present

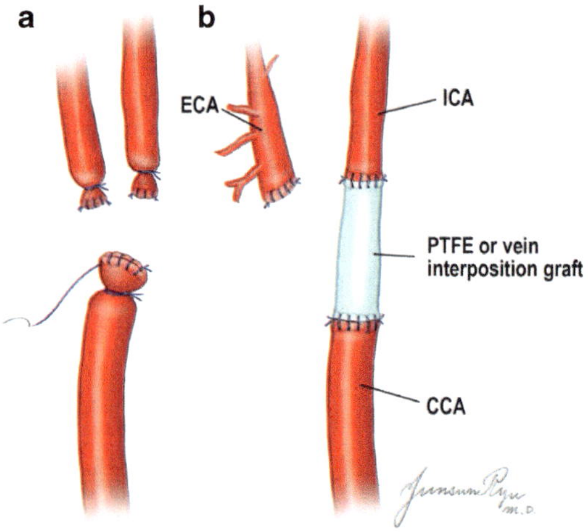

Fig. 19.9 Schematic pictures of carotid artery ligation for carotid blow-out. (**a**) Ligation of the internal carotid artery and common carotid artery. (**b**) Ligation of the carotid artery with simultaneous interposition graft. ECA, external carotid artery; ICA, internal carotid artery; PTFE, polytetrafluoroethylene; CCA, common carotid artery

Within the treatment framework, ligation becomes a viable option when managing a patient with an unstable condition, with type III carotid blow-out (active carotid blow-out), or when the patient is incapable of being transported to a facility with interventional radiology capabilities. In such urgent situations, medical personnel often apply numerous dressings to the wound without exerting focused pressure on the bleeding site, potentially leading to ongoing blood loss. A more effective approach involves using a gloved finger to apply pressure and temporarily controlling the bleeding until definitive treatment can be administered. To summarize, addressing bleeding using active and appropriate resuscitation measures is imperative. The risk of complications associated with ligation increases significantly when accompanied by hypotension, which is the primary predictor of unfavorable outcomes in the acute management of carotid blow-out syndrome.

Endovascular embolization is feasible for bleeding from the external carotid artery (ECA) trunk or its branches. Following endovascular embolization of the ECA, the occurrence of surgical stroke is less than 2%, while the rebleeding rate ranges from 30% to 35%. Factors contributing to rebleeding include potential issues such as inadequate identification of the target vessel, reflux triggered by the well-developed ECA collateral circulation, regeneration of the tumor vascular bed, and the emergence of new ECA branches [14–16].

In cases of common carotid artery (CCA) or internal carotid artery (ICA) bleeding, the decision to resect, reconstruct, or ligate the artery is compounded in the emergency setting of a carotid blow-out. Life-threatening arterial disruption secondary to radiation arteriopathy usually requires concomitant exposure to the source of bacterial contamination, and ligation may be the ideal choice for preventing recurrent hemorrhage [17] (Fig. 19.9a). In addition to the inherent challenges posed by performing surgery within an infected and necrotic wound surrounded by fibrotic irradiated tissue, the reconstruction process in this surgical area is prone to interpositional graft rupture or the formation of pseudoaneurysms [18]. Therefore, in situations of disease recurrence involving the carotid artery, excising the vessel could be the exclusive surgical avenue for potentially achieving a cure or providing palliation [19]. When surgery is deemed necessary, the surgeon must proceed to the operating room while applying accurate pressure to the bleeding site using a gloved finger. An incision should be made around the bleeding site to attempt the dissection and exposure of the internal jugular and vagus nerves. The dissection can be extended 5 cm above and below the bleeding site to facilitate ligation. Subsequently, the proximal and distal portions of the carotid artery should be identified, and vessel clamps and ties should be applied. After resection of the injured portion of the carotid artery, both sides of the vessel lumen should be oversewn with running sutures using prolene 5-0.

Expert Opinion
Bleeding often emerges through defects in the pharyngeal wall and into the mouth. While adequate compression is crucial, it can be challenging to achieve effective pressure. In such cases, the risk of pulmonary aspiration or airway complications is high. Therefore, securing the airway through endotracheal intubation or tracheostomy is often essential. (Yuh S Jung)

Vascular reconstruction using an interpositional graft following carotid artery resection should be considered if feasible. In such cases, either Dacron or polytetrafluoroethylene (PTFE) can be used, and autologous vein grafts may also be employed (Figs. 19.9b and 19.10). However, autologous vein grafts are reportedly inferior to prosthetics in terms of long-term patency [20]. Nevertheless, such carotid artery replacement is not always technically or physiologically possible, particularly when the area of tumor involvement along the internal carotid artery is situated near the skull base. In such cases, carotid bypass surgery accompanied by craniotomy may be an option. This entails performing a bypass using a graft from the contralateral or ipsilateral carotid artery to the middle cerebral artery (MCA) territory or from the subclavian and vertebral arteries [21]. If the external carotid artery is accessible and selective internal carotid artery ligation is feasible, a bypass procedure utilizing branches of the external carotid artery (e.g., the superficial temporal artery) in the MCA territory can be considered (Fig. 19.11). However, these vascular reconstruction methods are often not feasible in emergencies due to fibrotic changes or infected conditions around the surgical area and the unsta-

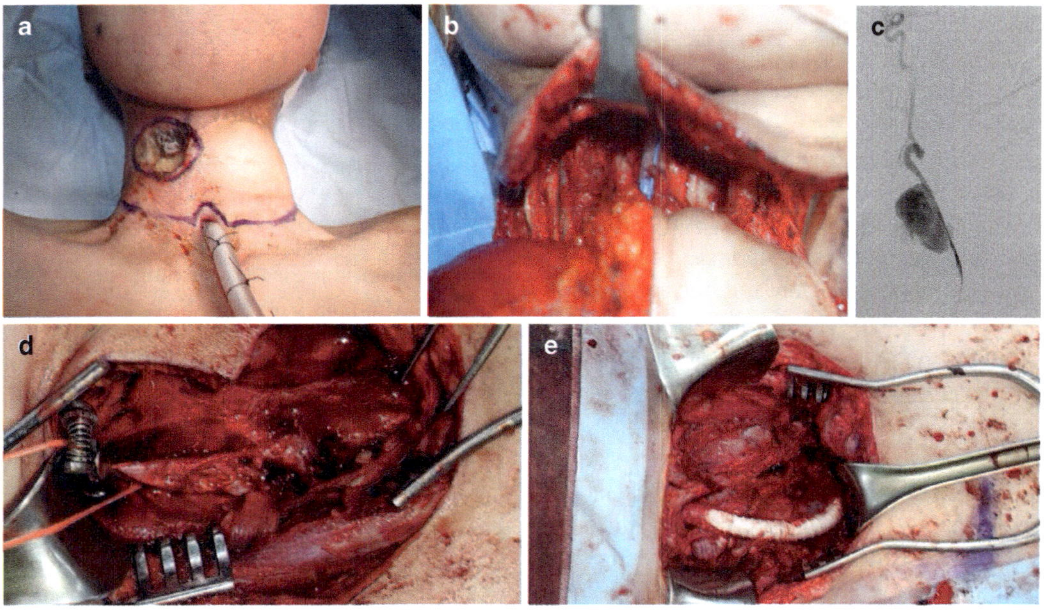

Fig. 19.10 Clinical photographs of carotid blow-out. (**a**) Skin necrosis after radiation therapy, (**b**) pharyngocutaneous fistula with carotid blow-out, (**c**) angiography of carotid blow-out in common carotid artery, (**d**) after clamping common carotid artery, and (**e**) interposition graft from the subclavian artery to the internal carotid artery

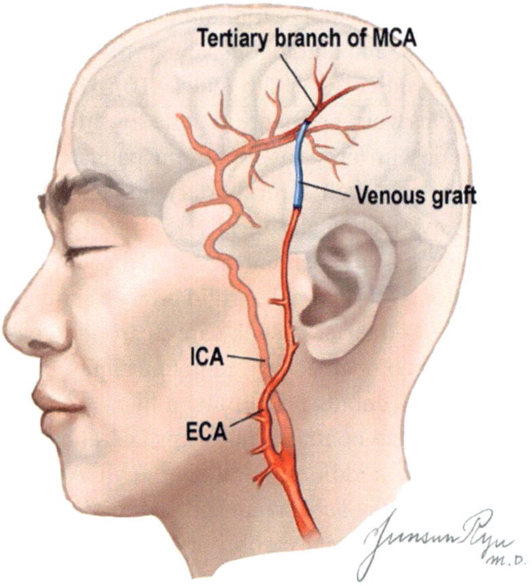

Fig. 19.11 Carotid artery ligation with bypass surgery. Bypass from the superficial temporal artery to the MCA territory using an autologous venous graft. MCA, middle cerebral artery; ICA, internal carotid artery; ECA, external carotid artery

ble condition of the patient. Furthermore, the risk of rebleeding following surgery remains. Therefore, these should be considered only under limited circumstances.

Expert Opinion
Vascular reconstruction should be undertaken only on very select patients in whom there is no overt infection, salivary fistula, or recurrent tumor. Coverage of the entire graft and anastomotic sites with vascularized tissue are imperative to minimize the risk of anastomotic rupture. (David Eisele)

After managing the affected carotid artery, any infected and necrotic tissue must be removed, existing fistulas must be addressed, arterial coverage must be provided, soft tissue interposed, and the wound site reconstructed. Dermal and facial grafts do not have an independent blood supply; thus, they are unreliable for infected and contaminated wounds and have limited use in carotid coverage. Although local tissue flaps are commonly accessible, they may not provide sufficient healthy tissue to address coverage concerns reliably in irradiated patients. The most effective solution involves using myocutaneous flaps, which provide self-sustaining vascular pedicles, healthy tissues, and local availability. These flaps create an optimal environment for wound healing, arterial protection, and redirection of salivary flow. If the fistula remains unclosed, it should be managed by rerouting salivary flow over the external surface of the flap and away from the previously exposed carotid artery. If available, pectoralis major, deltopectoral, latissimus dorsi, and trapezius flaps can be considered. Free flap reconstruction can also be considered for wound healing. However, in cases where carotid ligation has been performed, vessels from the contralateral side or the use of a long pedicle may be necessary. Additionally, because most patients with carotid blow-outs often have vessel-depleted situations, caution is necessary when deciding to proceed with free flap reconstruction.

◆ Protocol for surgical management of carotid blow-out

① Maintain pressure (digital, balloon tamponade) on the bleeding vessel
② Maintain normotension with mean arterial pressure > 60 mmHg
③ Maintain hemoglobin levels > 10 g/dL
④ Maintain oxygen saturation > 95%
⑤ Perform proximal and distal artery ligation
⑥ Debride and irrigate the wound, excise persistent malignant disease
⑦ Close salivary fistulae
⑧ Perform flap coverage of exposed arteries with non-irradiated, well-vascularized tissue

Expert Opinion
Rebleeding following definitive surgery is not uncommon, particularly in the setting of disease progression or associated pharyngocutaneous fistula. (David Eisele)

References

1. Alterio D, Turturici I, Volpe S, Ferrari S, Russell-Edu SW, Vischioni B, et al. Carotid blowout syndrome after reirradiation for head and neck malignancies: a comprehensive systematic review for a pragmatic multidisciplinary approach. Crit Rev Oncol Hematol. 2020;155:103088.
2. Suárez C, Fernández-Alvarez V, Hamoir M, Mendenhall WM, Strojan P, Quer M, et al. Carotid blowout syndrome: modern trends in management. Review Cancer Manag Res. 2018;10:5617–28.
3. Lipe DN, Viets-Upchurch J, Hanna EY, Reyes-Gibby C, Chen SR, Elsayem A, et al. Carotid blowout syndrome in the emergency department: a case report and review of the literature. Review J Emerg Med. 2022;62(3):e29–34.
4. Slijepcevic AA, Roh J, Pipkorn P, Lipsey K, Bradley JP. Carotid blowout syndrome in head and neck cancer patients: management of patients at risk for CBS. Laryngoscope. 2023;133(3):576–87.
5. Dixon L, Warriner D. Carotid blowout. Review Br J Hosp Med (Lond). 2012;73(7):C98–100.
6. American Society of Interventional and Therapeutic Neuroradiology. Carotid artery balloon test occlusion. AJNR Am J Neuroradiol. 2001;22(8 Suppl):S8–9.
7. Wu PA, Yuan GY, Zhou RM, Ho WW, Lu ZQ, Cai JF, et al. Extracranial/intracranial vascular bypass in the treatment of head and neck cancer—related carotid blowout syndrome. Laryngoscope. 2021;131(7):1548–56. https://doi.org/10.1002/lary.29427.
8. Wu CJ, Lin WC, Hsu JS, Han IT, Hsieh TJ, Liu GC, et al. Follow-up for covered stent treatment of carotid blow-out syndrome in patients with head and neck cancer. Br J Radiol. 2016;89(1058):20150136. https://doi.org/10.1259/bjr.20150136.
9. McCready RA, Divelbiss JL, Bryant MA, Denardo AJ, Scott JA. Endoluminal repair of carotid artery pseudoaneurysms: a word of caution. J Vasc Surg. 2004;40(5):1020–3. https://doi.org/10.1016/j.jvs.2004.07.034.
10. Wong DJY, Donaldson C, Lai LT, Coleman A, Giddings C, Slater LA, et al. Safety and effectiveness of endovascular embolization or stent-graft reconstruction for treatment of acute carotid blowout syndrome in patients with head and neck cancer: case series and systematic review of observational studies. Head Neck. 2018;40(4):846–54. https://doi.org/10.1002/hed.25018.
11. Chaloupka JC, Putman CM, Citardi MJ, Ross DA, Sasaki CT. Endovascular therapy for the carotid blowout syndrome in head and neck surgical patients: diagnostic and managerial considerations. AJNR Am J Neuroradiol. 1996;17(5):843–52.
12. Powitzky R, Vasan N, Krempl G, Medina J. Carotid blowout in patients with head and neck cancer. Ann Otol Rhinol Laryngol. 2010;119(7):476–84.
13. McDonald MW, Moore MG, Johnstone PA. Risk of carotid blowout after reirradiation of the head and neck: a systematic review. Int J Radiat Oncol Biol Phys. 2012;82(3):1083–9.
14. Wong DJY, Donaldson C, Lai LT, Coleman A, Giddings C, Slater LA, et al. Safety and effectiveness of endovascular embolization or stent-graft reconstruction for treatment of acute carotid blowout syndrome in patients with head and neck cancer: case series and systematic review of observational studies. Head Neck. 2018;40(4):846–54.
15. Chang FC, Luo CB, Lirng JF, Lin CJ, Lee HJ, Wu CC, et al. Endovascular management of post-irradiated carotid blowout syndrome. PLoS One. 2015;10(10):e0139821.
16. Liang NL, Guedes BD, Duvvuri U, Singh MJ, Chaer RA, Makaroun MS, et al. Outcomes of interventions for carotid blowout syndrome in patients with head and neck cancer. J Vasc Surg. 2016;63(6):1525–30.
17. Katras T, Baltazar U, Colvett K, Rush D, Dunn J, Stanton P Jr. Radiation-related arterial disease. Am Surg. 1999;65(12):1176–9.
18. Witz M, Korzets Z, Shnaker A, Lehmann JM, Ophir D. Delayed carotid artery rupture in advanced cervical cancer--a dilemma in emergency management. Eur Arch Otorhinolaryngol. 2002;259(1):37–9.
19. Okamoto Y, Inugami A, Matsuzaki Z, Yokomizo M, Konno A, Togawa K, et al. Carotid artery resection for head and neck cancer. Surgery. 1996;120(1):54–9.
20. Ziomek S, Quiñones-Baldrich WJ, Busuttil RW, Baker JD, Machleder HI, Moore WS. The superiority of synthetic arterial grafts over autologous veins in carotid-subclavian bypass. J Vasc Surg. 1986;3(1):140–5.
21. Hecht N, Wessels L, Fekonja L, von Weitzel-Mudersbach P, Vajkoczy P. Bypass strategies for common carotid artery occlusion. Acta Neurochir (Wien). 2019;161(10):1993–2002.

Radiation-Induced Osteoradionecrosis

20

Kang-Min Ahn and Yoon Se Lee

20.1 KQ 20.1. How to Prevent and Manage Osteoradionecrosis

Kang-Min Ahn

20.1.1 Prevention

Prevention of osteoradionecrosis (ORN) consists of two parts. The first part is dental prophylactics that should be administered before radiation therapy (RT). ORN prevention begins with thorough dental screening before RT [1]. Oral examinations by oral and maxillofacial specialists using panoramic radiography are mandatory. Damaged teeth with periodontal disease or severe dental caries should be extracted at least 2 weeks before RT [2]. Extraction depends on the location of the target radiation and the condition of the involved tooth. Fully impacted teeth without clinical symptoms do not need to be extracted. A partially impacted wisdom tooth, which is a candidate for the treatment of pericoronitis, needs to be extracted. Usually, postoperative RT is initiated 6–8 weeks after surgery, and dental extraction during cancer surgery is ideal. Dental scaling should be performed at least 1 week before RT. Periodontal treatment every 6 months is recommended for patients undergoing RT.

The second step in ORN prevention is dental management after RT. Radiation caries and xerostomia are the two most common complications of the oral cavity after radiation therapy (Fig. 20.1). Periodic fluoride coating using individual trays and tooth brushing with fluoride-containing toothpaste can prevent radiation caries. Xerostomia can also cause radiation-induced caries. Artificial saliva and pilocarpine may help relieve the symptoms.

Advanced dental caries and retained roots can induce periapical lesions, which are one of the primary causes of ORN. Extraction and curettage of lesions are required to prevent ORN. When extraction is required, the wound should be primarily closed as well as possible. When complete primary suturing is not possible, a collagen plug graft is recommended to prevent alveolar bone exposure during the healing period (Fig. 20.2).

◆ Prevention of ORN consists of dental prophylactics before radiotherapy and dental management after radiotherapy.

K.-M. Ahn (✉)
Department of Oral and Maxillofacial Surgery, Asan Medical Center, College of Medicine, University of Ulsan, Seoul, Republic of Korea

Y. S. Lee (✉)
Department of Otolaryngology—Head and Neck Surgery, Asan Medical Center, University of Ulsan, College of Medicine, Seoul, Republic of Korea
e-mail: yselee@amc.seoul.kr

K.-J. Cho, J.-O. Park (eds.), *Management of Head and Neck Surgery Complications*,
https://doi.org/10.1007/978-981-96-1860-6_20

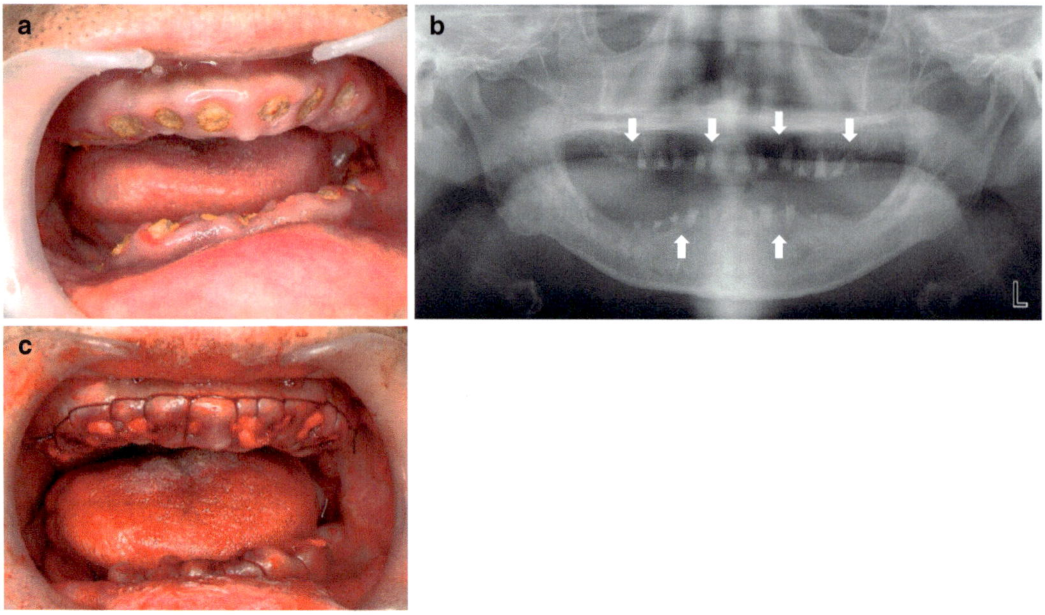

Fig. 20.1 Multiple retained roots due to radiation caries after radiation therapy. (**a**) Intraoral photograph showing fracture of the crowns. (**b**) Panoramic radiograph showing rest of the multiple roots (arrows). (**c**) Full extraction and socket preservation with a collagen plug

20.1.2 Management

The management of ORN is markedly diverse, and decision-making is difficult. It mainly depends on the stage, site involved, and general condition of the patient [3]. Lifestyle modifications (e.g., smoking cessation), medications (e.g., antibiotics, antioxidants, and antifibrotics), non-surgical interventions (e.g., hyperbaric oxygen therapy [HBO] and ultrasound therapy), and minor and major surgical options (ranging from debridement to free tissue transfer) have been suggested for the treatment of ORN. Although no consensus about the stages of ORN has been established, we usually use the classifications by Notani et al. [4] or those of Schwartz and Kagan [5]. These classifications are useful for the application of treatment options. Management options for ORN are divided into conservative and surgical treatments (minor or major).

20.1.2.1 Conservative Treatment

Conservative treatment includes medication, a mouthwash containing chlorohexidine, local curettage, simple debridement, and HBO. ORN grade I (a state of a small amount of exposed bone limited to the alveolar bone) requires conservative treatment (Fig. 20.3). Medication includes antibiotics, antioxidants, and antifibrotics, according to the PENTOCLO (pentoxifylline + tocopherol + clodronate) protocol [6]. The mobile sequestrum can be easily removed. No further surgical procedures are required when granulation tissue is present in the sequestrum.

20.1.2.2 Minor Surgical Treatment

ORN grade II indicates that ORN has extended into the bone marrow, and the lesions are located at both the alveolar level and above the level of the mandibular alveolar canal in the mandible. Maxillary lesions extending below the inferior orbital nerve are classified as ORN grade II. Minor surgical treatments include sequestrectomy or alveolectomy with primary closure.

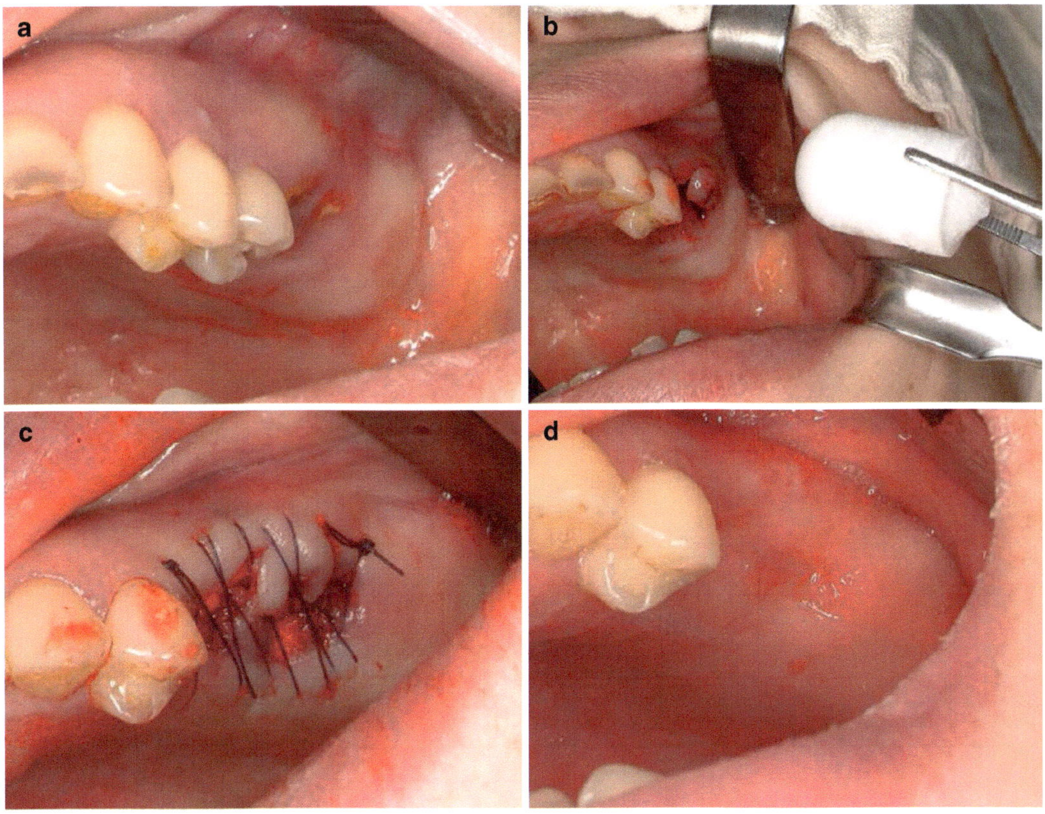

Fig. 20.2 Treatment of retained roots after radiation therapy. (**a**) Retained root and exposed maxillary alveolar bone. (**b**) Removal of the retained root, alveolar bone, and collagen plug graft. (**c**) Tight suture with absorbable suture material. (**d**) Healed gingiva 2 months after extraction

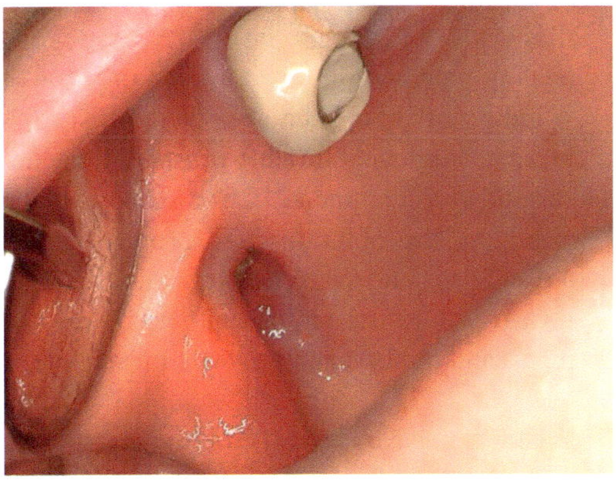

Fig. 20.3 Exposed bone in the right maxilla without any signs of infection, indicating osteoradionecrosis grade I. Conservative treatment is indicated

Expert Opinion

The role of hyperbaric oxygen therapy in the prevention or treatment of osteoradionecrosis remains controversial. (Man Ki Chung)

- **Sequestrectomy and primary closure**: When the jawbone exposure is <1 cm without any nasal and maxillary sinus communication or inferior alveolar nerve involvement, it could be primarily closed (Fig. 20.4). In cases with a risk of bone exposure in the posterior maxilla

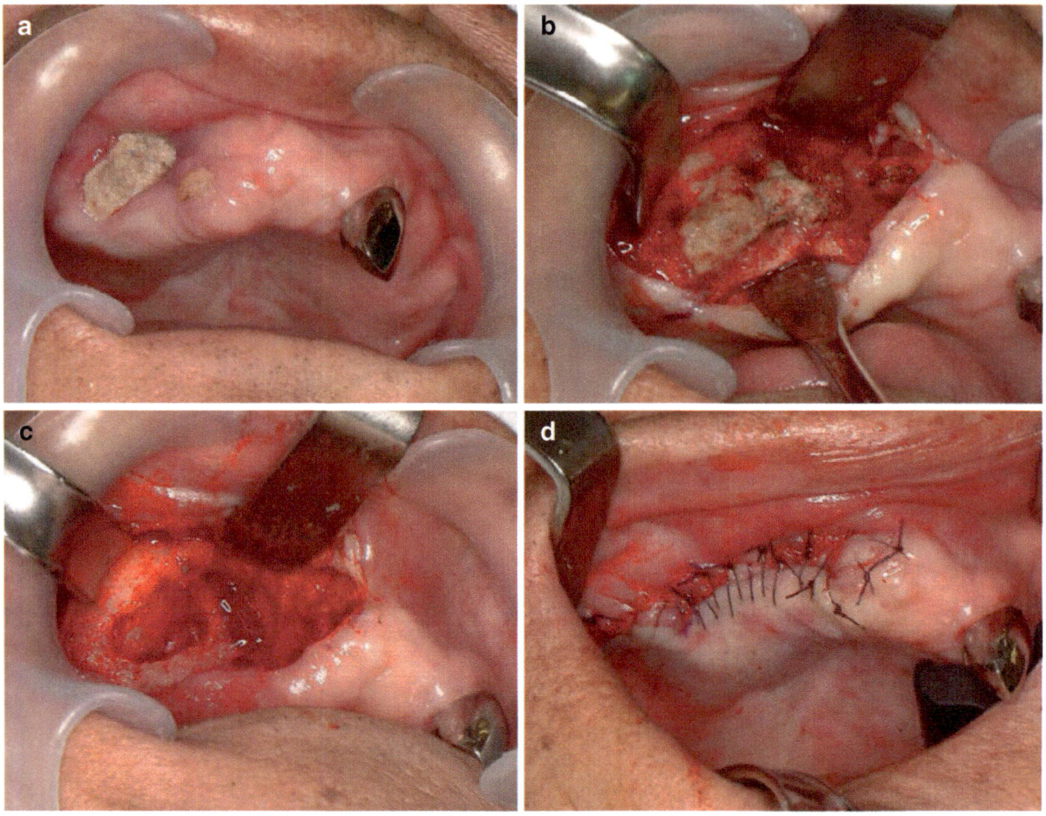

Fig. 20.4 Osteoradionecrosis of the right maxilla. (**a**) Exposed necrotic bone. (**b**) Flap elevation and exposing necrotic bone. (**c**) Granulation tissue under the sequestrum. (**d**) Suture and primary closure

and mandible, a buccal fat graft is useful for covering the exposed bone (Fig. 20.5).

20.1.2.3 Major Surgical Treatment

Major surgical treatments include segmental resection of the mandible or partial/total maxillectomy, with or without reconstruction. ORN grade III, which includes lesions that extend to the mandible below the level of the mandibular alveolar canal with a skin fistula and/or pathological fracture, is indicated for major surgical treatment. Grade III ORN in the maxilla includes total necrosis of the maxilla involving the inferior orbital nerve and midpalatal area.

- **Partial maxillectomy and obturator**: An oroantral fistula can develop after partial maxillectomy if extensive ORN occurs in the maxilla. Although buccal fat grafts have good healing potential, they are limited in terms of volume and site. When an oroantral fistula is present, surgical obturation or free-flap reconstruction is recommended. Compared with the free flap, the obturator flap provides many advantages (Fig. 20.6). In particular, it is less invasive, does not require surgery, is easy to repair and modify, and provides lip support.

When extensive necrosis of the maxilla or mandible occurs, free-flap reconstruction is necessary (Fig. 20.7). The most versatile flap is the fibular free flap, which can simultaneously reconstruct soft and hard tissues. A detailed description is provided in KQ 20.2.

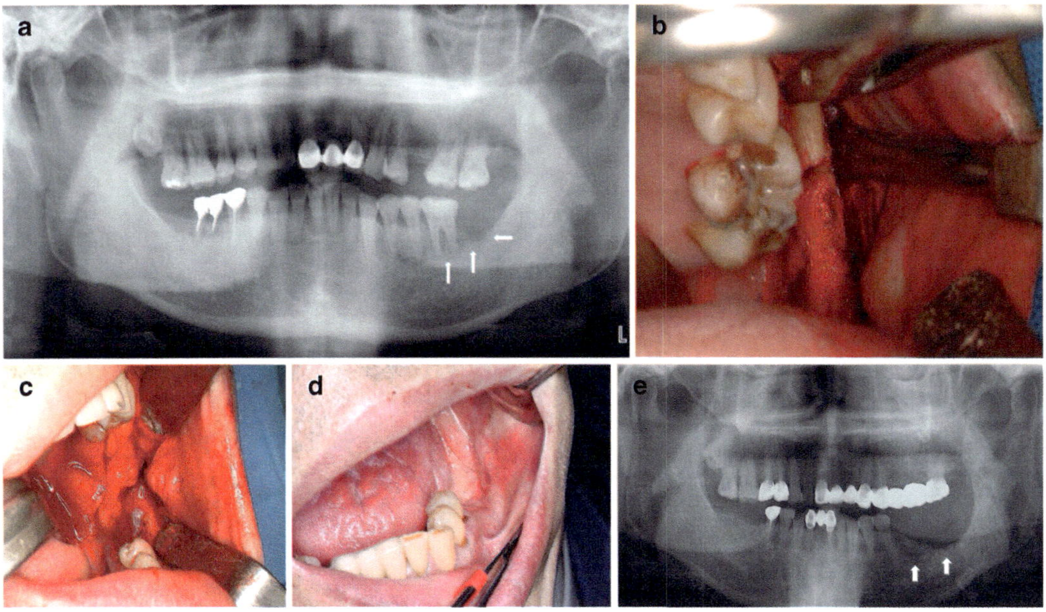

Fig. 20.5 Osteoradionecrosis of the mandible (grade II). (**a**) Osteoradionecrosis of the left mandible showing bone destruction in the left first molar and second molar area (arrows). (**b**) Extraction of the first molar and marginal mandibulectomy. (**c**) Buccal fat graft for primary closure. (**d**) Ten years follow-up showing a good healing state. (**e**) Panoramic radiograph showing a good healing state in the left mandible ten years post-operation (arrows)

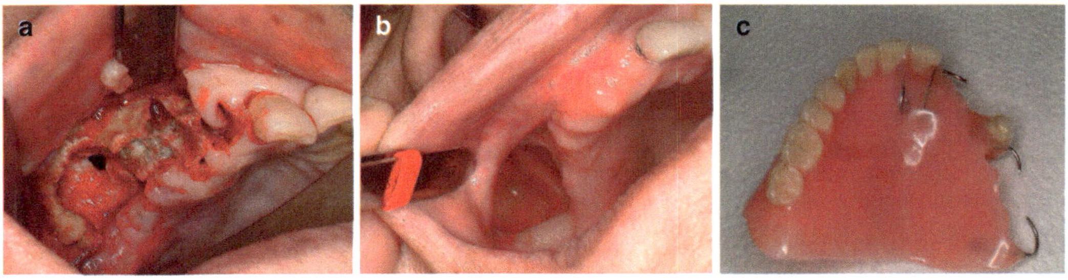

Fig. 20.6 Osteoradionecrosis of the right maxilla (grade II). (**a**) Necrotic bone involving the maxilla. (**b**) Healing at 6 months postoperatively. (**c**) Obturator functioning partial denture

Expert Opinion

In the case of ORN, free flap reconstruction may not always proceed as described in the literature. Unless the patient is experiencing severe pain due to a fracture or similar conditions, conservative treatment, minor surgical procedures, or soft tissue flaps may be more appropriate than a fibular free flap. (Eun-Jae Chung)

A summary of the treatments for maxillary and mandibular ORN is presented in Table 20.1.

Key Points

ORN of the jawbone is a rare complication associated with head and neck RT. ORN is difficult to treat and is sometimes refractory to conservative therapy. Prevention is better than cure; however, its spontaneous occurrence makes it difficult to predict ORN. ORN prevention consists of pre- and post-RT management.

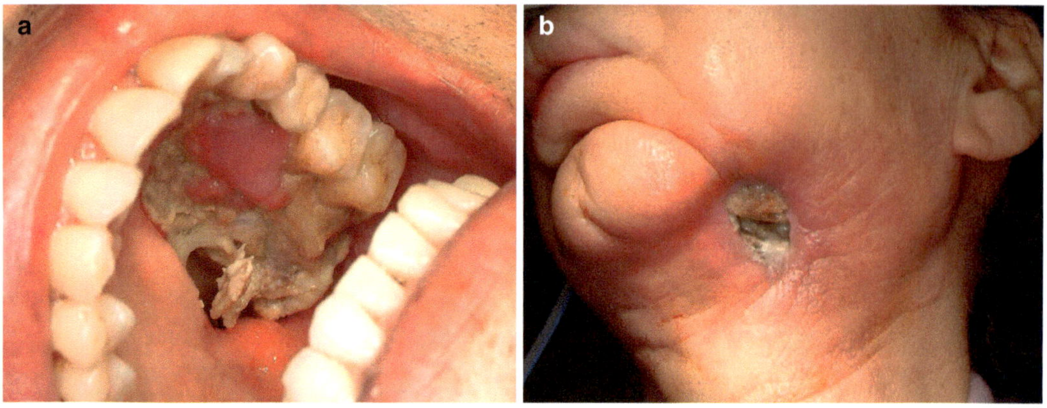

Fig. 20.7 Severe osteoradionecrosis of the jawbone (grade III) requiring major surgical treatment. (**a**) Palatal and maxillary bone necrosis with oronasal and oro-antral fistulas. (**b**) Exposed mandible with pathological fracture and skin fistula

Table 20.1 Treatment of the osteoradionecrosis by sites and stages [17]

Stage	Sign	Treatment	Methods
Treatment of Osteoradionecrosis in the mandible			
Stage I	Exposed alveolar bone	Conservative	Medication, mouthwash, local curettage, and HBO
Stage II	Invasion into bone marrow	Minor surgical treatment	Sequestrectomy and local flap
Stage II	Skin fistula or pathologic fracture	Major surgical treatment	Mandibulectomy with/without free flap reconstruction
Treatment of Osteoradionecrosis in the maxilla			
Stage I	Exposed alveolar bone	Conservative	Medication, mouthwash, local curettage and HBO
Stage II	Invasion into bone marrow	Minor surgical treatment	Sequestrectomy and buccal fat graft
Stage II	Skin fistula or major sequestra	Major surgical treatment	Maxillectomy with/without free flap reconstruction

HBO, hyperbaric oxygen therapy

Extraction of damaged teeth and removal of the oral infection nidus should be performed at least 12 weeks before the start of RT. Patients who undergo RT require cautious dental treatment. The extraction of teeth in the radiation field requires socket preservation with collagen or a bone-containing plug. The management of ORN depends on the stage. Stage I requires conservative therapy, which includes medication, mouthwash, HBO, and sequestrum curettage. Surgical treatment is required when ORN is refractive to conservative treatment or when definite ORN progression is evident. Surgical treatment is so diverse that proper planning should be performed according to the stage of ORN, the patient's general condition, and the involved site. Fibular free-flap reconstruction is the flap of choice for the reconstruction of the maxilla and mandible. Dental implant-supported prostheses should be considered to restore mastication and swallowing functions.

◆ Management of ORN starts with conservative therapy, followed by minor and major surgery. Conservative therapy includes medication, mouthwash with chlorohexidine, local curettage, simple debridement, and hyperbaric oxygen therapy. Minor and major surgery depends on the stage of ORN.

20.2 KQ 20.2. What Are the Reconstruction Options for Osteoradionecrosis Management?

Kang-Min Ahn

Reconstruction options after ORN resection depend on the defect site, size of the tissue defect, and patient's condition [7]. Because many methods for jaw reconstruction are available, they should be selected according to individual requirements. Maxillary reconstruction is indicated when partial or total maxillectomy results in oronasal or oroantral fistulas that cannot be covered by an obturator. Mandibular reconstruction is indicated when segmental or total mandibulectomy is performed.

20.2.1 Maxilla Reconstruction

- **Pedicled flap**: A partial maxillectomy results in an oronasal or oroantral fistula. Soft tissue flaps or obturators can be used to close oral communication. The most versatile pedicled flaps are pedicled buccal fat grafts or temporal fascial flaps [8]. If the defect is located between the premolar and molars, a pedicled buccal fat graft can be used for primary closure of the wound. If soft tissue is lacking, the pedicled temporal fascia can be used to alternate between the mucosa and gingiva.
- **Soft tissue free flap**: Free-flap reconstruction is indicated when defects are > 5 cm in size. The forearm or lateral arm free flap and anterior lateral thigh free flap can be used successfully [9].
- **Osteocutaneous free flap for dental implants**: A fibular free flap is indicated if a dental implant is planned. The fibular-free flap is the most versatile for maxilla reconstruction (Fig. 20.8).

◆ Reconstruction of the maxilla with ORN involves the use of a pedicle flap, soft tissue-free flap, or osteocutaneous flap. Dental implant restoration is ideal for ORN patients.

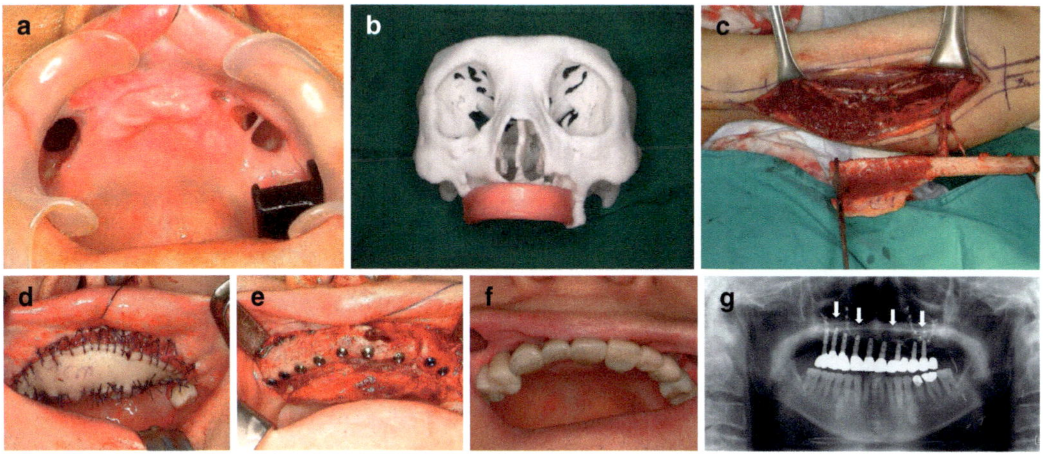

Fig. 20.8 Reconstruction of the maxilla with the fibular free flap and dental implant in patients with osteoradionecrosis. (**a**) Bilateral oroantral fistula after partial maxillectomy. (**b**) Rapid prototype model and simulation of fibular reconstruction. (**c**) Harvesting the osteocutaneous fibular flap. (**d**) Intraoral suture of fibular skin paddle. (**e**) Dental implant installation in the reconstructed maxilla. (**f**) Definite dental prosthesis. (**g**) Panoramic radiograph showing the reconstructed maxilla and dental implant (arrows)

Expert Opinion
For severe maxillary ORN requiring a fibular free flap, significant soft tissue reconstruction is often necessary. In such cases, a chimeric flap using the scapula tip and latissimus dorsi muscle can be an excellent option. (Eun-Jae Chung)

20.2.2 Mandible Reconstruction

Expert Opinion
To avoid issues like residual problematic tissue, skin fistulas caused by reconstruction plates, plate exposure, and pathologic fractures, it is crucial to collaborate closely with oral and maxillofacial surgeons and carefully select patients. (Eun-Jae Chung)

- **Segmental mandibulectomy with reconstruction plate (R-plate)**: If the ORN defect in the mandible is <4 cm with good skin condition, partial mandibulectomy and R-plate application can be successfully performed. Intact intraoral mucosa is a prerequisite for R-plate reconstruction (Fig. 20.9).
- **Segmental mandibulectomy with free autogenous bone graft:** If no soft tissue defect is present in the oral mucosa or skin, an iliac crest-free bone graft can be successfully utilized. Both ends of the mandibular bone should be healthy and contain viable bone cells. If soft tissue dehiscence occurs during the healing period, the free bone graft will be resorbed or fail.
- **Segmental resection with osteocutaneous free-flap reconstruction**: If the mandibular defect after ORN resection is >4 cm and the soft tissue condition is poor, free-flap reconstruction is the first choice. The fibular flap is the most popular free flap for mandibular reconstruction because both soft and hard tissue reconstruction is possible (Fig. 20.10) [10]. Owing to the high likelihood of a vessel-depleted neck at the ORN site, selection of a fibular flap is important [11]. When an oral mucosal defect is present on the ipsilateral side, a fibular graft is required.
- **Distraction osteogenesis**: When free-flap reconstruction is not possible, distraction osteogenesis may be the next option [12]. The surgical procedure included corticotomy with an initial gap of 0–2 mm and internal distraction device fixation. After a 7–10-day latency period, distraction is performed at a rate of 0.25–1 mm/day.

Expert Opinion
Always be prepared for through-and-through defects of the external skin and oral mucosa. Chimeric flaps are a good option, and when harvesting a free fibula flap, designing a wide skin paddle allows simultaneous coverage of both internal and external areas. (Eun-Jae Chung)

◆ Reconstruction of the mandible with ORN consists of titanium plate application, free autogenous bone graft, and osteocutaneous flap. Dental implant restoration is ideal for ORN patients.

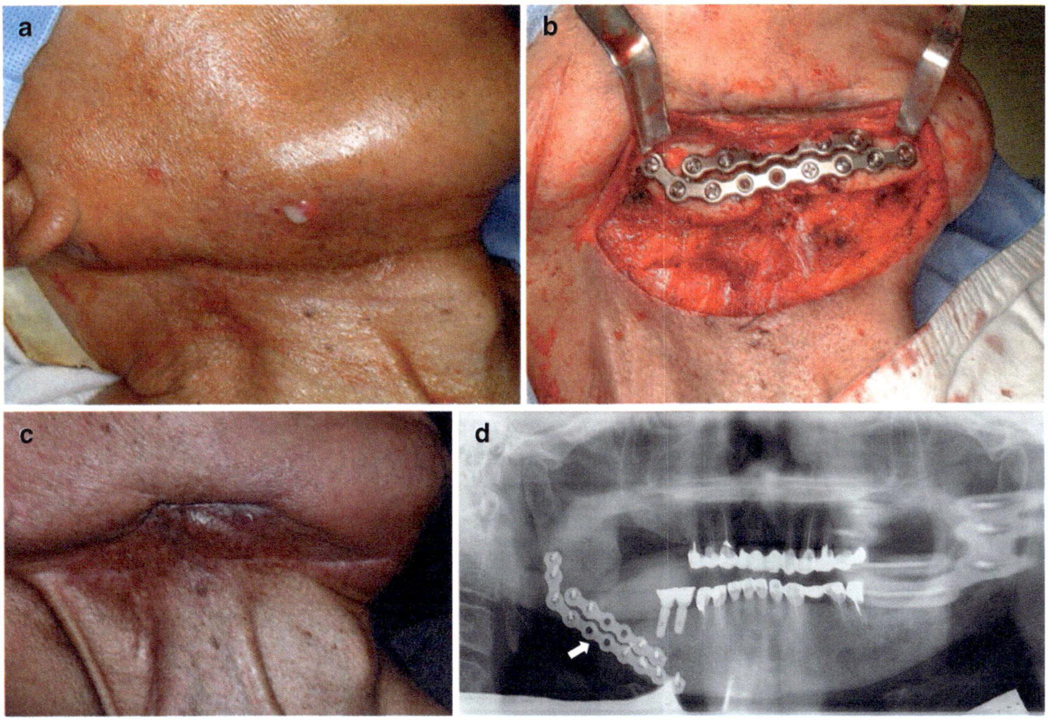

Fig. 20.9 Osteoradionecrosis of the mandible reconstructed with reconstruction titanium plate. (**a**) Skin fistula and pus discharge due to osteoradionecrosis of the mandible. (**b**) Skin flap elevation, partial mandibulectomy, and application of a titanium plate. (**c**) Healed skin one year after the operation. (**d**) Panoramic radiograph showing two titanium plates applied to the partially resected mandible (arrow)

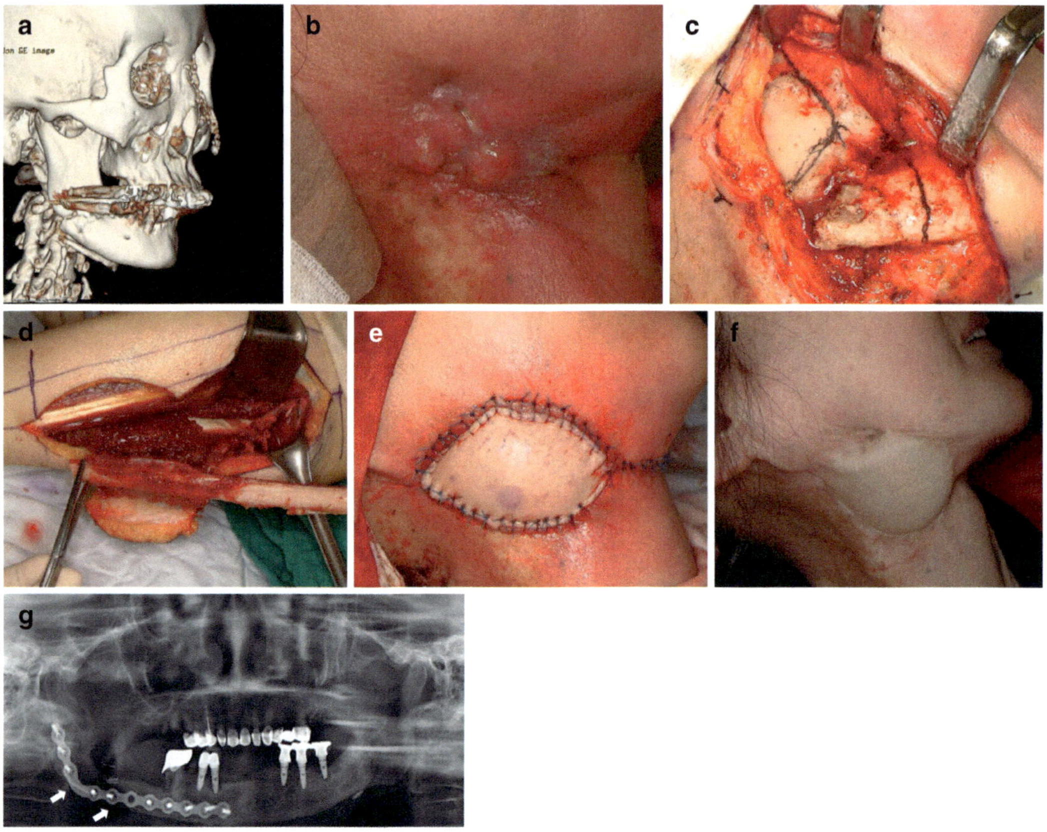

Fig. 20.10 Osteoradionecrosis of the mandible reconstructed with the free fibular flap. (**a**) Pathological fracture of the right mandibular angle due to advanced osteoradionecrosis. (**b**) Skin fistula with pus discharge. (**c**) Flap elevation and marking for partial mandibulectomy. (**d**) Harvesting the osteocutaneous fibular flap. (**e**) Suture of the cutaneous flap on the extraoral side. (**f**) Healed skin flap 5 years postoperatively. (**g**) Panoramic radiograph showing the reconstructed mandible with a fibular flap (arrow)

20.3 KQ 20.3. How Can Hyperbaric Oxygen Therapy Be Used to Manage Osteoradionecrosis?

Yoon Se Lee

20.3.1 The Indications of Hyperbaric Oxygen Therapy for Osteoradionecrosis

Osteoradionecrosis (ORN) is a complex complication of radiation treatment. Risk factors include high radiation dose (> 60 Gy), advanced stage, old age, smoking habits, systemic diseases (diabetes mellitus, hypertension, and collagen vascular diseases), and poor nutritional status [13]. In patients with head and neck cancer, ORN usually occurs in the mandible, cervical spine, or skull base. The mandible is the most frequently involved bone, and active periodontal disease or tooth extraction after radiation therapy increases the risk of ORN. Thus, most studies on ORN in the head and neck region have focused on ORN occurring in the mandible.

◆ ORN usually occurs in the mandible.

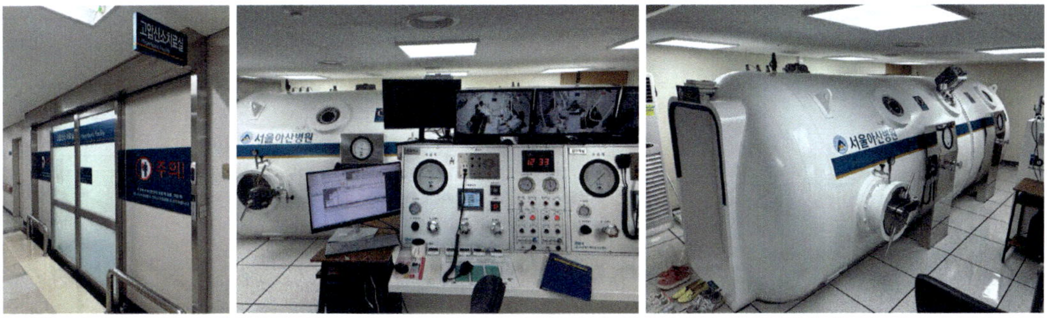

Fig. 20.11 Hyperbaric oxygen chamber for multiple patients

Given that the hypoxic–hypocellular–hypovascular theory is one of the pathophysiologies of ORN, hyperbaric oxygen therapy (HBOT) has been regarded as the mainstay of nonsurgical treatment for ORN, particularly in the early stages, as it corrects the hypoxic–hypocellular–hypovascular status of the tissue (Fig. 20.11) [14]. HBOT increases dissolved oxygen in tissues and blood, which leads to the delivery of up to 20 times the normal levels of oxygen into the tissues [15]. HBOT is used in combination with other medical treatments, such as antibiotics, steroids, and antioxidants, although its efficacy remains controversial [16].

◆ The concept underlying HBOT is that delivering high-pressure oxygen can alleviate the hypoxic condition in tissues compromised by radiation-induced hypoxia.

A few staging and classification systems are used for ORN, although the first classification proposed by Marx et al. has been widely used to determine treatment modalities (Table 20.2) [17]. Regardless of the classification system used, conservative and medical treatments, rather than surgical debridement, are indicated in the early stages. In these stages, lesions of a short length are confined to the alveolar bone or to the exposed alveolar bone without pathological fracture [18]. Either dental sepsis or loose and necrotic bone is an indication for surgical treatment in addition to medication treatment, including HBOT. Recognition of the early stages of ORN is important for improving treatment outcomes and avoiding surgical resection.

◆ Various staging systems of ORN have been suggested. In the early stages, nonsurgical treatments combined with HBOT are recommended.

20.3.2 Suggested Protocols and Therapeutic Efficacy

Effective burn wound healing was observed with HBOT, which enhanced capillary angiogenesis, fibroblast proliferation, and collagen synthesis [21]. Based on the idea that HBOT may improve vascularity and fibroblastic cellular density, which are disrupted in ORN, HBOT was used as a treatment for ORN. Since the introduction of the Wilford Hall protocol for HBOT for refractory ORN, successful treatment results have been reported according to variations in protocols [22, 23]. However, adequate protocols of HBOT remain poorly elucidated due to the rarity of randomized trials evaluating the therapeutic benefit of HBOT. Initially, the protocol of Marx et al. consisted of 30 sessions before and 10 sessions after operations involving bone, at 2.4 atmospheres in 90-min sessions, to prevent ORN. Most British Hyperbaric Association (BHA) members prefer to

Table. 20.2 Classification of osteoradionecrosis

Author	Classification	
Marx [17]	Stage I	Exposed alveolar bone without pathological fracture which responds to hyperbaric oxygen therapy
	Stage II	No response to HOT, and requires sequestrectomy and saucerization
	Stage III	Pathologic fracture, orocutaneous fistula, radiographic evidence of resorption to the inferior border and requires resection and reconstruction with free tissue
Notani et al. [19]	Stage I	Confined to alveolar bone
	Stage II	Limited to alveolar bone and/or the mandible above the level of mandibular cana
	Stage III	Extended to mandible under the level of mandibular canal with skin fistula or pathological fracture
Lyons et al. [20]	Stage I	<2.5 cm length of bone affected (damaged or exposed)
	Stage II	>2.5 cm length of bone; asymptomatic, including pathological fracture or involvement of inferior dental nerve or both. Medical treatment only unless dental sepsis or loose, necrotic bone is observed
	Stage III	>2.5 cm length of bone; symptomatic, but with no other features despite medical treatment
	Stage IV	2.5 cm length of bone; pathological fracture, involvement of inferior dental nerve, orocutaneous fistula, or a combination of both

use the Marx protocol in its original form or with modifications. The US Navy protocol, composed of three sessions of hyperbaric oxygen for 30 min, with 5-min intervals between sessions, is also currently used. The success rate of reconstruction of previously irradiated mandibles was reported to be as high as 93% in selected patients, whereas that of surgery varied from 50% to 60% [17, 23, 24]. These studies were not based on randomized controlled trials. The hyperbaric oxygen for the prevention of osteoradionecrosis (HOPON) trial was conducted to assess the benefit of HBOT in the prevention of ORN during dental extraction or implant placement in previously irradiated mandibles [25]. This randomized controlled, phase 3 trial showed that the incidence of ORN and late pain did not differ between the HBOT and control groups. Patients in the HBOT arm exhibited fewer acute symptoms.

◆ Duration of HBOT ranges from 30–90 min per session. The therapeutic efficacy of HBOT remains to be elucidated.

HBOT is typically used as adjuvant therapy for advanced ORN. Multinational and multicenter randomized clinical trials have shown that the healing rate of surgical debridement of necrotic mandibular bone treated with HBOT was slightly better (70%) than that of the surgery-only group (51%). Although the treatment outcomes were not statistically significantly different, HBOT may potentially have some benefit for ORN. Studies evaluating the therapeutic effect of HBOT for ORN are warranted after refining selected patients to avoid type II errors.

◆ Although the therapeutic efficacy of HBOT for ORN remains controversial, a certain degree of therapeutic or prophylactic effect of HBOT is anticipated as an adjuvant treatment.

20.3.3 Complications of HBOT

Oxygen pressure should not exceed 3 atm, and the treatment sessions should be limited to a maximum of 120 min. Despite the use of this protocol, adverse effects are unavoidable. Barotrauma to the ear causes otitis media, which is relieved by ventilation tube insertion. Increased oxygen concentration in the eyes due to HBOT can cause reversible myopia, cataracts, and keratoconus. Pneumothorax, pleural effusion, and seizures are rare [26]. During HBOT, visual disturbances, eyeball pain, and headaches should be evaluated, and all ophthalmic or chest surgeries should be delayed. HBOT cannot be administered to patients with claustrophobia.

◆ Barotrauma by high-pressure oxygen even <3 atm can occur in the ear, eye, and thorax. Before and after HBOT, complications should be consulted and evaluated.

References

1. Dumoulin S, van Maanen A, Magremanne M. Dental prevention of maxillo-mandibular osteoradionecrosis: a ten-year retrospective study. J Stomatol Oral Maxillofac Surg. 2021;122(2):127–34.
2. Wang TH, Liu CJ, Chao TF, Chen TJ, Hu YW. Risk factors for and the role of dental extractions in osteoradionecrosis of the jaws: a national-based cohort study. Head Neck. 2017;39(7):1313–21.
3. Chrcanovic BR, Reher P, Sousa AA, Harris M. Osteoradionecrosis of the jaws--a current overview--Part 2: dental management and therapeutic options for treatment. Oral Maxillofac Surg. 2010;14(2):81–95.
4. Notani K, Yamazaki Y, Kitada H, Sakakibara N, Fukuda H, Omori K, et al. Management of mandibular osteoradionecrosis corresponding to the severity of osteoradionecrosis and the method of radiotherapy. Head Neck. 2003;25(3):181–6.
5. Schwartz HC, Kagan AR. Osteoradionecrosis of the mandible: scientific basis for clinical staging. Am J Clin Oncol. 2002;25(2):168–71.
6. Rice N, Polyzois I, Ekanayake K, Omer O, Stassen LF. The management of osteoradionecrosis of the jaws--a review. Surgeon. 2015;13(2):101–9.
7. Md JBM, Md EZ, Md MAF, Md PJC. Overview and emerging trends in the treatment of osteoradionecrosis. Curr Treat Options Oncol. 2021;22(12):115.
8. Zenga J, Nussenbaum B, Rich JT, Sclaroff A, Diaz JA. Reconstruction of composite oral cavity defects with temporalis flaps after prior treatment. Am J Otolaryngol. 2015;36(1):97–102.
9. Meleca JB, Kerr RP, Prendes BL, Fritz MA. Anterolateral thigh fascia lata rescue flap: a new weapon in the battle aagainst osteoradionecrosis. Laryngoscope. 2021;131(12):2688–93.
10. Kim MG, Lee ST, Park JY, Choi SW. Reconstruction with fibular osteocutaneous free flap in patients with mandibular osteoradionecrosis. Maxillofac Plast Reconstr Surg. 2015;37(1):7.
11. Kim JW, Hwang JH, Ahn KM. Fibular flap for mandible reconstruction in osteoradionecrosis of the jaw: selection criteria of fibula flap. Maxillofac Plast Reconstr Surg. 2016;38(1):46.
12. Raghoebar GM, Jansma J, Vissink A, Roodenburg JL. Distraction osteogenesis in the irradiated mandible. A case report. J Craniomaxillofac Surg. 2005;33(4):246–50.
13. Caparrotti F, Huang SH, Lu L, Bratman SV, Ringash J, Bayley A, et al. Osteoradionecrosis of the mandible in patients with oropharyngeal carcinoma treated with intensity-modulated radiotherapy. Cancer. 2017;123(19):3691–700.
14. Nadella KR, Kodali RM, Guttikonda LK, Jonnalagadda A. Osteoradionecrosis of the jaws: clinico-therapeutic management: a literature review and update. J Maxillofac Oral Surg. 2015;14(4):891–901.
15. Oguz H, Sobaci G. The use of hyperbaric oxygen therapy in ophthalmology. Surv Ophthalmol. 2008;53(2):112–20.
16. Costa DA, Costa TP, Netto EC, Joaquim N, Ventura I, Pratas AC, et al. New perspectives on the conservative management of osteoradionecrosis of the mandible: a literature review. Head Neck. 2016;38(11):1708–16.
17. Marx RE. Osteoradionecrosis: a new concept of its pathophysiology. J Oral Maxillofac Surg. 1983;41(5):283–8.
18. Rice N, Polyzois I, Ekanayake K, Omer O, Stassen LF. The management of osteoradionecrosis of the jaws--A review. Surgeon. 2015;13(2):101–9.
19. Ki N, Yamazaki Y, Kitada H, Sakakibara N, Fukuda H, Omori K, Nakamura M. Management of mandibular osteoradionecrosis corresponding to the severity of osteoradionecrosis and the method of radiotherapy. Head & Neck. 2003;25(3):181–6.
20. Lyons A, Osher J, Warner E, Kumar R, Brennan PA. Osteoradionecrosis—a review of current concepts in defining the extent of the disease and a new classification proposal. Br J Oral Maxillofac Surg. 2014;52(5):392–5.
21. Jereczek-Fossa BA, Orecchia R. Radiotherapy-induced mandibular bone complications. Cancer Treat Rev. 2002;28(1):65–74.
22. Myers RA, Marx RE. Use of hyperbaric oxygen in postradiation head and neck surgery. NCI Monogr. 1990;9:151–7.

23. Tibbles PM, Edelsberg JS. Hyperbaric-oxygen therapy. N Engl J Med. 1996;334(25):1642–8.
24. Mainous EG, Boyne PJ. Hyperbaric oxygen in total rehabilitation of patients with mandibular osteoradionecrosis. Int J Oral Surg. 1974;3(5):279–301.
25. Shaw RJ, Butterworth CJ, Silcocks P, Tesfaye BT, Bickerstaff M, Jackson R, et al. HOPON (Hyperbaric Oxygen for the Prevention of Osteoradionecrosis): a randomized controlled trial of hyperbaric oxygen to prevent osteoradionecrosis of the irradiated mandible after dentoalveolar surgery. Int J Rad Oncol Biol Phys. 2019;104(3):530–9.
26. Riley DJ, Kerr JS, Shiu YY, Berg RA, Edelman NH. Pulmonary oxygen toxicity connective tissue changes during injury and repair. Chest. 1983;83(5):98S–9S.

GPSR Compliance

The European Union's (EU) General Product Safety Regulation (GPSR) is a set of rules that requires consumer products to be safe and our obligations to ensure this.

If you have any concerns about our products, you can contact us on ProductSafety@springernature.com

In case Publisher is established outside the EU, the EU authorized representative is:

Springer Nature Customer Service Center GmbH
Europaplatz 3
69115 Heidelberg, Germany

Batch number: 10731395

Printed by Printforce, the Netherlands